Pathology of the Cardiomyopathies

To my wife Eileen, without whose help and encouragement this book could not have been written

Pathology of the Cardiomyopathies

Brian McKinney
M.D., M.R.C.Path.

Wellcome Trust Research Fellow;
Honorary Lecturer in Pathology,
Royal Free Hospital, London

Butterworths

ENGLAND: BUTTERWORTH & CO. (PUBLISHERS) LTD.
                LONDON: 88 Kingsway, WC2B 6AB

AUSTRALIA: BUTTERWORTHS PTY. LTD.
                SYDNEY: 586 Pacific Highway 2067
                MELBOURNE: 343 Little Collins Street, 3000
                BRISBANE: 240 Queen Street, 4000

CANADA: BUTTERWORTH & CO. (CANADA) LTD.
                TORONTO: 14 Curity Avenue, 374

NEW ZEALAND: BUTTERWORTHS OF NEW ZEALAND LTD.
                WELLINGTON: 26–28 Waring Taylor Street, 1

SOUTH AFRICA: BUTTERWORTH & CO. (SOUTH AFRICA) (PTY.) LTD.
                DURBAN: 152–154 Gale Street

Suggested U.D.C. Number: 616·127

ISBN: 0 407 62000 1

Printed in Great Britain by
The Pitman Press, Bath

Contents

Foreword

This book on the pathology of the cardiomyopathies by Dr. Brian McKinney is an important contribution to the medical literature. The cardiomyopathies constitute a significant portion of diseases of the heart. They are being recognized more throughout the world as physicians learn about diseases of the myocardium. McKinney has had a profound interest in diseases of the myocardium for many years. His interest has not been limited entirely to pathology but has also included the related clinical manifestations of, and research devoted to, cardiomyopathies. The chapters of this book reflect his extensive knowledge. Students of heart disease will readily find the presentations to reflect these many interests and personal contributions to the field. The clinician as well as the pathologist will appreciate this book and learn a great deal from it.

McKinney has included most, if not all, of the causes of heart muscle disease in his monograph. He has used the term 'cardiomyopathy' literally, i.e. as the term implies: heart muscle pathology. His general approach to the pathology of cardiomyopathies is certainly helpful to the physician. Regardless of cause, the clinical manifestations that follow damage to the myocardium are quite similar. There are some cardiologists who limit the term 'cardiomyopathy' to disease of the myocardium of unknown cause. This relatively narrow or limited approach seems to me to be less effective in the management of all the cardiomyopathies of known cause, many preventable and many curable if recognized early. For example, myocardial disease due to hyperthyroidism or anaemia is certainly preventable and many are curable if recognized early. McKinney's concepts and approach to heart disease emphasize prevention and cure. The importance of prevention and cure is even more appreciated when it is realized that cardiomyopathy is disease of the myocardium itself, i.e. the tissue that does the work. The health of the power source of the pump must be preserved for good health.

The book is clearly written, the illustrations are excellent and the bibliographies supporting each disease entity are well selected. McKinney has properly devoted more pages in his book to the more common types of cardiomyopathies without neglecting the less common ones.

McKinney has rendered a great service to cardiology and medicine in general. This is an important book in pathology and is concerned with an organ responsible for the most deaths in many nations of the world. The clinician must understand the pathological basis of the diseases he treats. This book provides an excellent and much needed source of this information. McKinney is to be thanked and congratulated—he has produced a good book.

GEORGE E. BURCH

Preface

Since first becoming interested in endomyo cardial fibrosis in Uganda in 1959, I found that I was unable to obtain any book which was devoted entirely to a complete survey of cardiomyopathies, either clinically or pathologically. Much information on these diseases has been published but it is widely scattered in reports of symposia which have been held in different parts of the world, and in odd chapters and sections in textbooks on cardiology and cardiovascular pathology.

Subsequently, I found that many other people were faced with a similar problem. Pathologists or cardiologists, particularly those working for higher examinations, have often asked me to recommend a suitable book and I have had to say that there appears to be none available.

I was, therefore, very pleased when the opportunity to write such a book presented itself to me in 1970, particularly as, by then, I had amassed a great deal of material on cardiomyopathies and had become acquainted with many pathologists and cardiologists who were, like myself, particularly interested in this subject.

I should like to thank the many pathologists who have lent me slides and photographs of some of their specimens to use as illustrations in this book. These workers are listed in detail on the following pages. I am also deeply grateful to the following pathologists who have read and criticized sections of the manuscript of this book before it was finally submitted for publication:

Professor Norman Woody of Tulane University, New Orleans—Chagas' disease. Professor George Burch, also of Tulane University, New Orleans—Alcoholic cardiomyopathy. Professor Charlos Arribada of Chile—Cardiac toxoplasmosis. Dr Merton Sandler, London—Carcinoid heart disease. Dr Peter Hopper, London—Bacterial and viral infections. Dr Joyce Skinner, London—Fungal diseases and the remaining parasitic diseases. The late Professor E. Bajusz, McGill University—Hereditary cardiomyopathies in hamsters. Professor

P. J. Pretorius, Potchefstroomse, South Africa—The ovine cardio-myopathy: gousiekte. Professor George Rona, McGill University, for much of the remainder of this book, and whose stimulating advice and criticism have proved almost essential for its completion.

I should also like to thank my secretary, Mrs Sheila Meering, for dealing with the great amount of correspondence with very many people, which this book has entailed; Miss Linda Turney, for typing the manuscript; Mr George Brocklebank for much of the technical work; and Mr Cedric Gilson and the other members of the photo-graphic department of the Royal Free Hospital who spent much time and energy in taking and printing photographs for me.

Lastly, I would like to thank the British Heart Foundation for a grant to allow me to obtain specimens of many of the tropical cardiomyopathies and another grant so that I could buy a Vickers Patholux microscope, with which I was able to take many of the photographs that are included in this book; and the Wellcome Trust for personal support over many years and without whose help this work could not have been carried out.

B. McK.

Illustration
Acknowledgements

The author would like to thank the following authors and editors for permission to reproduce the illustrations from their articles and journals.

Figures 2.5, 2.6 and 2.9: Zoltawska (1971); *Journal of Clinical Pathology*

Figures 3.11–3.16: Takatsu *et al.* (1968); *American Heart Journal*

Figures 4.5–4.10: Ferrans *et al.* (1972); *Acta pathologica et microbiologica scandinavica*

Figures 5.1, 5.10 and 5.11: Spach *et al.* (1966); *American Heart Journal*

Figures 5.2, 5.5 and 5.6: Rattenberg *et al.* (1964); *American Heart Journal*

Figures 5.3, 5.4, 5.7, 5.8 and 5.9: Nihill, Wilson and Hugh-Jones (1970); *Archives of Disease in Childhood*

Figures 5.14–5.16: Arnason *et al.* (1964); *Acta medica scandinavica*

Figures 11.6–11.8, and 11.12: Koberle (1968); *Cardiologia*

Figures 11.9–11.11, and 11.13: Anselmi *et al.* (1966); *American Heart Journal*

Figures 12.2–12.9: Roberts, Liegler and Carbone (1969); *American Journal of Medicine*

Figures 13.1, 13.3 and 13.4: Pomerance (1965); *British Heart Journal*

Figures 13.18, 13.20 and 13.21: O'Donnell and Mann (1966); *American Heart Journal*

Figures 14.1–14.5: Rubler and Fleischer (1967) and Fleischer and Rubler (1968); *American Journal of Cardiology*

Figures 14.10–14.12: Engel, Erlandson and Smith (1964); *Circulation*

Figures 15.11–15.14: Ferrans *et al.* (1965); *American Heart Journal*

Figures 16.3, 16.4 and 16.6: Skause, Berg and Westfelt (1959); *Acta medica scandinavica*

Figures 16.1, 16.5 and 16.9: Sterns *et al.* (1966); *British Heart Journal*

Figures 16.14–16.18: Fine and Morales (1971); *Archives of Pathology*
Figures 16.23, 16.24, 16.26 and 16.27: Aikat and Nirodi (1971); *Journal of Pathology and Bacteriology*
Figures 17.1–17.4, 17.10, 17.11, 17.14 and 17.16: Deodhar and Chatty (1969); *Archives of Pathology*
Figures 17.13, 17.15 and 17.17: Bonenfant, Miller and Roy (1967); *Canadian Medical Association Journal*
Figures 18.5, 18.6, 18.8–18.10: Bajusz (1969); *American Heart Journal*

One

Introduction

During the past twenty-five years the importance of heart disease of unknown or unusual origin has become obvious. Previously the only agents commonly regarded as causing damage to the myocardium were coronary artery obstruction, causing myocardial infarction, or rheumatic myocarditis.

Many cases of cardiac disease have since been recognized which are not due to either of these causes. This originally became evident probably because of reports of idiopathic cardiac disease arising from all parts of the world, but chiefly, from differing parts of Africa. Although cases of cardiac failure (due to various causes such as alcohol) have been known for many years, this has not been generally appreciated and it is only recently that it has become evident that many cases of heart failure are due to a cardiomyopathy—involvement of the heart muscle; and not due to an infarct, ischaemic heart disease or rheumatic carditis. The terms most frequently applied in description of heart muscle disease of unknown or unusual origin are: idiopathic myocardial hypertrophy, idiopathic cardiomegaly, cardiomyopathy and/or myocardiopathy, although there are many other even more non-specific terms such as myocardioses (commonly used by many continental writers).

All these terms may be misleading. In general pathology 'cardiac hypertrophy' implies that the cardiac enlargement has been caused by an increase in the size of the cardiac muscle fibres. According to this definition many obscure heart diseases, such as some cases of endomyocardial fibrosis, must be excluded.

The myocardium may be affected by a number of inflammatory, degenerative or neoplastic processes; the principal manifestations of which may, however, be located in other parts of the body.

This book will be limited to describing conditions where the disease involving the myocardium is of such clinical significance as to produce cardiac enlargement, congestive heart failure or both. The term commonly accepted for the description of this type of cardiac disease is *cardiomyopathy*.

DEFINITION

The word cardiomyopathy simply means disease of the heart muscle, and was first used by Brigden (1957) in his St Cyres Lecture. He went further, however, in confining his description to that group of diseases of the myocardium which were of unknown aetiology and did not have a basis of coronary occlusion as their principal aetiological origin.

Goodwin *et al.* (1961) describe cardiomyopathies as 'sub-acute or chronic disorder of the heart muscle of unknown or obscure aetiology, often with associated endocardial and sometimes with pericardial involvement but not atherosclerotic in origin'.

Robin (1961), however, calls them 'a broad group of diseases of diverse etiology, that specifically involve the myocardium to produce abnormalities of structure, abnormalities of function or both. The end result of many of these diseases may be the development of myocardial fibrosis'.

The definition accepted by the WHO study group on cardiomyopathies states that: 'the name indicates conditions of different— frequently, unknown or unclear, etiology in which the dominant feature is cardiomegaly, and cardiac failure. It excludes heart diseases resulting from damage to the valvular strictures of the heart, and from disorder of coronary, systemic or pulmonary vessels.'

This definition deliberately omits reference to the duration of the disease process in view of the inadequate knowledge of their natural history.

At present there are three descriptions of the cardiomyopathies which are commonly accepted by different groups of cardiologists and pathologists.

(1) Goodwin (1966) divides all types of cardiomyopathies into four groups (*Figure 1.1*).

The largest group of cases, for which he uses the descriptive term 'congestive cardiomyopathy', include all those types of cardiomyopathy which present, clinically, in congestive cardiac failure with a large heart, gallop rhythm and often with evidence of valvular insufficiency (Goodwin *et al.*, 1961). Most cases of idiopathic cardiomegaly will present in this way, but not all cases presenting as 'congestive cardiomyopathy' will consist of patients with this disease.

The second most common type is *hypertrophic obstructive cardiomyopathy* (in North America this is known as idiopathic hypertrophic subaortic stenosis); this being an inherited disorder characterized by marked ventricular hypertrophy without dilatation.

The third type, *constrictive (restrictive) cardiomyopathy*, resembles constrictive pericarditis with diastolic filling, difficulty due to myocardial rigidity, infiltration and often endocardial involvement. This type of cardiomyopathy is rare; the most common cause being amyloid infiltration.

The last type, *obliterative cardiomyopathy*, describes disorders in which obliteration of the cavities of the ventricles is associated with

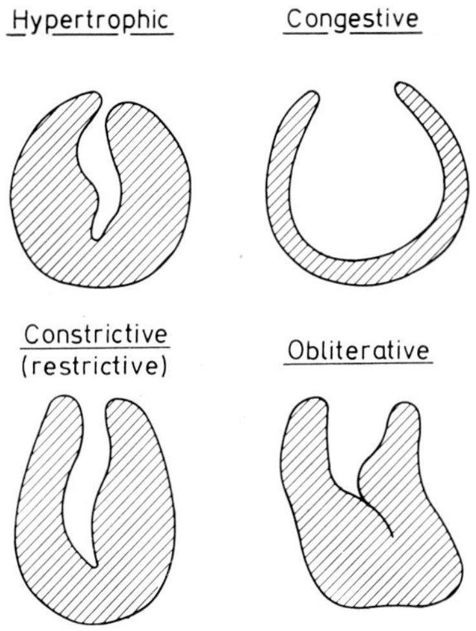

Hypertrophic　　　　Congestive

Figure 1.1. Diagram to show gross differences in ventricular form in four types of cardiomyopathy (Goodwin, 1970)

Constrictive
(restrictive)　　　　Obliterative

atrioventricular valve regurgitations as in endomyocardial fibrosis (Davies, 1948) and in Loeffler's (1936) eosinophilic fibroplastic endocarditis.

(2) Hudson (1970) has proposed that the definitions of the terms for cardiomyopathy should include all diseases of the endocardium, pericardium and myocardium, irrespective of functional characteristics and whether or not of recognized origin.

(3) Mattingly (1965) uses the term cardiomyopathies to include all disease of the myocardium alone, whether or not of recognized aetiology but, of course, not including that due to coronary artery disease. This is the definition which is generally accepted by most North American and European workers in this field.

CLASSIFICATION

The many conditions, which fall into the broad category of cardiomyopathies, make it very difficult to construct a simple system for
classification.

Several classifications have been proposed, some of them depending on aetiology (Emmanuel, 1970), some on clinical or
pathological features (Carlisle, 1971); or whether the disease involves
primarily processes affecting other organs as well as, and often
before, the heart (Fejfar, 1970).

One group of workers employs the term 'primary myocardial
disease' as inclusive not only of the idiopathic disorders of the
myocardium but also of more generalized diseases when the myocardium is the principle site of involvement. In other classifications
(Fowler, 1964) the term primary myocardial disease is used only to
refer to the idiopathic disorder which, in actual fact, probably
represents a heterogeneous group of diseases which, in many
instances, begin as myocarditis.

In the classification proposed below, the cardiomyopathies are
divided into those which are thought to be 'primary', i.e., those in
which the disease process involves the heart alone and those which
are 'secondary', i.e., the cardiomyopathy is part of a generalized
disease process which affects other parts of the body, either before or
after the heart is involved. This definition, of course, excludes the
changes which may be found in the body which have been caused
by congestive cardiac failure.

A certain group of heart diseases of unknown aetiology, for
example, some types of cardiomyopathies producing symptoms or
signs of obstruction, show no cardiac muscle hypertrophy or enlargement. This fact does not seem to fit with the term 'myocardiopathy'. Finally, 'cardiomyopathy' means a disorder of the
heart muscle and therefore it is unfit to include those forms of heart
disease where the lesion is principally of the endocardium or valves—
as, for example, in a case of bacterial endocarditis.

In considering all these terms, I suggest the use of the word
'cardiomyopathy'. This term is not completely satisfactory as it
means any disorder of the heart. However, if the word has a definite
meaning, others will know to what one is referring. In this respect I
do not think the definition proposed by Korb (1973) can be improved
upon. 'Cardiomyopathies are heart diseases of unknown or unusual
etiology, associated with pathological processes within the myocardium or endocardium or both and including certain lesions of
the conduction system.' This definition excludes such common

aetiological categories as coronary, valvular, hypertensive and pulmonary heart disease. Constrictive pericarditis and other forms of pericardial disease, and cardiac malformations, should also not be included. Concerning the classification, it seems reasonable to start by dividing cardiomyopathies into primary and secondary forms. A *primary cardiomyopathy* means that the heart alone is affected by a disease process of either known or unknown aetiology, while *secondary cardiomyopathies* comprise a group of conditions where the heart is involved as part of a generalized underlying disease process. Additionally, one must include heart diseases of unusual or unknown aetiology involving the heart only, for example, primary tumours of the endocardium or myocardium.

From the viewpoint of clinicians the best classification is that proposed by Goodwin (1966) where, as stated above, he divided the cardiomyopathies into the following four groups: (1) congestive cardiomyopathies; (2) hypertrophic cardiomyopathies, with and without obstruction; (3) constrictive cardiomyopathies; and (4) obliterative cardiomyopathies.

The classification given below does not consider clinical aspects purposely, because it seems impossible to mix morphological, geographical and functional concepts of a disease.

This classification of myocardial disease—cardiomyopathies—includes such common aetiological categories as the following.

PRIMARY CARDIOMYOPATHIES

(1) Endocardial fibro-elastosis
(2) Hypertrophic obstructive cardiomyopathy
(3) Primary myocardial disease
(4) Familial cardiomyopathies

   (a) Metabolic storage disease

      (i) Pompe's disease (glycogen)
      (ii) Refsum's disease (phytannic acid)
      (iii) Fabry–Anderson's disease (glycolipid)
      (iv) Hurler's syndrome, i.e., gargoylism (mucopolysaccharidosis)
      (v) Haemochromatosis (iron)
      (vi) Oxalosis (calcium oxalate)
     (vii) Pseudoxanthoma elasticum

   (b) The muscular dystrophies and myotonia congenita
   (c) Friederich's ataxia
   (d) Sickle-cell anaemia

(5) Tropical cardiomyopathies. The term includes both endo-
     myocardial fibrosis and cardiomegaly of unknown origin
(6) Peri-partal and post-partal cardiomyopathies

SECONDARY CARDIOMYOPATHIES

(1) Inflammatory

   (a) Viral infection: Coxsackie, psittacosis, rubella, rubeola,
smallpox, vaccinia, infectious mononucleosis, infectious hepatitis,
varicella, mumps, rabies, yellow fever, atypical pneumonia, herpes
zoster, cytomegalic inclusion body disease
   (b) Rickettsial infection: typhus, scrub typhus, Q fever,
Bartonelliasis
   (c) Bacterial infection: infections of the upper respiratory
tract, diphtheria, streptococcal infections, infections of the lower
respiratory tract, meningococcal, haemophilus, salmonellosis,
brucellosis, tetanus, tuberculosis, clostridia, gonococcal, tularaemia
   (d) Spirochaetal infection: leptospirosis, syphilis
   (e) Fungal infection: aspergillosis, actinomycosis, histoplasmosis, blastomycosis, cryptococcosis, candidiasis, coccidioidomycosis
   (f) Parasitic infection:

      (i) *Protozoal*—Chagas' disease (*Trypanosoma cruzi*), African
   trypanosomiasis (*T. gambiense* and *T. rhodesiense*), toxoplasmosis, malaria
      (ii) *Metazoal*—cysticercosis, trichiniasis, schistosomiasis,
   filariasis, ascariasis, strongyloidiasis, visceral larva migrans,
   heterophydiasis, paragonimiasis

(2) 'Collagen' diseases

   (a) Rheumatic heart disease
   (b) Rheumatoid arthritis
   (c) Ankylosing spondilitis
   (d) Scleroderma
   (e) Systemic lupus erythematosus
   (f) Myasthenia gravis
   (g) 'Loeffler's disease'
   (h) Periarteritis nodosa
   (i) Dermatomyositis

(3) Idiopathic

   (a) Sarcoidosis

  (b) Giant-cell myocarditis
  (c) Amyloidosis

(4) Endocrine abnormalities

  (a) Thyrotoxicosis
  (b) Myxoedema
  (c) Phaeochromocytoma
  (d) Acromegaly
  (e) Hyperparathyroidism producing myocardial calcification

(5) Nutritional causes

  (a) Starvation and malnutrition (including kwashiorkor)
  (b) Anaemia
  (c) Beriberi

(6) Alcoholic heart disease

(7) Poisons

  (a) Carbon monoxide
  (b) Scorpion sting
  (c) Snake bite
  (d) *Argemone mexicana* (epidemic dropsy)
  (e) Cobalt
  (f) Arsenic
  (g) Antimony

(8) Drugs

  (a) Immunosuppressive drugs, i.e., Methotrexate
  (b) Daunrubicin
  (c) Emetine
  (d) Phenylbutazone
  (e) Sulphonamides
  (f) Antibiotics
  (g) Paracetamol
  (h) Other anaesthetic agents
  (i) Phenylthiazine and derivatives
  (j) Lithium carbonate
  (k) Adrenaline, noradrenaline and isoproterenol

(9) Physical trauma

  (a) Temperature and humidity
  (b) Radiant energy
  (c) Electricity
  (d) Ionizing radiation

(10) Tumours

   (a) Benign—myxoma, rhabdomyoma, fibroma, lipoma or teratoma
   (b) Malignant—(i) Primary—sarcoma, fibrosarcoma, rhabdomyosarcoma, neurosarcoma, reticulum cell sarcoma and lymphosarcoma, angiosarcoma, Kaposi's sarcoma, mesothelioma
        (ii) Secondary—from non-cardiac primary tumours, i.e., Kaposi's sarcoma or leukaemia

In conclusion, it can be said that (1) the diagnosis of a cardiomyopathy, either primary or secondary, depends to a great extent on excluding conditions, such as an old myocardial infarction, which are not cardiomyopathies; (2) necropsy is the last court of appeal; and (3) the end stage, which is most frequently seen, often consists of only a dilated or hypertrophied heart which has undergone much muscle destruction with ensuing fibrous tissue replacement. The final diagnosis is often very inconclusive.

References

Brigden, W. (1957). 'Uncommon myocardial diseases, the non-coronary cardiomyopathies.' *Lancet* **2**, 1179 and 1243

Carlisle, R. (1971). 'A classification for the cardiomyopathies.' *Am. J. Cardiol.* **28**, 242

Davies, J. N. P. (1948). 'Endocardial fibrosis in the African native.' *E. Afr. med. J.* **25**, 454

Emmanuel, R. (1970). 'Classification of the cardiomyopathies.' *Am. J. Cardiol.* **26**, 438

Fejfar, Z. (1970). 'Definition and classification of the cardiomyopathies.' *Pathologia Microbiol.* **35**, 17

Fowler, N. D. (1964). 'Classification and differential diagnosis of the myocardiopathies.' *Prog. cardiovasc. Dis.* **7**, 1

Goodwin, J. F. (1966). 'The cardiomyopathies.' *Royal College of Physicians Symposium*, Edinburgh. p. 76.

— (1970). 'Congestive and hypertrophic cardiomyopathies.' *Lancet* **1**, 731

— Gordon, H., Hollman, A. and Bishop, M. B. (1961). 'Clinical aspects of cardiomyopathy.' *Br. med. J.* **1**, 69

Hudson, R. E. (1970). 'The cardiomyopathies: order from chaos.' *Am. J. Cardiol.* **25**, 70

Korb, G. (1973). *Pathologia Microbiol.* (In press)

Loeffler, W. (1936). 'Endocarditis parietalic fibroplastica mit Blutensinophilia.' *Schweiz. med. Wschr.* **66**, 817

Mattingly, T. W. (1965). 'Changing concepts of myocardial disease.' *J. Am. med. Ass.* **191**, 33

Robin, E. D. (1961). 'Cardiovascular disease: Myocardiopathies.' *Ann. Rev. Med.* **12**, 55

Part One

Primary Cardiomyopathies

Two

Endocardial fibro-elastosis

The term endocardial fibro-elastosis indicates a cardiomyopathy which consists of diffuse endocardial thickening of one or more cardiac chambers: the chamber most often involved being the left ventricle, and, to a lesser degree, the left atrium. The endocardial thickening consists largely of layers of collagenous fibrous tissue, between which are a large number of long and straight, or slightly twisted elastic fibres.

PATHOLOGY

Endocardial fibro-elastosis has been called by a variety of other names, particularly 'endocardial sclerosis' (Blumburg and Lyon, 1952) and endomyocardial fibro-elastosis (Halliday, 1954).

This disease is usually divided into two forms: primary and secondary. The *primary form* where the disease is not associated with any other congenital cardiac or metabolic abnormalities, may be subdivided on the basis of the size of the left ventricular chamber (Edwards, 1952), as seen at autopsy. In the 'dilated' type (*Figure 2.1*) the left ventricular cavity is enlarged and the wall hypertrophied with diffuse endocardial fibro-elastosis. It is not associated with lesions preventing or obstructing the outflow of blood from the left ventricle, septal defects or anomalous origin of a coronary artery. In the 'constricted' type (*Figure 2.2*), which is much less common, the left ventricular cavity is normal or diminished in size; the right ventricle is enlarged and both have diffuse fibro-elastosis (Farber and Hubbard, 1953). This pathological classification divides primary fibro-elastosis into two distinct types with dissimilar clinical findings.

The *secondary form* of fibro-elastosis is associated with other malformations (Kelly and Anderson, 1956), such as aortic stenosis, coarctation of the aorta, a ventricular septal defect, or an anomalous origin of the left coronary artery from the pulmonary artery; and when the left ventricle and ascending aorta are hypoplastic.

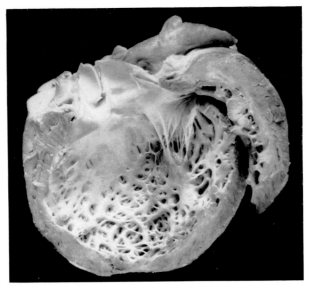

Figure 2.1. The heart in endocardinal fibro-elastosis—the dilated type (By courtesy of Dr Jesse E. Edwards)

Secondary fibro-elastosis is also commonly associated with defects of the myocardium itself—thus it is commonly seen in cases of glycogen storage disease (type II glycogenosis—Pompe's disease) involving the heart.

AGE, SEX AND RACIAL INCIDENCE

Panke and Rottino (1955) found that of 129 cases 78 per cent had died before reaching the age of 12 months but that the incidence of death in older children and adults became much less (Smith and Forth, 1943; White and Fennell, 1954; Thomas *et al.*, 1954; Panke and Rottino, 1955).

Forter *et al.* (1964) reported their experiences with 72 babies suffering from fibro-elastosis seen in the Royal Hospital for Sick Children in Edinburgh during the period 1948–62—the series constituting 17 per cent of the 433 cases of congenital heart disease seen in this time. In those cases which were primary, 37 per cent died within three months and 75 per cent within a year; while in the secondary cases, of which there were 56, 15 per cent died within three months and 95 per cent within a year.

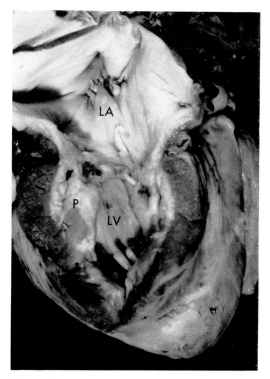

Figure 2.2. Gross appearance of the heart in the constricted type of fibro-elastosis (LA—left auricle: LV—left ventricle: P—pulmonary valve). (Reproduced from Fixler et al. (1970) by courtesy of Dr Foster Paul and the Editor of the American Journal of Cardiology)

In the series of 47 cases published by Moller *et al.* (1964) 42 had enlarged left ventricles. In 23 cases (8 males and 15 females aged from birth to 3½ years) the condition was primary and death occurred at 3 hours and up to 16 years. In 8 cases (4 males and 4 females dying between 3 and 18 months) aortic stenosis was present while in a further 8 (6 males and 2 females dying between 2½ and 3¾ years) aortic coarctation was present. In another 3 (1 male and 2 females dying between 2 and 22 months) an anomalous origin of the left coronary artery from the pulmonary artery was the cause.

Five patients (4 males and 1 female—dying between 2 days and 14 months) had a hypoplastic left ventricle; this was primary or part of the hypoplastic left heart syndrome.

There are several reports of cases of fibro-elastosis living into adolescence or adult life, or being discovered only at autopsy. Some of these cases (such as the cases reported by Van Buchan, Arends and Schroder (1959) who were aged 13, 16, 18, 26 and 46, and the 39 year old woman reported by Yoshida *et al.* (1967)) appear to be true cases of fibro-elastosis but others are much more doubtful: such as the case of a 71 year old male reported by White and Fennel (1954) and the cases of fibro-elastosis reported by Dyson, Burton and Decker (1958). These latter cases are probably due to coronary vessel disease but the presence of fibro-elastosis is, it seems to me, also confused with some tropical cardiomyopathies, as cases of what appear to be adult fibro-elastosis have been reported as endomyocardial fibrosis (Ogan, 1962).

Most reported descriptions of cases of fibro-elastosis have been in white (Caucasian) children but the disease has been found in Negro children (Peale and Lucchesi, 1942); while Lintermans *et al.* (1966) also describe the disease in an American Indian girl as well as reporting fibro-elastosis in three Negro children.

McLoughlin, Schiebler and Knovetz (1966) think that, in discussing the incidence of fibro-elastosis in Negro children, they may be dealing with a different entity, as fibro-elastosis has never been described in a Negro child in the newborn period.

This disease is most commonly found in boys. Moller and associates give a 2:1 predominance over girls in their series (Moller *et al.*, 1964). The ages at which this disease most commonly presents itself is between 3 and 6 months, but the child may present much later in life when perhaps it is one or two years of age, or even much later when in its teens (Van Buchan, Arends and Schroder, 1959). Some of the children may present with the disease at a much earlier age or even be born with symptoms of the disease (Moller *et al.*, 1966). The oldest reported patient is a girl aged 22 (Moller *et al.*, 1966).

There are numerous reports of the occurrence of this disease in siblings (Weinberg and Himelfarb, 1943; Winter *et al.*, 1960; Nielson, 1965). In a few cases this disease is found in two generations of a family (Fixler *et al.*, 1970) while in the remarkable case described by Moller *et al.* (1966) the disease is reported in a mother and son, both of whom died soon after the infant was born.

CLINICAL HISTORY

ONSET

The child is usually noticed to be perfectly well at birth but after some months develops congestive heart failure, usually insidiously and often associated with an upper respiratory tract infection. The age of onset of symptoms can vary considerably and has been described all through the paediatric age-range. However, by far the greatest number present with clinical difficulties in the first year of life and, if not by then, almost uniformly, by the end of the second year (Sellers, Keith and Manning, 1964).

Most patients complain originally of shortness of breath on exertion but, in some patients, dizziness seems to be of greater importance. Other cases may present with the Stokes–Adams syndrome due to complete interventricular block, while a few patients may have attacks of angina and others complain of attacks of palpitations. The symptomatology is basically that of congestive heart failure of the 'low output' type. The onset of symptoms may be abrupt and fulminating, or develop over the course of several weeks, or insidious and spread over several months (Sellers, Keith and Manning, 1964). Some patients may have no complaints and the diagnosis may be made only during routine examination, while others may die suddenly, without any apparent cause and, in them, the cause of death is probably due to the onset of a cardiac arrhythmia (Zoltowska, 1971).

All patients are found to have enlarged hearts radiologically; the cardiothoracic ratio being usually between 60 and 75 per cent or even greater. The hearts are usually globular in shape and may show extensive intracardiac calcification, especially in the adult cases of this disease (Van Buchan, Arends and Schroder, 1959). Similar changes of intracardiac calcification have also been noted in infants, although these are usually less marked.

PROGRESS

It has been assumed that the thickened left ventricular endocardium behaves like a constrictive pericarditis to limit the left ventricular output, and that the left ventricle is incapable of maintaining a normal stroke volume and a normal cardiac output. This assumption has been based largely upon the findings of radiography, which has revealed little difference between the systolic and diastolic volume of the left ventricle (Linde, Adams and O'Loughlin, 1958; Hoffman, 1960). As Black-Schaffer (1957) has pointed out, with the increase of the size of the left ventricle diminished linear excursion of the left ventricular wall is needed to maintain a normal cardiac output.

Observations by Moller et al. (1969) indicate that in children with endocardial fibro-elastosis, the stroke volume is normal. These authors believe that many of the clinical and laboratory manifestations of endocardial fibro-elastosis, can be attributed to mitral valve insufficiency. When endocardial fibro-elastosis is associated with aortic stenosis, or coarctation of the aorta, the resulting cardiac function is the summation of the behaviour of any associated anomalies and of mitral valve insufficiency.

The onset of congestive heart failure often seems to be preceded by an upper respiratory infection. In this country, the patients, although initially responding well to conservative treatment of congestive heart failure, later progressively become worse and die in congestive heart failure.

PATHOLOGICAL FINDINGS

The heart is usually much enlarged and increased in weight. The myocardium, especially the wall of the left ventricle, is thickened and hypertrophied. The apex of the ventricles is rounded so that the heart often assumes a globular shape. The pericardium has been normal in the great majority of reported cases, although patchy thickening and adhesions between visceral and parietal layers has been described. The endocardium of the affected chamber or chambers is diffusely covered by a thick greyish-white layer of fibrous tissue and has a porcelain-like appearance.

In almost all instances the left ventricle is most involved and has this characteristic appearance. Sometimes the endocardial thickening is most pronounced, just below the aortic valve. It may be diffuse in the left ventricle and patchy in the other chambers or diffuse throughout all the chambers. Sometimes ante-mortem thrombi may also be present in the auricular appendages. Another striking feature is of the appearance of the mitral valve. Deformities of the mitral and aortic valves are present in about 50 per cent of cases, while involvement of the pulmonary and tricuspid valves are less frequent. The valve leaflets are thickened and opaque, while their edges are often 'rolled'. Fusion of the cusps may occur and the chordae tendineae may be thickened so that stenosis results. 'Myxomatous nodules', each 1–3 mm in diameter and projecting from the free edges of the mitral and triscuspid leaflets, may often be seen.

In every case reviewed by Moller et al. (1964) the valve was rendered inefficient by certain alterations of the papillary muscles, and chordae tendineae. The papillary muscles, instead of originating from the junction of the lower and middle thirds of the left ventricle, arose from a higher level; short chordae tendineae extended from the apices of the papillary muscles into the leaflets of the mitral valve and the chordae were disposed horizontally with respect to the long axis of the left ventricle, instead of in their normal vertical arrangement.

Several anatomical features are present which support the clinical impression that mitral insufficiency frequently exists during life. The free margin of the anterior leaflet of the mitral valve is thickened and rolled, a finding often associated with mitral regurgitation. On the endocardium of the posterior wall of the left atrium, jet lesions occur at the site of impact of the regurgitant stream; the left atrium is nearly always enlarged and the foramen ovale is sealed at an earlier age than normally happens.

HISTOLOGICAL FACTORS

Histologically the endocardium is increased in thickness and is largely composed of collagenous fibres (*Figure 2.3*), which often extend into the underlying myocardial sinusoids (*Figure 2.4*) while in most instances the underlying myocardium is normal. Sometimes some muscle fibres are found in the thickened endocardium (*Figure 2.5*), but it is uncertain whether these cells have arisen from the muscle fibres normally present in the endocardium, or whether they are only small groups of subendocardial muscle cells which have become incorporated in the endocardium by the development of a layer of fibrous tissue between these cells and the underlying myocardium. Sometimes, however, much larger groups of muscle fibres are isolated by the development of large areas of fibrotic tissue surrounding and separating them from the rest of the myocardium.

Occasionally, evidence of focal chronic inflammation has been observed but this is uncommon. Sometimes small foci of fibrosis, deep within the myocardium itself are also seen (*Figure 2.6*).

Very often the endocardial surface is covered with a thin layer of fibrin, but sometimes these fibrin thrombi are fairly large and may even be obvious to the naked eye. They can usually be demonstrated by fibrin stains (*Figure 2.7*) and it is thought that they are eventually incorporated into the thickened endocardium.

When the endocardium is stained to demonstrate elastic tissue, the thickened endocardium usually contains many large and often closely packed elastic tissue fibres, as illustrated in *Figure 2.8*. Sometimes the more superficial parts of the thickened endocardium contain no elastic tissue or only a few fine strands or fragments of elastic tissue. The reason for this seems to be that the endocardial thickening is caused by the organization of overlying thrombi, but, in these regions elastic tissue fibres have not yet been laid down.

In fibro-elastosis the endothelium is usually intact, except where thrombus has been deposited but the cells may be swollen and prominent. Between the endothelium and the myocardium is a thick

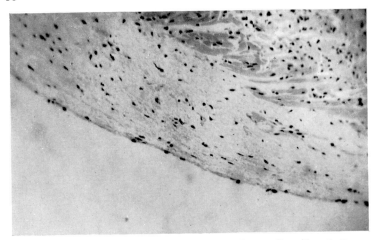

Figure 2.3.   Illustration to show thickened endocardium in fibro-elastosis (haematoxylin and eosin × 50, reduced to 2/3)

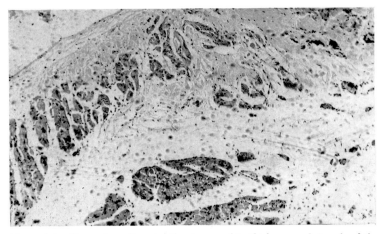

Figure 2.4.   The endocardium is often increased in thickness and strands of the collagenous tissue often extend into the underlying myocardium (haematoxylin and eosin × 256, reduced to 2/3)

layer composed of collagenous and elastic fibres mainly disposed parallel to the surface. A moderate number of fibrocytes are scattered between these fibres, but inflammatory cells are usually absent. Blood vessels are scanty and are confined to the deeper part of the thickened endocardium. The smooth muscle cells may or may not

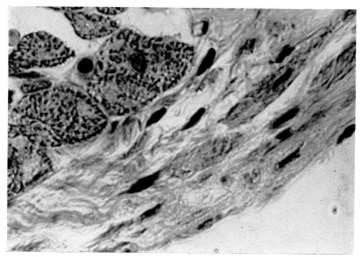

Figure 2.5. Showing single myocardial cells preserved in the thickened endocardium (haematoxylin and eosin × 256) (Zoltowska, 1971)

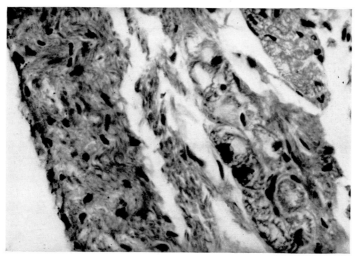

Figure 2.6. Muscle cells without nuclei and with rarefied sarcoplasm and vacuolar degeneration. Some of these degenerate muscle cells are being replaced by fibrous tissue (haematoxylin and eosin × 300) (Zoltowska, 1971)

still be visible, but sometimes they are pronounced and appear hypertrophied. Fibrous tissue bands from the endocardium may penetrate into the myocardium for a short distance and link up with

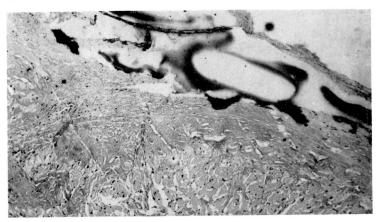

Figure 2.7.   Fibrin thrombi overlying the thickened endocardial surface in a case of fibro-elastosis (Martius' scarlet blue × 256, reduced to 2/3)

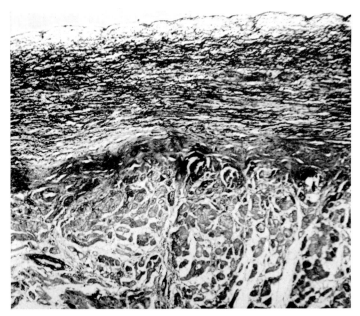

Figure 2.8.   Showing the presence of many elastic tissue fibres within the thickened endocardium (Verhoeff and van Gieson × 160, reduced to 3/4)

other strands of connective tissue surrounding degenerate muscle
fibres.

The histological appearance of the thickened valves differs from
that of the mural endocardium. There are an increased number of
spindle-shaped and stellate connective tissue cells, with an accumulation of much basophilic ground substance so that the cusps
are swollen and mucoid. Increased collagen may appear in lesions of

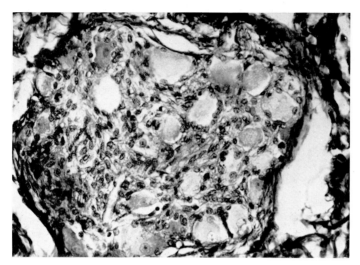

*Figure 2.9. Cell shadows and empty spaces of vanished ganglioh cells
surrounded by wreath of excessively proliferating amphicytes and fibroblasts
(haematoxylin and eosin × 90) (Zoltowska, 1971)*

longer-standing but elastic tissue is often scanty. Various changes
have been described in the myocardium but they are not constant,
and their severity does not seem to parallel the degree of endocardial
thickening. The myocardial lesions are usually most marked in the
layers adjacent to the endocardium, including the papillary muscles.
Hydropic and fatty degeneration (Prior and Wyatt, 1950), acute
necrosis and patchy calcification (Cosgrove and Kaump, 1946),
fibrosis and lymphatic infiltration (Stohr, 1934; Mahon, 1936) have
all been reported. Sometimes the muscle fibres in the affected areas
contain an excess of glycogen as demonstrated by Best's carmine
stain. It has recently been shown that cases of fibro-elastosis usually
show diffuse degenerative changes in the cells of the cardiac ganglia
(Zoltowska, 1971) (*Figure 2.9*). No changes were found in the
conduction tissues of these hearts. It was suggested that cardiac ganglia

are partly responsible for the normal functioning of the conducting tissue in the heart and that these abnormalities might be responsible for the high incidence of arrhythmias and sudden death in fibro-elastosis. The coronary arteries are usually normal. In some instances, however, they have shown histological abnormalities including perivascular fibrosis (Kugel and Stoloff, 1933), medial hypertrophy and calcification (Craig, 1949).

AETIOLOGICAL FACTORS

Of the many factors suggested as being responsible for the causation of endocardial fibro-elastosis, including anoxia (Johnson, 1952), foetal endocarditis (Farber and Hubbard, 1953), 'collagen disease' (Hill and Reilly, 1951) and many others (Rosahn, 1955), four seem worthy of serious consideration.

INHERENT CHANGES IN THE MYOCARDIUM

The primary abnormality may result from changes in the myocardium itself. Black-Schaffer (1957) and Black-Schaffer and Turner (1958) regarded the underlying condition as an *idiopathic myocardial hypertrophy* with dilatation of the left ventricular chamber. In response to dilatation of the left ventricle the endocardium becomes thickened in order to provide internal support to the chamber. Kelly and Anderson (1956) in an earlier report expressed the opinion that myocardial disease, possibly of metabolic origin, may underlie endocardial fibro-elastosis; as supporting evidence they pointed out that endocardial fibro-elastosis may occur in more than one member of a family. Hübschmann (1917), who supplied other evidence supporting the possible role of a myocardial defect, reported the occurrence of left ventricular endocardial fibro-elastosis in instances of diphtheritic myocarditis. Lynfield et al. (1960), on the basis of angiocardiographic and pathological data, have also contended that idiopathic myocardial hypertrophy may be the underlying disease process. This discussion of changes in the myocardial muscle is supported also by the numerous reports of the disease in siblings (Weinberg and Himelfarb, 1943; Nielsen, 1965; Hallidie-Smith and Olsen, 1968), while it has also been reported to have occurred at the same time in a mother and her infant (Moller et al., 1966). These factors do not, however, show definitely that the disease is congenital in origin but may, perhaps, only be due to the same extraneous factors acting on two or more siblings or mother and child.

CARDIAC LYMPHATICS

Another new observation regarding the pathogenesis of endocardial fibro-elastosis, is that furnished by the investigations of Miller *et al.* (1963) concerning the role played by cardiac lymphatics in this disease. Following interruption of cardiac lymphatic drainage, these observers noticed endocardial fibro-elastosis principally of the left ventricle. The histological appearance of the left ventricular endocardium in their experimental animals was identical to that of primary endocardial fibro-elastosis of man. Kline *et al.* (1964) have proposed that the obstruction of cardiac lymph flow produces an aseptic necrosis of some of the myocardial fibres underlying the

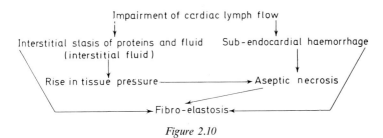

Figure 2.10

endocardium, and then their replacement by fibrous tissue, in which elastic tissue subsequently develops. A schematic outline of this process is given in *Figure 2.10* (Kline *et al.*, 1964).

Kline *et al.* (1964) have also shown at necropsy on two subjects, aged 6 months and 52 years respectively, who suffered from fibro-elastosis, the presence of chronic impairment of cardiac lymphatic drainage. The emphasis upon the possibility that lymphatic obstruction contributes to endocardial fibro-elastosis awaits confirmation by further similar studies.

POSSIBLE RELATIONSHIP OF MUMPS

A possible relationship of mumps infection to primary endocardial fibro-elastosis is commonly put forward, this viral infection being the primary causative factor. This was originally reported by Noren, Adams and Anderson (1963), who noticed a high incidence of positive reactions to the mumps skin test among children who suffered from primary endocardial fibro-elastosis. Subsequently, Sellers, Keith and Manning (1964) and Vosburgh *et al.* (1965) made similar observations. On the contrary, among patients with secondary endocardial fibro-elastosis coexisting with aortic stenosis or coarctation of the aorta, the incidence of positive skin tests is no greater than among those with other congenital manifestations not associated with endocardial fibro-elastosis. The aetiological relationship, between the mumps virus and primary endocardial fibro-elastosis, is not clear. Despite their frequent positive response to the mumps antigen skin test, children with primary endocardial fibro-elastosis rarely have serologically demonstrable circulating antibodies against mumps virus. There may be no aetiological relationship between mumps infection and fibro-elastosis as demonstrated by the study of Chen, Thompson and Rose (1971), who have demonstrated that, although many patients with fibro-elastosis have a positive reaction to mumps antigen, none can be demonstrated in their serum. St Geme, Noren and Adams (1964) reported that several mothers who either had developed clinical mumps or had been exposed to mumps during early pregnancy, subsequently delivered children with endocardial fibro-elastosis. On the other hand a perspective study of mumps infection by Korones *et al.* (1970) detected no case of fibro-elastosis in the children of 18 mothers in whom mumps virus infection had been demonstrated during pregnancy.

It has also been suggested that fibro-elastosis may be due to infection with other types of virus. Thus, Mehrizi *et al.* (1965) described two infants dying of heart failure following enterovirus infection, one at 37 months from poliovirus type II and the other at 22 months from Coxsackie B5 infection. At autopsy both hearts showed endocardial fibro-elastosis; no virus was isolated from either heart. Brown and Evans (1967) found serological evidence that Coxsackie virus infection in the first trimester was related to congenital heart disease.

METABOLIC AND CONGENITAL ABNORMALITIES

It should also be noted here that some metabolic disease, i.e., glycogen storage disease, may exhibit secondary fibro-elastosis. The mechanism for this is not understood.

Similarly other congenital cardiac abnormalities such as left ventricular hypoplasia may be associated with fibro-elastosis, but to me this relationship does not seem clear and infers only that the aetiology is purely mechanical.

CONCLUSIONS

In conclusion, although we do not know the cause of fibro-elastosis it seems relatively certain that the endocardial thickening is due to two separate factors. (1) The organization of small fibrin thrombi which are laid down on the endocardial surface (2). The proliferation of mesenchymal cells below the endocardium, in a similar manner to that which has been shown to cause subintimal thickening of the coronary arteries in children (Schornagel, 1956).

It is uncertain as to whether inheritance plays any part in the development of this disease, although there are about 11 case reports in the literature of relatives being affected. This work of Chen appears to show that there is a family relationship. Thus in a study of 119 families with fibro-elastosis, 7 had 2 siblings affected and 2 had 3. It may well be that cases of mother and child being affected, as in the case reported by Moller *et al.* (1966), are due to both having been exposed simultaneously to the same stress.

PROGNOSIS

Although death during the neonatal period is uncommon, most children fail to live longer than four or five years of age. In the 23 cases of primary endocardial fibro-elastosis, of the dilated type studied by Moller *et al.* (1966) the age of death ranged from 7 hours to 16 years. Fifteen of these patients survived the first year of life.

References

Black-Schaffer, B. (1957). 'Infantile endocardial fibro-elastosis—a suggested etiology.' *Archs Path.* **63**, 281
— and Turner, M. E. (1958). 'Hyperplastic infantile cardiomegaly; a form of "idiopathic hypertrophy" with or without endocardial fibro-elastosis; and a comment on cardiac atrophy.' *Am. J. Path.* **34**, 745
Blumberg, R. W. and Lyon, R. A. (1952). 'Endocardial sclerosis'. *Am. J. Dis. Child.* **84**, 291
Brown, G. C. and Evans, T. N. (1967). 'Serologic evidence of Coxsackie virus etiology of congenital heart disease.' *J. Am. Med. Ass.* **199**, 151
Chen, S. C., Thompson, M. W. and Rose, Vera (1971). 'Endocardial fibro-elastosis: family studies with special reference to counselling.' *J. Pediat.* **79**, 385
Cosgrove, G. E. and Kaump, D. H. (1946). 'Endocardial sclerosis in infants and children.' *Am. J. clin. Path.* **16**, 322
Craig, J. M. (1949). 'Congenital endocardial sclerosis.' *Bull. int. Ass. med. Mus.* **30**, 15
Dyson, A., Burton, C. and Decker, J. P. (1958). 'Endocardial fibro-elastosis in the adult.' *Br. Heart J.* **66**, 190
Edwards, J. E. (1953). 'Congenital malformations of the heart and great vessels.' In *Pathology of the Heart.* Ed. by S. E. Gould p. 420. Springfield, Ill: Thomas

Farber, S. and Hubbard, J. (1953). 'Fetal endomyocardial intrauterine infection as the cause of congenital cardiac anomalies.' *Am. J. med. Sci.* **186**, 705

Fixler, D. E., Cole, R. B., Paul, M. H., Lev, M. and Girod, D. A. (1970). 'Familial occurrence of the contracted form of endocardial fibroelastosis.' *Am. J. Cardiol.* **26**, 208

Forter, J. O., Miller, R. A., Bein, A. D. and McCloed, W. (1964). 'Endocardial fibro-elastosis.' *Br. med. J.* **2**, 7

Hallidie-Smith, K. A. and Olsen, E. G. J. (1968). 'Endocardial fibroelastosis, mitral incompetence and coarctation of the abdominal aorta.' *Br. Heart J.* **30**, 850

Halliday, W. R. (1954). 'Endomyocardial fibro-elastosis. A study of thirty cases.' *Dis. Chest* **26**, 27

Hill, W. T. and Reilly, W. A. (1951). 'Endocardial fibro-elastosis.' *Am. J. Dis. Child.* **82**, 579

Hoffman, F. G. (1960). 'Adult endocardial fibro-elastosis associated with dextro-cardia and situs inversus.' *Circulation*, **22**, 437

Hübschmann, P. (1917). 'Über Myokarditis und andere Pathologische— anatomische Baspachturgen bei Diphthire.' *München med. Wschr.* **64**, 73

Johnson, F. R. (1952). 'Anoxia as a cause of endocardial fibro-elastosis in infancy.' *Archs Path.* **54**, 237

Kelly, J. and Anderson, D. H. (1956). 'Congenital endocardial fibroelastosis; Clinical and pathologic investigation of those cases without associated cardiac malformations including report of 2 familial instances.' *Pediatrics, Springfield* **18**, 539

Kline, I. K., Miller, A. J., Pick, R. and Katz, L. N. (1964). 'The relationship between human endocardial fibro-elastosis and obstruction of the cardiac lymphatics.' *Circulation* **30**, 728

Korones, S. B., Todaro, J., Roane, J. A. and Sever, J. L. (1970). 'Maternal virus infection after the first trimester of pregnancy and status of offspring to 4 years of age in a predominantly Negro population.' *J. Pediat.* **77**, 245

Kugel, M. A. and Stoloff, E. G. (1933). 'Dilatation and hypertrophy of heart in infants and in young children with myocardial degeneration and fibrosis (so-called congenital idiopathic hypertrophy).' *Am. J. Dis. Child.* **45**, 828

Linde, L. M., Adams, F. H. and O'Loughlin, B. J. (1958). 'Endocardial fibro-elastosis. Angiocardiographic studies.' *Circulation* **17**, 40

Lintermans, J. P., Kaplan, E. L., Morgan, B. C., Baum, D. and Guntheroth, W. G. (1966). 'Infection patterns in endocardial fibro-elastosis.' *Circulation* **33**, 202

Lynfield, J., Gasul, R. M., Luan, L. L. and Dillon, R. K. (1960). 'Right and left heart cathaterisation and angiocardiographic findings in idiopathic cardiac hypertrophy with endocardial fibro-elastosis.' *Circulation* **21**, 386

McLoughlin, T. G., Schiebler, G. L. and Knovetz, L. J. (1966). 'Endocardial fibro-elastosis in American Negro children, a distinct entity?' *Am. Heart J.* **71**, 748

Mahon, G. S. (1936). 'Idiopathic hypertrophy of the heart with endo-cardial fibrosis: Report of 2 cases.' *Am. Heart J.* **12**, 608

Mehrizi, A. I., Hutchins, G. M., Medearis, D. N. Jnr. and Rowe, R. D. (1965). 'Enterovirus infection and endocardial fibro-elastosis.' *Circulation* suppl. II, 31, 27, 150

Miller, A. J., Pick, Ruth and Katz, L. N. (1963). 'Ventricular endomyocardial changes after impairment of cardiac lymph flow in dogs.' *Br. Heart J.* **25**, 182

Moller, J. H., Fisch, R. O., From, A. H. L. and Edwards, J. E. (1966). 'Endocardial fibro-elastosis occurring in a mother and son.' *Pediatrics*, *Springfield* **38**, 918

— Luces, R. V., Jnr, Adams, P., Jnr, Anderson, R. C., Jorgans, J. and Edwards, J. E. (1964). 'Endocardial fibro-elastosis. A clinical and anatomic study of 47 patients with emphasis on its relationship to mitral insufficiency.' *Circulation* **30**, 759

Nielson, J. S. (1965). 'Primary endocardial fibro-elastosis in three siblings.' *Acta med. scand.* **177**, 195

Noren, G. R., Adams, P. and Anderson, R. C. (1963). 'Positive skin reactivity to mumps virus antigen in endocardial fibro-elastosis.' *J. Pediat.* **62**, 604

Ogan, H. (1960). 'Diffuse endomyocardial sclerosis (a report of a case diagnosed during life).' *Bull. Soc. int. Chir.* **19**, 469

Panke, W. and Rottino, A. (1955). 'Endocardial fibro-elastosis occurring in the adult.' *Am. Heart J.* **49**, 89

Peale, A. R. and Lucchesi, P. F. (1942). 'Report of case of measles encephalitis complicated by so-called "fetal endocarditis and gonorrheal pyosalpinx".' *Am. J. clin. Path.* **12**, 357

Prior, J. T. and Wyatt, T. C. (1950). 'Endocardial fibro-elastosis. A study of eight cases.' *Am. J. Path.* **26**, 969

Rosahn, P. D. (1955). 'Endocardial fibro-elastosis—old and new concepts.' *Bull. N.Y. Acad. Med.* **31**, 453

Schornagel, H. E. (1956). 'Intimal thickening in coronary arteries in infants.' *J. Am. med. Ass.* **62**, 427

Sellers, F. J., Keith, J. D. and Manning, J. A. (1964). 'The diagnosis of primary endocardial fibro-elastosis.' *Circulation* **29**, 49

Smith, J. J. and Forth, J. (1943). 'Fibrosis of the endocardium and myocardium with mural thrombosis.' *Archs intern. Med.* **71**, 602

Stohr, Grete (1934). 'Malformations of the heart of the new-born; congenital lesions suggestive of inflammatory origin.' *Archs Path.* **17**, 311

St Geme, J. W., Noren, G. R. and Adams, P. (1964). 'Some immunologic and virologic aspects of apparent intrauterine mumps virus infection and subsequent primary endocardial fibroelastosis (obstruct).' *J. Pediat.* **65**, 1111

Thomas, W. A., Randall, R. V., Bland, E. F. and Castleman, B. (1954). 'Endocardial fibro-elastosis.' *New Engl. J. Med.* **251**, 327

Van Buchan, F. S. P., Arends, A. and Schroder, E. A. (1959). 'Endocardial fibro-elastosis in adolescents and adults.' *Br. Heart J.* **21**, 229

Vosburgh, J. B., Diehl, A. M., Liu, C., Lauer, R. M. and Fabiyi, A. (1965). 'Relationship of mumps to endocardial fibro-elastosis.' *Am. J. Dis. Child.* **109**, 67

Weinberg, T. and Himelfarb, A. J. (1943). 'Endocardial fibro-elastosis (so called fetal endocarditis); report of 2 cases occurring in siblings.' *Bull. Johns Hopkins Hosp.* **72**, 299

White, P. P. and Fennell, R. H. Jnr (1954). 'Endocardial fibro-elastosis with marked cardiac enlargement and failure in a man of 71, dying at the age of 71 after 15 years of angina pectoris and two years of congestive heart failure.' *Archs intern. Med.* **41**, 333

Winter, S. T., Moses, W. S., Cohen, N. J. and Naftalin, J. M. (1960). 'Primary endocardial fibro-elastosis in two sisters.' *Am. J. Dis. Child.* **99**, 529

Yoshida, T., Nimura, Y., Sakakebara, H., Matsutani, K., Nishizaki, K. and Nakata, T. (1964). 'A diffuse endocardial fibro-elastosis with markedly dilated right atrium observed in an adult.' *Jap. Heart J.* **5**, 85

Zoltowska, Albina (1971). 'Endocardial fibro-elastosis in children with special reference to the lesions of cardiac ganglia.' *J. clin. Path.* **24**, 263

Three

Primary myocardial disease

Disorders which affect the myocardium have been classified in several different ways. Mattingly (1961) employs the term 'primary myocardial disease' as inclusive not only of the idiopathic disorders, but also of more generalized disorders when the myocardium is the principal site of involvement. He then goes further and defines it as: 'a cardiac disease which specifically affects the heart muscle but spares other anatomical structures within the cardiovascular system.' For greater clarity I prefer a different classification. Here the term 'primary myocardial disease' refers only to that group of idiopathic cardiomyopathies which are characterized by dilatation and hypertrophy of the whole heart and slight endocardial thickening, which commonly underlies a mural thrombus. Josserand and Gallavardin (1901) appear to have been the first to describe this disease when they reported three cases; two had cardiomegaly, myocardial fibrosis, mural thrombus at the apex and pulmonary emboli; the third patient presented similarly, but also showed degeneration of some myocardial fibres. Such terms as myocardiosis (Blankenhorn and Gall, 1956), idiopathic cardiac hypertrophy (Levy and Von Glahn, 1944) and idiopathic cardiomyopathy (Goodwin et al., 1961) are probably equivalent terms for describing primary myocardial disease.

This primary form of idiopathic cardiomyopathy almost certainly represents a heterogeneous group of disorders of varying aetiological causes and in some instances may include cardiomyopathies which are discussed in this work under some other titles such as the familial cardiomyopathies described by Evans (1957).

INCIDENCE

Employing commonly used aetiological classifications of heart disease there will be left about a half per cent of cases which do not fit into any of the known causes of cardiac disease, and which present with signs of myocardial insufficiency of unknown origin (Storstein, 1964).

There are only a few large series of patients with primary myo-cardial disease where the sex is given, but it appears that about two-thirds of the patients reported are men (Storstein, 1964).

CLINICAL PRESENTATION

Dyspnoea is the most common way in which these patients present themselves but the symptoms of this heart disease are sometimes discovered accidentally. Thus, for instance, a patient may be found to have an enlarged heart on routine radiography, but about half the cases present first with congestive heart failure.

It is very important to recognize the role which respiratory involvement may play in the development of congestive heart failure in primary myocardial disease. Thus, in the paper by Goodwin (1970) 13 out of the 74 cases of primary congestive cardiac myopathy described were preceded by attacks of respiratory infection.

AGE OF ONSET

The most common age for this disease to present is between 40 and 50, but it can be found in the young adult, thus two of the cases of Parameswaran, Meadows and Sharp (1969) were males aged between 30 and 33 or even children (Harris, Rodin and Ngheim, 1968). That the cardiac enlargement found in these patients is not present from birth or childhood can be shown to be correct by a study of the records of military personnel who have died with this disease. For example, Norris and Pote (1946) described four cases of primary myocardial disease from the Philadelphia Naval Hospital and showed that 20 per cent of them had normal-sized hearts two to four years before the disease was detected. In the 9 cases, reported by Muehsam, Pschibul and Scerbo (1964), who died from primary myocardial disease, all had normal-sized hearts in routine chest x-ray taken between 7 and 17 years beforehand. In one patient where the diagnosis of cardiomegaly was made by mass radiography, before the onset of congestive heart failure, the time interval between the last documented evidence of a normal-sized heart and the diagnosis of 'congestive cardiomyopathy' was four years. It is not clear from the description given if primary myocardial disease does occur in children, but Hill and Reilly (1968) describe 8 cases of what they call idiopathic non-obstructive cardiomegaly; and 7 of their cases appear to be so with patchy endocardial thickening, containing both fibrous and to a lesser extent elastic tissue which affected the inflow more than the outflow tract. Some of these hearts were considerably enlarged, the largest weighing 890 g.

PATHOLOGY

The hearts of these patients are enlarged in almost all cases and are usually in the range of 500–700 g, although weights of up to 1,040 g (Muehsam, Pschibul and Scerbo, 1964) have been recorded. The ventricles are usually dilatated (*Figure 3.1*) and the myocardium is often flabby. *Figure 3.2* shows the heart weights and ventricular wall

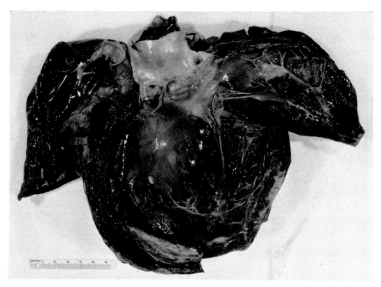

Figure 3.1. The left ventricle has been opened through the aortic valve. A flat organized thrombus overlies the endocardium in the region of the apex. The adjacent ventricular wall has scarred areas of thick grey fibrosis. (Reproduced from Harris, Rodin and Nghiem (1968) by courtesy of the authors and Editor of the American Journal of Cardiology)

thickness as found in the series of patients described as cases of 'congestive cardiomyopathy' by Goodwin (1970). Most of this series were cases of primary myocardial disease, although some were probably cases of alcoholic cardiomyopathy or peri-partal cardiomyopathy.

The heart is usually enlarged, the ventricles being dilated. The left ventricular wall retains, in most cases, its normal thickness but often the wall of the right ventricle becomes considerably thickened.

On opening the heart, the endocardium lining both the atria and ventricles is seen to be greyish-white in colour and slightly thickened (*Figure 3.3*).

This endocardial thickening is not usually so great as to interfere with the normal functioning of any cardiac valves, papillary muscles or chordae tendineae. Overlying the thickened endocardium there is

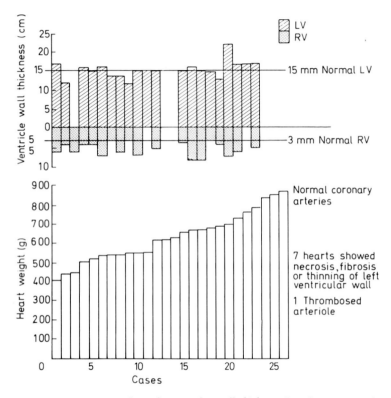

Figure 3.2. Heart weight and ventricular wall thickness in primary congestive cardiomyopathy. (*Reproduced from Goodwin (1970) by courtesy of the author and Editor of the* Lancet)

very often thrombus which is commonly situated at one or both of the ventricular apices. However, heart weights are above normal in almost all cases, confirming the fact that hypertrophy does indeed occur; the lack of increase in wall thickness usually observed is due to dilatation of the cavity. Coronary artery atherosclerosis is absent in the majority of cases or, if present, is only minimal in extent.

Microscopically, the endocardium is usually found to be only slightly thickened (*Figure 3.4*). In some places thin strands of fibrous tissue are seen extending down from the endocardium into the underlying myocardium, sometimes for considerable distances. Small areas of perivascular fibrosis are often seen in the myocardium around small intramyocardial blood vessels. Also sometimes present are

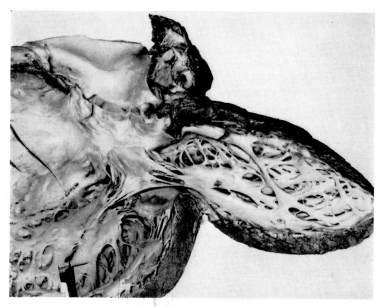

Figure 3.3. Gross appearance of a primary myocardial diseased heart from a 60 year old female who died in intractable cardiac failure. Note that all the endocardium is diffusely thickened and that there is slight speckling of the cut myocardium due to diffuse infiltration with fibrotic tissue

small foci of fibrosis, seeming possibly to be small infarcts in the myocardium.

Patchy myocardial fibrosis is present in about half the hearts described. These fibrous areas most commonly involve the myocardium immediately below the endocardium of the left ventricle and less commonly the right ventricle or interventricular septum. This fibrosis is diffuse in about a third of the cases but the fibrous tissue usually seems to have a function to replace myocardial tissue, although it may be focal in distribution. Small foci of degeneration with decreased cell size and nuclear pyknosis are also seen (*Figure 3.5*).

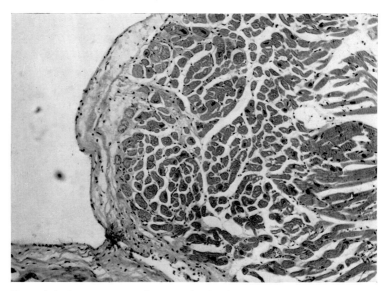

Figure 3.4   In congestive cardiomyopathy the photograph shows slight thickening of the endocardium and a few strands of fibrous tissue passing into the underlying myocardium. In this section a scattering of lymphocytes may be seen together with the fact that a few of the myocardial nuclei are distorted and 'staghorn' shaped (haematoxylin and eosin × 40, reduced to 2/3)

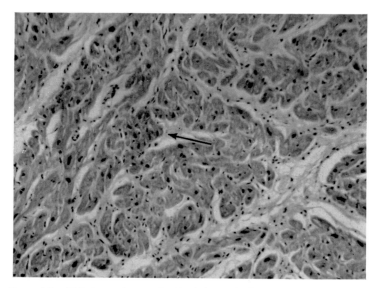

Figure 3.5.   This is a micrograph of a left ventricular myocardium. Interstitial areas are increased in width and exhibit a fine fibrous reaction. The arrow points to a focus of degeneration with decreased cell size, increased cytoplasmic density and nuclear pyknosis (haematoxylin and eosin × 120, reduced to 9/10). (Reproduced from Harris, Rodin and Ngheim (1968) by courtesy of the authors and Editor of the American Journal of Cardiology)

There is often an infiltration of the myocardium with chronic inflammatory cells, which are chiefly lymphocytes together with a smaller number of monocytes. Eosinophils and plasma cells are not usually present. In the myocardium immediately adjacent to the pericardium this lymphocytic infiltrate may be increased if a pericardial effusion is also present. This cellular infiltration of the myocardium is usually focal in distribution.

The myocardial cells are not usually hypertrophied, but there is a considerable variation in their size and intensity of staining. These myocardial cells often do not appear to have nuclei or, if present, these are often pyknotic or abnormally shaped. Almost all the myocardial cells are diffusely separated by thin strands of fibrous tissue (*Figure 3.6*).

Infrequently, small intracytoplasmic vacuoles may also be present. The cell nuclei are often pyknotic and distorted in shape, taking up abnormal forms such as those likened to a 'staghorn'. Less commonly, some of these nuclei may be enlarged and contain small vacuoles.

The intramyocardial blood vessels are normal but may be congested and dilatated, especially when congestive heart failure is present.

Fibrin stains less commonly show a thin layer of fibrin overlying the thickened endocardium (*Figure 3.7*). Larger fibrin clots may be seen much less commonly. In the thickened endocardium small deposits of fibrin are also sometimes present, having possibly originated from the incorporation of fibrin by organization. No fibrin deposits are seen elsewhere in the myocardium.

Elastic tissue stains demonstrate that the thickened endocardium always retains its normal basement layer. In the more superficial parts of the endocardium there are, commonly, many scattered and fragmented strands of elastic tissue, while in the area immediately below the cardiac cavity there is often another elastic tissue layer (*Figure 3.8*).

However, occasionally, the thickened endocardium contains little elastic tissue (*Figure 3.9*) or, much less commonly, a great deal. Some parts of the myocardium are replaced by fibrous tissue (*Figure 3.10*).

Apart from a slight increase in acid mucopolysaccharides present around foci of inflammatory cells, no other changes can be demonstrated with routine histological stains on material which is obtained after death.

Patchy myocardial fibrosis is present in about half the hearts described. These fibrous areas most commonly involve the myocardium immediately below the endocardium of the left septum. This fibrosis is diffuse in about a third of the cases but the fibrous

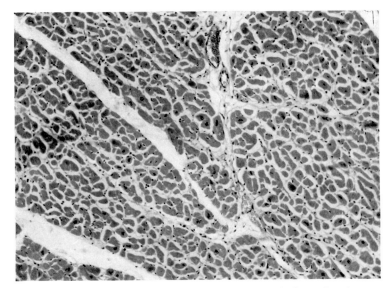

Figure 3.6. *In congestive cardiomyopathy the photograph shows that the myocardial cells are not hypertrophied but that there is a considerable variation in the size and staining of many myocardial cells, which often do not appear to have nuclei. Note that almost all the myocardial cells are diffusely separated by thin strands of fibrous tissues (haematoxylin and eosin × 40, reduced to 2/3)*

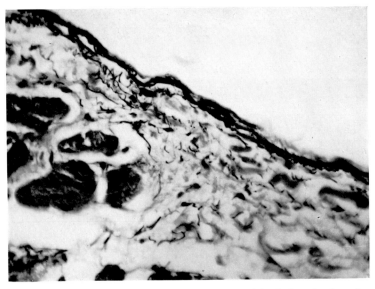

Figure 3.7. *A thin layer of fibrin seen on the surface of the thickened endocardium (Martius' scarlet blue × 120, reduced to 2/3)*

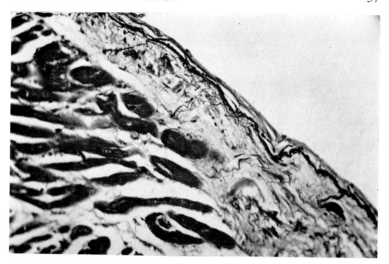

Figure 3.8. This micrograph shows many scattered elastic fibres in the thickened endocardium (Verhoeff and van Gieson × 750, reduced to 2/3)

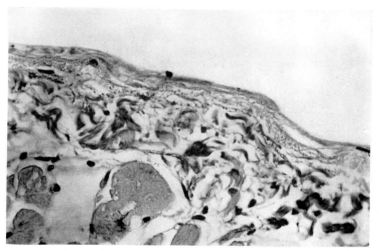

Figure 3.9. The endocardium containing little elastic tissue (Verhoeff and van Gieson × 756, reduced to 2/3)

tissue usually has a function to replace myocardial tissue, although it may sometimes be focal in nature.

ELECTRON MICROSCOPY

In a few cases of primary myocardial disease, where needle biopsies of the heart have been carried out during life, the following results have been described (Takatsu *et al.*, 1968). In these cases the biopsies were taken for the right and left ventricles. In almost all the muscle fibres present in the biopsies a diffusely-stained or granular substance of peculiar nature was seen. This substance was stored in the widened sarcoplasmic space, and often occupied the whole

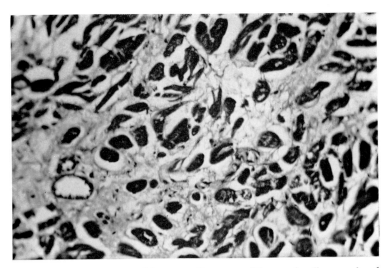

Figure 3.10.   In some parts of the myocardium many of the muscle cells are replaced or separated by fibrous tissue (haematoxylin and eosin × 250, reduced to 2/3)

section of a muscle fibre with apparent loss of myofibrils (*Figure 3.11*). This material was stained light red with eosin and blue with alcian blue, probably indicating that this material contained acid mucopolysaccharides. In cardiac muscle where the amount of fibrous tissue present is considerably greater, this curious eosinophilic or granular substance was still present (*Figure 3.12*).

Bulloch and Murphy (1967) studied needle biopsies of the interventricular septum of 10 patients, comparing the findings with control samples from patients undergoing open heart surgery and with needle biopsies from dogs. Light microscopy showed lesions in 5. Electron microscopy in 8 cases showed partial to complete loss of

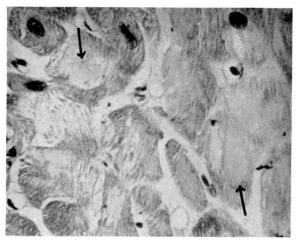

Figure 3.11. Right ventricular myocardium of biopsy specimen obtained by a Konno biopsy catheter, or 'biotome'. Note a diffusely stained or granular substance (arrows) in the widened sarcoplasmic space (haematoxylin and eosin × 320, reduced to 2/3). (Reproduced from Bulloch and Murphy (1967) by courtesy of the authors and the Editor of Circulation)

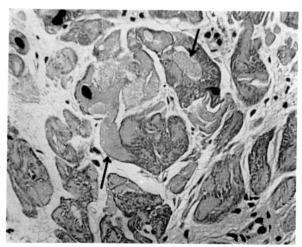

Figure 3.12. Left ventricular myocardium of needle biopsy specimen obtained during thoracotomy for implantation of an electric pacemaker. Arrows show the similar deposits seen in the muscle fibres of the right auricle (haematoxylin and eosin × 320, reduced to 2/3). (Reproduced from Bulloch and Murphy (1967) by courtesy of the authors and the Editor of Circulation)

cristae in the mitochondria. One showed unidentified particles in swollen mitochondria, some of which were ruptured, 5 showed dilatation of the sarcoplasmic reticulum and 3 showed an increase in glycogen. None showed any consistent lesion of the nuclei or sarcolemma. The authors suggested that the changes in mitochondria

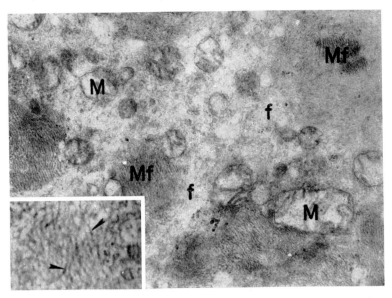

Figure 3.13.   Electron micrograph of left ventricular myocardium. Note peculiar fine fibrous structures (Mf) and definitely abnormal mitochondria (M) (× 20,000, reduced to 2/3). The peculiar fibrous structures at the higher magnification are shown at the left lower corner with arrows (× 100,000, reduced to 2/3). (Reproduced from Takatsu et al. (1968) by courtesy of the authors and the Editor of the American Heart Journal)

and sarcoplasmic reticulum represented defects of energy production and of exertation-contraction.

Takatsu *et al.* (1968) also carried out electron microscopic studies on their cardiac biopsy material. In many of the sarcoplasmic spaces there were peculiar, fine fibrous structures running in various directions (*Figure 3.13*). At higher magnification the fibrous structures revealed a tubular appearance measuring approximately 50–80 Å in diameter and were tightly tangled together in the sarcoplasm. Besides the fibrous structures, pigment granules consisting of a number of spherical osmophilic bodies of varying size were found in the sarcoplasm (*Figure 3.14*).

In all the specimens examined the myofibrils and mitochondria are found to be very scarce (*Figure 3.15*). Most of the mitochondria are definitely abnormal. Some are small, whereas others are swollen or have few or no cristae. Besides abnormal mitochondria and pigment granules, there are numerous vesicular formations in the area of sarcoplasm where no myofibrils are seen.

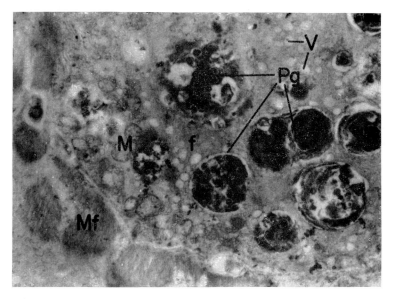

Figure 3.14.   Pigment granules (Pg) consisting of a number of spherical osmiophilic materials of varying size in the left ventricular myocardium. Abnormal mitochondria (M) and vesicular structures (V) are seen. Peculiar fibrous structures (f) are also present in the sarcoplasm where myofibrils (Mf) are very scarce (× 12,500, reduced to 2/3. (Reproduced from Takatsu et al. (1968) by courtesy of the authors and the Editor of the American Heart Journal)

In this study these workers found an increased number of glycogen granules (*Figure 3.16*).

The morphological features of the peculiar deposits found in the myocardial fibres described above resemble those of the deposits of a fibrillary polysaccharide material reported by Ferrans *et al.* (1966).

All the work carried out on the fine fibrous structures and pigment granules suggest some degradation process resulting from abnormal metabolism and functions of the myocardial cells.

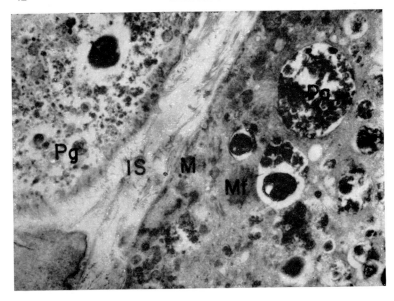

Figure 3.15. In the left ventricular myocardium some of the pigment granules (Pg) *are limited by the membraneous structure, while others are not. Some of the constituents of the pigment granules are dispersed into the cytoplasm. The myofibrils* (Mf) *are extremely scarce* (M—*mitochondria;* IS—*interstitial space:* × *12,500, reduced to 2/3*). (*Reproduced from Takatsu* et al. (*1968*) *by courtesy of the authors and the Editor of the* American Heart Journal)

MODE OF DEATH

Many of these patients die of congestive heart failure, but there is a high incidence of thrombo-embolic episodes, the thrombi usually arising from the left and right ventricles particularly their apices. There also seems to be an appreciable number of cases where the cause of death is myocardial infarction, due to obstruction of a coronary artery by an embolus arising in the heart (Gau *et al.*, 1969; Parameswaran, Meadows and Sharp, 1969).

AETIOLOGY OF UNIDENTIFIED AGENTS

It has long been suspected that the aetiological cause for this disease may be infectious in origin. This view has been given some support by the studies of Braimbridge *et al.* (1967).

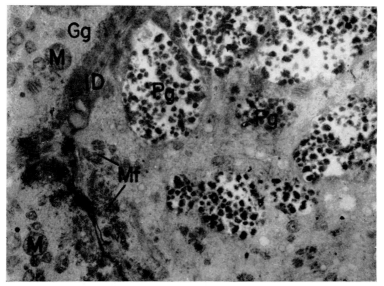

Figure 3.16. Glycogen granules (Gg) *in the ventricular myocardium seem to be increased in number. Pigment granules* (Pg), *myofibrils* (Mf), *mitochondria* (M) *of varying sizes and intercalated discs* (ID) *are indicated* (× *12,500, reduced to 2/3*). (*Reproduced from Takatsu et al.* (*1968*) *by courtesy of the authors and the Editor of the* American Heart Journal)

UNIDENTIFIED INFECTIOUS AGENTS

Braimbridge *et al.* (1967) claimed to have isolated a possible infectious agent from 7 patients (6 males and 1 female aged 20–60 years) with congestive cardiomyopathy; 6 in myocardial drill biopsies (obtained by Braimbridge) and 1 from a necropsy heart; in 2 cases both sources were used. The tissues were frozen at −70°C in hexane; cryostat sections were cut at −30°C, fixed in a picrate-formaline solution and stained with 0·1 per cent toluidine blue in 0·2 M acetate buffer at pH 4·2; this stained nuclei and the infective agent presented as large pink so-called 'mark' bodies up to 40 × 20 μ in size, being amorphous, granular or segmented, often resembling round nuclei. There were also numerous pink, purple or greenish granules measuring 1 μ in diameter. These structures also stained with Giemsa but were not seen in ordinary paraffin sections. They were not lipofuchsine, amyloid or glycogen and enzymes studied, especially cytochrome oxidase and dopa-oxidase, indicated foreign living matter. No growth was obtained on blood agar, or nutrient broth or in the peritoneum of mice, but proliferation occurred in four days, in the synthetic median T8, containing chloramphenicol, adenosine diphosphate (ADP) or nicotinamide-adenime dinucleotide (NAD) plus NADphosphate in an atmosphere of 95 per cent oxygen and 5 per cent carbon dioxide.

Cultures injected into mice caused dyspnoea, stridor and paralysis in 5 hours, and death in 18; the metachromatic particles were found in the brain, nerves and skeletal muscles mainly, but also in the heart and liver. Mice receiving normal myocardium preparations were unaffected. Braimbridge claimed that the agent fulfilled Koch's postulates. Naturally this work came under criticism. Grist (1967) said that intracellular bodies could be produced by a wide variety of toxic and non-physiological influences and that the rapid death of the mice suggested a toxic effect.

Until this work can be reproduced and the ability of this agent to be further passaged in mice, together with its more precise identity established, this work remains a matter of speculation.

VIRAL

Several studies for viral antibodies have been carried out—the most detailed being that of Fletcher et al. (1968) who studied 34 patients with primary myocardial disease. Neutralizing antibodies to Coxsackie viruses B1–6 and ECHO viruses 6 and 9 were sought as well as complement-fixing antibodies to influenza A and B, mumps soluble antigen, mumps viral antigen, herpes simplex and psittacosis. There were 34 patients and the average duration of illness was 72 months.

Antibody titres did not differ significantly when compared with an age- and sex-matched control group. There was also no significant difference between the sexes or in patients aged more or less than 50 years. This does not, however, exclude an aetiological role for a previous viral infection in myocardial disease. In chronic situations auto-immune mechanisms initiated by a previous viral infection may no longer be detected by the estimation of antibody titres.

AUTO-IMMUNE MECHANISMS

Fletcher and Wenger (1968) have carried out heart immuno-fluorescent antibody tests, the complement-fixation test for Chagas' disease, the haemagglutination test for toxoplasmosis and the latex flocculation test for rheumatoid disease in 34 patients with primary myocardial disease. There was no difference in the incidence of elevated titres when compared with the control group of any of these tests. This study, however, is limited in that it gives no information about an agent or mechanism for primary myocardial disease, which is no longer demonstrable by serological tests; particularly since the patients with primary myocardial disease were studied, on average, six years after the onset of symptoms.

They have, however, demonstrated that there is no serological evidence associating the parasites or immunological responses studied with the symptoms of primary myocardial disease. In another earlier study Gardner *et al.* (1967) of Los Angeles, California, observed cytoplasmic virus-like particles in the cells of an apical cardiac biopsy from a man of 27 years with idiopathic cardiomyopathy, who never recovered properly from an influenza-like illness several months previously. Electron microscopy showed spherical and oval particles 50–100 μ in diameter with dense centres, a limiting membrane and an outer envelope. The involved cells were interstitial cells and they showed cytolytic damage and also numerous fine, beaded cytoplasmic filaments which were not obviously related to the virus particles, the latter replicated by budding. Sanders (1963) in an earlier study carried out extensive virological studies on a large group of cases of 'primary myocardial disease', but all of which were negative.

ARTERIOPATHY

It was suggested by James (1962), when he reviewed his several publications concerning medial necrosis of the small coronary and pulmonary arteries in several inherited cardiomyopathies (such as Marfan's syndrome), that a similar pathology might underlie non-specific cardiomyopathies (primary myocardial disease). The author, however, has never seen any arterial changes in cases of primary myocardial disease and, in this, is supported by the work of Gau *et al.* (1969) who, having studied the coronary arteries in 32 patients with congestive cardiomyopathy found the vessels in all cases to be normal at autopsy. In 12 of these patients coronary angiography had been used in addition and this also revealed a normal vascular pattern.

ENZYME DEFICIENCY

Wendt *et al.* (1962) have also demonstrated increased glycolysis in the hearts of patients with primary myocardial disease and greater activity of malic dehydrogenase and aldolase in coronary venous rather than arterial blood suggesting increased permeability of the myocardial cell. This effect is, however, noted in other cardiomyopathies and is probably non-specific. Kobernick *et al.* (1963) reported the deficiencies of succinic dehydrogenase in cases of primary myocardial disease but no further studies have since been carried out in this field and the value of the observations is unclear.

ISCHAEMIC CARDIOMYOPATHY

This disease has many similarities with primary myocardial disease and these two conditions may very easily be confused (Raftery, Banks and Oram, 1969). It is most commonly seen in the 50–60 age group but may be found in younger patients (Burch and Giles, 1972). The primary cause is usually atherosclerosis of the smaller intramyocardial arteries causing impairment or obstruction of blood flow into the myocardium.

The hearts are dilated, flabby and hypertrophied weighing 500 g or more. The coronary arteries show diffuse arteriosclerotic disease. Scarring of the myocardium is seen and is mostly, but not always, limited to the left ventricle. Histological examination shows diffuse, scattered areas of fibrosis and myocardial degeneration and atrophy. Hypertrophy of myocardial fibres is seen, some with markedly abnormal nuclei. Myocytolysis is evident throughout but occasional areas of the myocardium appear relatively normal when seen with the light microscope. However, extensive cellular damage is evident in these areas when examined with the electron microscope.

References

Blankenhorn, M. A. and Gall, E. A. (1956). 'Myocarditis and myocardosis.' *Circulation* **13**, 217

Braimbridge, M. V., Darracott, Sally, Chayen, J., Bitensky, Lucille and Poulter, L. W. (1967). 'Possibility of a new infective aetiological agent in congestive cardiomyopathy.' *Lancet* **1**, 171

Bulloch, R. T. and Murphy, M. L. (1967). 'Electron microscopic changes in primary myocardial disease.' *Circulation*, Suppl. II, **36**, 78

Burch, G. E. and Giles, T. D. (1972). 'Ischaemic cardiomyopathy: diagnostic, pathophysiologic and therapeutic considerations.' *Cardiovasc. Clins.* **4**, 204.

Evans, B. (1957). 'Obscure cardiopathy.' *Br. Heart J.* **19**, 164

Ferrans, V. J., Hibbs, R. G., Walsch, J. J. and Burch, G. E. (1966). 'Cardiomyopathy, cirrhosis of the liver and deposits of a fibrillar polysaccharide. Report of a case with histochemical and microscopic studies.' *Am. J. Cardiol.* **17**, 457

Fletcher, G. F. and Wenger, N. K. (1968). 'Autoimmune studies in patients with primary myocardial disease.' *Circulation* **37**, 1032

— Coleman, M. T., Feorino, P. M., Marne, W. H. and Wenger, N. K. (1968). 'Viral antibodies in patients with primary myocardial disease.' *Am. J. Cardiol.* **21**, 6

Gardner, M. B., Lee, P. V., Norris, J. C., Phillips, E. and Caponegro, P. (1967). 'Virus like particles in cardiac biopsy.' *Lancet* **2**, 95

Gau, G., Goodwin, J. F., Oakley, C., Raphael, M. J. and Steiner, R. E. (1969). 'Q waves and coronary angiography in cardiomyopathy.' Proceedings of the British Cardiac Society. *Br. Heart J.* **32**, 554

Goodwin, J. F. (1970). 'Congestive and hypertrophic cardiomyopathies— A decade of study.' *Lancet* **1**, 731

— Gordon, H., Hollman, A. and Bishop, M. B. (1961). 'Clinical aspects of cardiomyopathy.' *Br. med. J.* **1**, 69

Grist, N. R. (1967). 'Aetiology of congestive cardiomyopathy.' *Lancet* **1**, 395

Harris, L. C., Rodin, A. E. and Nghiem, Q. X. (1968). 'Idiopathic nonobstructive cardiomyopathy in children.' *Am. J. Cardiol.* **21**, 153

Hill, W. T. and Reilly, W. A. (1957). 'Endocardial fibro-elastosis.' *Am. J. Dis. Child.* **82**, 579

James, T. N. (1962). 'Observations on the cardiovascular involvement, including the cardiac conduction system, in progressive muscular dystrophy.' *Am. Heart J.* **65**, 148

Josserand, E. and Gallavardin, L. (1901). 'De l'asystolie progressive des jeunes sujets par myocardite subaigue primative.' *Archs gén. Méd.* NS. **6**, II, 513

Kobernick, S. D., Mandell, G. H., Zirkin, R. M. and Hashimoto, Y. (1963). 'Succinic dehydrogenase deficiency in idiopathic cardiomegaly.' *Am. J. Path.* **43**, 661

Levy, R. L. and Von Glahn, W. C. (1944). 'Cardiac hypertrophy of unknown cause.' *Am. Heart J.* **28**, 714

Mattingly, T. W. (1961). 'Clinical features and diagnosis of primary myocardial disease. Part I.' *Mod. Concepts cardiovasc. Dis. Baltimore* **30**, 677

Muehsam, G. E., Pschibul, F. and Scerbo, J. E. (1964). 'The natural history of idiopathic cardiomegaly.' *Am. Heart J.* **67**, 173

Norris, R. F. and Pote, H. H. (1946). 'Hypertrophy of the heart of unknown etiology in young adults: report of four cases with autopsies.' *Am. Heart J.* **32**, 599

Parameswaran, R., Meadows, W. R. and Sharp, J. T. (1969). 'Coronary embolism in primary myocardial disease.' *Am. Heart J.* **78**, 682

Raftery, E. B., Banks, D. C. and Oram, S. (1969). 'Occlusive disease of the coronary arteries presenting as primary congestive cardiomyopathy.' *Lancet* **2**, 1147.

Sanders, V. (1963). 'Idiopathic disease of the myocardium. A prospective study.' *Archs intern. Med.* **112**, 661

Storstein, O. (1964). 'Primary myocardial disease.' *Acta med. scand.* **176**, 731

Takatsu, T., Kawai, C., Tsutsumi, J. and Inoue, K. (1968). 'A case of idiopathic myocardiopathy with deposits of a peculiar substance in the myocardium: diagnosis by endomyocardial biopsy.' *Am. Heart J.* **76**, 93

Wendt, V. E., Stock, T. B., Hayden, R. O., Bruce, T. A., Gubbjarnason, S. and Bing, R. J. (1962). 'The hemodynamics and cardiac metabolism in cardiomyopathies.' *Med. Clins N. Am.* **46**, 1445

Four

Hypertrophic obstructive cardiomyopathy

Many other names have been assigned to hypertrophic obstructive cardiomyopathy which is characterized by ventricular hypertrophy and abnormal function; and which is often associated with obstruction of the inflow of the left ventricle. Goodwin *et al.* (1960) first proposed the term 'obstructive cardiomyopathy' in order to emphasize the generalized nature of this heart muscle disease. Later the word 'hypertrophic' was added to the description by Cohen *et al.* (1964) to emphasize that, in some cases, obstruction may not be present, despite massive ventricular hypertrophy. This condition first received general recognition following the paper by Teare (1958) on cases of sudden death in young adults with idiopathic hypertrophied hearts.

Braunwald *et al.* (1964) have defined this disease as being characterized by marked hypertrophy of the left ventricle, especially of the interventricular septum and outflow, which often narrows in systole.

The typical patient with this disease has massive asymmetrical hypertrophy of the outflow tract of the left ventricle and diffuse hypertrophy of the ventricular walls.

AGE AND SEX INCIDENCE

Conflicting reports on this disease make it impossible to establish what its exact age and sex incidence is.

This disease may become manifest in individuals of practically any age. Hudson (1970) cites the case of an infant aged three months in which the disease was found. Cases have been described at all ages ranging from $2\frac{1}{2}$ to 55 years by Goodwin (1970), while this condition rarely may be present at birth. The report of Neufeld, Ongley and Edwards (1960) of two infants—one a stillborn—might suggest a challenge to the diagnostician to make an intrauterine diagnosis.

At the other end of the age spectrum are those patients who have a past history of superior athletic accomplishments and negative results of previous physical examinations and who develop the disability in the fifth or sixth decades of life.

In some patients there is a familial incidence as in the cases reported by Walther, Madoff and Zinner (1960) where a family of three siblings were found to have the disease. Taking account of all patients with this disease, the sex incidence is found to be approximately equal (Goodwin, 1970). There is, however, a sex difference in incidences when the cases are divided into those with and without a familial incidence.

TABLE 4.1

	Familial	Sporadic
Number of patients	40	86
Male/female ratio	1·2/1	2·6/1
Average age (years)	25·6	32·7
Sudden death	3	1
Electrocardiogram	Abnormal	Abnormal

Reproduced from Olsen (1971 by courtesy of the author and Messrs J. & A. Churchill.

In those patients suffering from hypertrophic subaortic stenosis, where no family history of the disease can be established or even suspected, there is usually a predominance of males (Braunwald et al., 1964). In patients with a family history of hypertrophic subaortic stenosis a predominance of females is found as in the family reported by Hollman et al. (1960).

Females usually present with the disease much earlier than in males and are also usually more severely disabled (Frank and Braunwald, 1968). The incidence of this disease among Africans and American Negroes is quite low (Wolstenholme and O'Connor, 1971). The disease may occur fairly commonly in some other racial groups in the tropics, such as the 55 cases of hypertrophic cardiomyopathy occurring among 101 members of 15 Ceylonese families reported by Wallooppillai et al. (1973).

CLINICAL HISTORY

The outstanding complaints of most patients when they present with this disease are dyspnoea or fatigue, closely followed by attacks of angina or effort syncope. Less common symptoms are arrhythmias, attacks of nocturnal dyspnoea, or palpitations which are predominantly associated with exercise—dyspnoea and fatigue often being mentioned together.

Prolonged episodes of atypical anginal pain are sometimes found in some patients. Female patients, who become pregnant initially, have an exacerbation of their symptoms but these settle down when pregnancy is over (Goodwin, 1970), and there is, therefore, no indication for terminating the pregnancy.

This disease is fairly commonly associated with other cardiac abnormalities such as coarctation of the aorta (McIntosh *et al.*, 1962), pulmonary valvular stenosis (Molthan, Paul and Lev, 1962) or ventricular septal defect (Lauer, du Shane and Edwards, 1960).

Although clinically the obstruction of the left ventricular outflow tract is capricious and may vary from day to day (Braunwald, 1962), the changes observed pathologically explain the obstructive part of the condition.

PATTERN OF PROGRESS

In some patients, inflow resistance steadily increases, the rate of ventricular filling is reduced and sudden death on effort may be due to this, together with tachycardia and loss of atrial contraction due to arrhythmia. Infective endocarditis may affect the mitral valve, usually in the phase of obstruction when mitral regurgitation is present (Vecht and Oakley, 1968). Progressive atrial stress and ventricular fibrosis, with a failing forward cardiac output, leads to congestive heart failure. The onset of atrial fibrillation may be associated with pulmonary oedema or systemic embolism. Finally, congestive heart failure completes the picture which is clinically almost indistinguishable from congestive cardiomyopathy except that in the hypertrophic type there may be a family history.

It appears that many patients remain stable for years, during which they may be symptom-free or have only dyspnoea and/or angina. Sudden death may occur without warning and is possibly the most common termination. There is, perhaps, a tendency for it to occur more usually in patients with a short history of symptoms rather than in those with a long, stable course (Braunwald *et al.*, 1970).

One hundred and six cases were followed for up to 12 years; the condition remained stable in 49 per cent, fluctuated in 17 per cent, improved in 5 per cent, deteriorated in 15 per cent and was fatal in 14 per cent of cases. Atrial fibrillation occurred in 8 per cent and AV conduction disturbances in 30 per cent; one-third developed disabling pulmonary hypertension.

COURSE

The course of this is very variable but progressive. At least three years usually elapse between the discovery of a murmur and the development of symptoms. Sometimes, however, symptoms never develop. Sudden death is more common in the familial form of the disease, the youngest death recorded being that of a boy aged 15 (Brunsden, 1967), who collapsed and died while running round a sports field.

EFFECTS OF PREGNANCY

Turner, Oakley and Dixon (1968) reported on 9 women with hypertrophic obstructive cardiomyopathy (familial in 5) who had 13 pregnancies. Natural delivery was best, aided by a β-adrenergic blocking drug during pregnancy and labour (the drug did no harm to the foetus), ergometrine at the end of the second stage, adequate blood transfusion and prophylaxis against bacterial infections; sudden death could occur.

AETIOLOGY

It seems likely that hypertrophic obstructive cardiomyopathy is an inherited disorder of ventricular muscle growth leading to irregular contraction and abnormal excessive hypertrophy and fibrosis, which is characterized by progressively increasing resistance to filling of the left ventricle and, in most patients, by incidental outflow tract obstruction.

The great majority of patients with hypertrophic obstructive cardiomyopathy have no other diseases of the heart or other system, and the disease is thus taken to be a primary one. In some cases, however, it is associated with, or secondary to, fixed outflow tract obstruction of the left ventricle, such as aortic valve or discrete subvalvular stenosis (Parker, Kaplan and Connolly, 1969); or to hypertension as originally described by Brock (1957).

The detection by Meerschwam (1969) of abnormalities in skeletal muscle raises the question of a more generalized muscle disorder, but the latter is still unresolved.

The studies of Van Noorden, Olsen and Pearse (1970) suggest that a spectrum of hypertrophic cardiomyopathy may exist. At one end of the spectrum is the typical asymmetrical hypertrophy of the septum, with abnormal fibres aggregated in one area, while at the other end of the spectrum, no microscopic changes are evident but some similar abnormal fibres are scattered throughout the myocardium.

It may be concluded, therefore, that in hypertrophic obstructive cardiomyopathy (HOCM) the following findings should be noted:

(1) A definite histological diagnosis is usually possible.

(2) Histology shows some overlap between cases of HOCM, other cardiomyopathies and normal cardiac tissue.

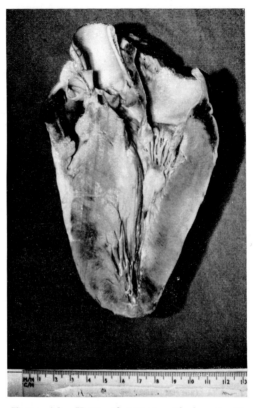

Figure 4.1. Heart of patient with hypertrophic obstructive cardiomyopathy showing marked hypertrophy of interventricular septum. Some of the papillary muscles are also hypertrophied. (Reproduced by courtesy of Professor Teare)

(3) The distribution of areas with abnormal fibres in HOCM indicates the use of needle biopsy as a useful diagnostic tool.

(4) A spectrum of hypertropic obstructive cardiomyopathy may exist.

PATHOLOGICAL PICTURE

The typical patient with obstruction shows massive asymmetrical hypertrophy of the outflow tract of the left ventricle and diffuse hypertrophy of the ventricular walls (Teare, 1958). The typical asymmetry of the septal hypertrophy has been observed in most cases

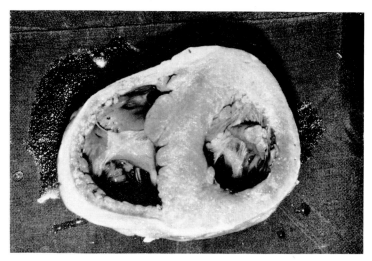

Figure 4.2. Transverse section through the heart of a patient with hypertrophic obstructive cardiomyopathy to show the marked interventricular septal hypertrophy which is found in this condition, due to obstruction of blood leaving the heart through the aortic valve. (Reproduced by courtesy of Professor Teare)

which have come to autopsy. The changes are best illustrated in *Figures 4.1* and *4.2* where extreme thickening of the septum is strikingly illustrated.

The anterior, lateral and posterior walls may show a moderate uniform hypertrophy. The papillary muscles and trabeculae carneae are enlarged and the 'aortic' cusp of the mitral valve is thickened. This disease may affect only the right side of the heart as in the case of Falcone, Moore and Lambert (1967) in a 14 year old boy, where septal hypertrophy had produced marked narrowing of the right ventricle.

There is also a group of patients who are difficult to classify clinically and who show little or no obstruction (Karatzas, Hamill and Sleight, 1968). In these cases there is usually dilatation of all chambers, endocardial thickening and occasionally thrombus

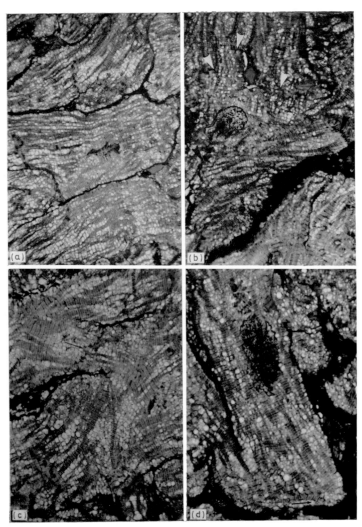

Figure 4.3. Light micrographs of semi-thin sections from left ventricular outflow tract (LVOT) of a case of hypertrophic obstruction cardiomyopathy. (a) A group of hypertrophic muscle cells with normally arranged myofibrils (× 800, reduced to 7/10). (b) Stellate-shaped muscle cell with myofibrils arranged in different directions. Cell outlines are indicated by arrowheads (× 1,000, reduced to 7/10). (c) Two muscle cells have obliquely and transversely orientated myofibrils and a side-to-side intercellular junction (arrow). Note the wide transverse diameter (55 µ) of the cell in the centre (× 1,000, reduced to 7/10). (d) Muscle cell in which myofibrils are normally orientated except in area (arrow) at the end of the cell, where myofibrils are orientated transversely (× 1,200, reduced to 7/10). (Reproduced from Ferrans, Morrow and Roberts (1972) by courtesy of the authors and Editor of Circulation)

formation in the apical region is seen. Myocardial hypertrophy is present, but is not striking, being marked by the dilatation. The hypertrophy is uniform. The appearance differs strikingly from that seen in classical cases of hypertrophic obstructive cardiomyopathy.

Similar gross pathological and histological appearances are seen in patients both with and without obstruction.

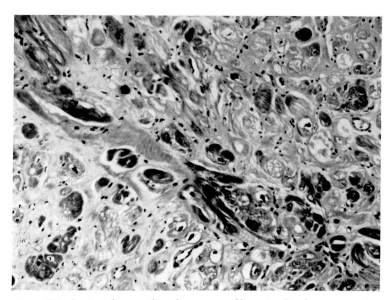

Figure 4.4   Section of myocardium from a case of hypertrophic obstructive cardio-myopathy showing the presence of many abnormally-shaped nuclei in some of the muscle fibres. The great increase is in the interstitial fibrous tissue and the perinuclear haloes around some of the muscle fibre nuclei (haematoxylin and eosin × 200, reduced to 2/3). (Reproduced by courtesy of Dr Olsen)

Histologically disorientation of muscle fibres is seen in the affected parts of the heart.

Individually, these fibres show extreme hypertrophy (*Figure 4.3*), and values up to 60 μm are not unusual, whereas in left ventricular hypertrophy, due to other causes, fibres 20–25 μm wide (normal value 5–12 μm) are the largest seen.

There may also be abnormalities of the nuclei (Kristinsson, 1969).

Bizarre-shaped nuclei are observed within spaces referred to as nuclei haloes. These appearances are typical in this condition. The myocardial fibres adjacent to the perinuclear haloes have a moth-eaten appearance.

The presence of the endothelial-lined spaces described by Teare in 1958 has been confirmed by other workers (Olsen, 1971), but these are not helpful in diagnosis. Interruption of the abnormal myocardial fibres by fibrous tissue is typically seen in these cases.

Serial sections of these areas show that the fibrous tissue arises within the myocardial fibres and spreads towards the surface, replacing a variable amount of muscle tissue (*Figure 4.4*); this results in the observed shortening of the fibre and its termination in collagen tissue.

Some of the fibres have lost their striations and others contain small vacuoles in their cytoplasm, although not usually containing lipid.

An additional point is the tendency for the myocardial bundles, sometimes, to form small 'whorls'. This finding is also said (Olsen, 1971) to be a fairly reliable guide to diagnosis.

HISTOLOGY

Changes similar to those described in classical HOCM are found in those cases showing no obstruction except that perinuclear haloes are not prominent but are present. Whereas in the classical type of HOCM abnormal fibres are aggregated in one area—usually but not always the septum and apex—in these cases areas varying between 2 and 3 cm. in size are scattered throughout the myocardium.

In order to evaluate the histological observations in HOCM and to assess their diagnostic reliability, Van Noorden, Olsen and Pearse (1971) have devised an index—the 'histological hypertrophic obstructive cardiomyopathy index' (HAI). This has been constructed by allowing points for each of the histological changes observed (fibrosis, bizarre nuclei, disappearing myocardial fibres with perinuclear spaces, whorls and short runs of fibres).

In their study of this index, material from known cases of HOCM was compared with material from other forms of heart disease. The results showed that some overlap occurred and that, in order to evaluate tissue fully, ample material is needed to make a diagnosis: if only two or three histological features are seen, the value of the index may be such that a reliable diagnosis is not possible.

ELECTRON MICROSCOPICAL STUDIES

Sonnenblick (1968) from studies of the ultrastructure of muscle in biopsies, found that the nuclei were enlarged and irregular and mitochondria increased. There was a great variation in sarcomere length; the 'I' bands sometimes being pulled out of the 'A' band to make a huge 'I' band; in other areas the sarcomeres were so short that there was no 'I' band; i.e., the thin filaments were 'right home' or even overlapping. There were zones where the myocardium could not develop tension. Lannigan (1965), from a necropsy study of the heart of a man who died suddenly of the disease, reported focal degenerative changes, muscle fibre hypertrophy, replacement fibrosis and some infiltration of the myocardium with mononuclear cells and lymphocytes.

The most detailed study on this disease has been that of Ferrans, Morrow and Roberts (1971), their findings being as follows.

(1) There is an abnormal arrangement and shape of muscle cells which are wider and often shorter than normal. Many bundles of muscle cells are severely disorganized, with muscle cells running in several directions instead of in parallel. Some cells are rectangular in shape and appear normally arranged; other cells, however, have irregular or stellate shapes and have several branches extending in different directions, so that they form intercellular junctions with several adjacent cells. Many muscle cells attain diameters (up to 80 μ) which are considerably larger than those found in other types of cardiomyopathies.

(2) There is often an abnormal arrangement of myofibrils, which often course in several directions (*Figure 4.5*) within one given cell, although this abnormality does not occur in all cells. It is most pronounced in branched or stellate-shaped cells (*Figure 4.6*) but is found also, to a lesser extent (*Figure 4.7*) in cells with more normal shapes. When only a few myofibrils are affected in one cell, these alterations occur near the sarcolemma and intercalated discs.

(3) An abnormal arrangement of myofilaments is seen in some areas of myofibrillar disarray, in which some of the myofilaments that originated from the Z band of a given myofibril are inserted into the Z band of an adjacent myofibril. These diverging myofilaments form a cross-woven appearance with those which are normally orientated. Actual branching of myofibrils is seen occasionally (*Figure 4.8*).

(4) Abnormal intercellular junctions which are unusually convoluted, more extensive than in usual cardiac muscle and which frequently have large areas of side-to-side apposition of the muscle cells instead of, or in addition to, end-to-end apposition are also sometimes seen (*Figure 4.9*).

(5) Abnormalities of Z bands, which are much more frequent and severe in patients with HOCM than in patients with other cardiomyopathies are also frequently seen. These abnormalities consist of

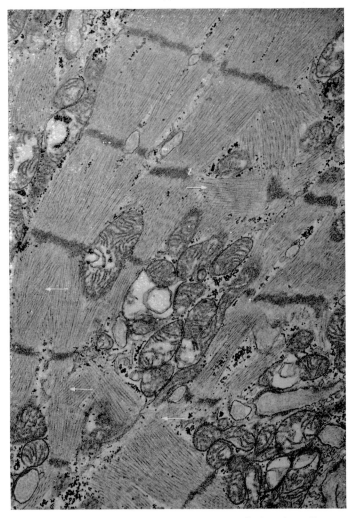

Figure 4.5.   Area of marked disorganization of myofibrils and myofilaments in muscle cell of patient with hypertrophic obstructive cardiomyopathy. A cross-woven arrangement of myofilaments is evident in several areas (arrows), and myofilaments that originate from single Z bands (Z) insert into several different myofibrils that course in various directions (× 21,900, reduced to 7/10) (Ferrans et al., 1972)

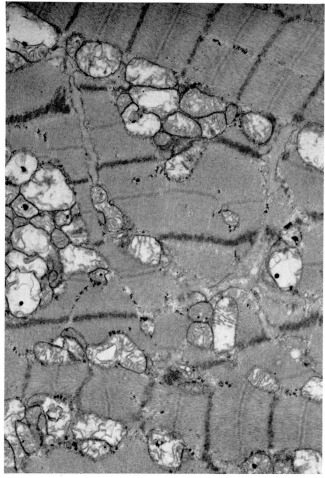

Figure 4.6. Myofibrils in this area of a muscle cell show marked variations in orientation (× 15,500, reduced to 7/10) (Ferrans et al., 1972)

irregular widening of Z bands (*Figures 3.5–4.8* and *Figure 4.10*); spreading of Z band material towards the centre of the sarcolemma; attachment of Z bands to the sarcolemma and T tubules, and the presence of increased amounts of Z band-like material at points of attachment of myofibrils to intercellular junctions (*Figure 4.9*). The extent to which these preceding features occur vary from one part of a section to another; however, all of these

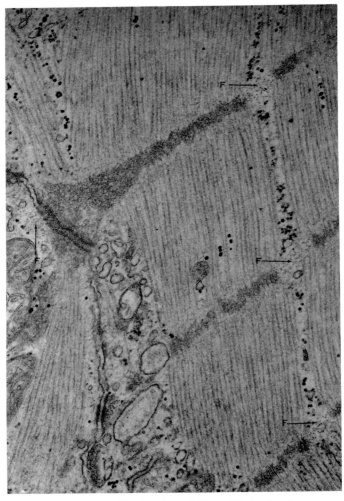

Figure 4.7. High magnification view of side-to-side junction between two muscle cells, showing cross sections of bundles of transversely orientated filaments (F) *at the level of Z bands and in the vicinity of the attachment of a widened Z band to the plasma membrane* (× *52,000, reduced to 7/10*) (*Ferrans* et al., *1972*)

abnormalities are seen in every HOCM heart which has been examined. Due to the increase in nuclear size, the myofibril-free pernicular area is much larger than in normal cardiac tissue and is filled with large masses of mitochondria and glycogen granules.

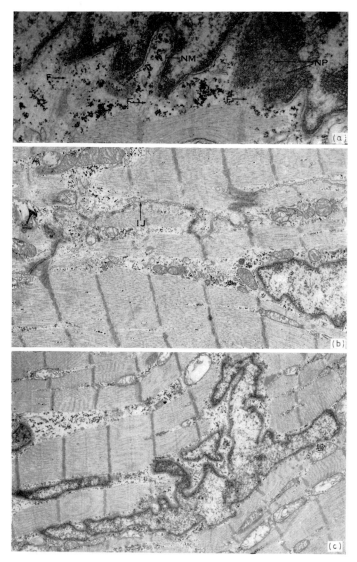

Figure 4.8. (a) *View of part of the nucleus of a muscle cell showing filaments* (F) *connecting Z bands of myofibrils to nuclear membranes* (NM). *Note the* en face *view of nuclear pores* (NP) (× *34,000, reduced to 7/10).* (b) *Longitudinal section of muscle cell showing bizarre-shaped nucleus* (× *11,250, reduced to 7/10).* (c) *Extensive side-to-side intercellular junction* (IJ) *between two muscle cells. Area on left is shown at higher magnification in* Figure 4.7 (× *13,500, reduced to 7/10) (Ferrans* et al., *1972)*

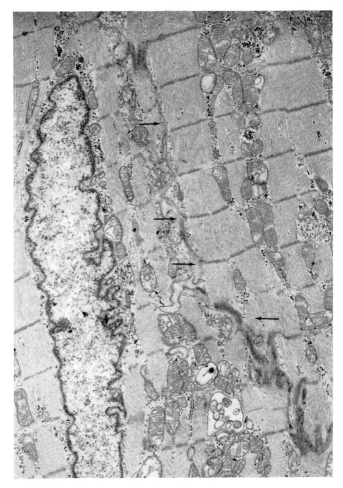

Figure 4.9. Tortuous, extensive side-to-side junction between two muscle cells is associated with material similar to Z bands. Note small areas of obliquely and transversely orientated myofibrils (arrows) (× 12,000, reduced to 7/10) (Ferrans et al., 1972)

(6)   Lipid droplets are rarely observed in muscle cells. Neural elements were not abnormally large or numerous.

Some degree of interstitial fibrosis, characterized by increased numbers of developing and mature collagen fibrils, is found in all patients. Examination of the apical myocardium from patients with

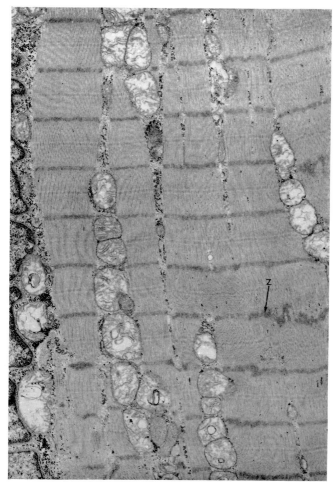

*Figure 4.10.   Muscle cell shows normally arranged myofibrils, irregular
widening of some Z bands (Z) and mitochondria damage (× 16,500,
reduced to 7/10) (Ferrans et al., 1972)*

HOCM shows myocardial cells which are hypertrophied but are
much more uniform in size, shape and arrangement than those in the
outflow tract.

Therefore, it is considered that this combination of abnormalities
constitutes a lesion that is characteristic of HOCM.

HISTOCHEMICAL STUDIES

It was originally thought, following the work of Pearse (1964), that there was an increased noradrenaline content and an increased sympathetic nerve supply to the interventricular myocardium in the cases of HOCM. Later work by Van Noorden, Olsen and Pearse

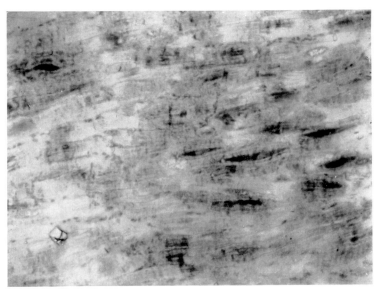

Figure 4.11. Sections of myocardium from a case of hypertrophic obstructive cardiomyopathy to show a perinuclear deposition of glycogen in many of the myocardial cells (× 200, reduced to 2/3). (Reproduced by courtesy of Dr Olsen)

(1971), who have been unable to substantiate these findings, have found that autofluorescence, of a similar colour and brightness to that of the formaldehyde-induced fluorescence of noradrenaline, is emitted by fibrous tissue in both HOCM and control hearts.

Although sections of myocardium from HOCM cases do tend to fluoresce more strongly than normal myocardium after treatment with formaldehyde, this is due to the fact that they contain more connective tissue. These workers could also not confirm the presence of noradrenaline by microspectrofluorimetric methods.

Pearse (1964) also claimed that the myocardium in HOCM contained increased numbers of nerve fibres; Van Noorden, Olsen and Pearse (1971) could also not confirm these findings in HOCM and found that the ethylamine silver oxalate stain behaved erratically and that frequently reticulin fibres rather than nervous fibres appeared to be stained.

In HOCM muscle, as previously described by Pearse (1964), accumulations of glycogen can often be seen around the nuclei in the affected areas of muscle (*Figure 4.11*), although glycogen levels are quite high in both HOCM and normal muscle; this pooling distribution is fairly typical of HOCM hearts, but not confined to them.

TABLE 4.2
Incidence and Degree of Glycogen Pooling

Glycogen pools	HOCM		Non-HOCM	
	No. of patients	*% of total*	*No. of patients*	*% age of total*
3+	9	56·2	3	8·8
2+	2	12·5	7	20·7
1+	4	25·0	4	11·7
0	1	6·3	20	58·8
Total cases	16		34	

(Reproduced from Van Noorden, Olsen and Pearse (1971) by courtesy of the authors and publishers)

In Table 4.2 the incidence and degree of glycogen pooling in the cases described by Van Noorden, Olsen and Pearse (1971) are shown.

References

Braunwald, E., Brockenbrough, E. C. and Morrow, A. G. (1962). 'Hypertrophic subaortic stenosis—a broadening concept.' *Circulation* **26**, 161
— Lambrew, C. T., Rockoff, S. D., Ross, J. and Morrow, A. G. (1964). 'Idiopathic hypertrophic sub-aortic stenosis. I: A description of the disease based upon an analysis of 64 patients.' *Circulation* **30**, Suppl. 4, 3.
Brock, R. C. (1957). 'Functional obstructions of the left ventricle (acquired sub-valvular stenosis).' *Guy's Hosp. Rep.* **106**, 221
Brunsdon, D. F. V. (1967). 'Hypertrophic obstructive cardiomyopathy as a cause of sudden death in a 15 year-old boy.' *Can. med. Ass. J.* **97**, 974
Cohen, J., Effet, H., Goodwin, J. F., Oakley, C. M. and Steiner, R. E. (1964). 'Hypertrophic obstructive cardiomyopathy.' *Br. Heart J.* **26**, 16
Falcone, D. M., Moore, D. and Lambert, E. C. (1967). 'Idiopathic hypertrophic cardiomyopathy involving the right ventricle.' *Am. J. Cardiol.* **19**, 735
Ferrans, V. J., Morrow, A. G. and Roberts, W. C. (1972). 'Myocardial ultrastructure in idiopathic hypertrophic sub-aortic stenosis. A study of operatively excised left ventricle outflow tract muscle in 14 patients.' *Circulation* **45**, 769

Frank, S. and Braunwald, E. (1967). 'Observations on the natural history of idiopathic hypertrophic sub-aortic stenosis.' *Circulation* **35**, Suppl. II; **36**, Suppl. II

—— (1968). 'Idiopathic hypertrophic sob-aortic stenosis. Clinical analysis of 126 patients with emphasis on the natural history.' *Circulation* **37**, 759

Goodwin, J. F. (1970). 'Congestive and hypertrophic cardiomyopathies—a decade of study.' *Lancet* **1**, 731

— Hollman, A., Cleland, W. P. and Teare, D. (1960). 'Obstructive cardiomyopathy simulating aortic stenosis.' *Br. Heart J.* **22**, 403

Hollman, A., Goodwin, J. F., Teare, D. and Renwick, J. W. (1960). 'A family with obstructive cardiomyopathy (asymmetrical hypertrophy).' *Br. Heart J.* **22**, 449

Hudson, R. E. B. (1970). 'Obstructive cardiomyopathy.' *Cardiovalvular Pathology*, Vol. 3, p. 474. London: Edward Arnold

Karatzas, N. B., Hamill, J. and Sleight, P. (1968). 'Hypertrophic cardiomyopathy.' *Br. Heart J.* **30**, 826

Kristinsson, A. (1969). 'Diagnosis, natural history and treatment of congestive cardiomyopathy.' Ph.D. Thesis, University of London

Lannigan, R. (1965). 'Hypertrophic sub-aortic stenosis with myocardial fibre degeneration.' *Br. Heart J.* **27**, 772

Lauer, R. M., Du Shane, J. W. and Edwards, J. E. (1960). 'Obstruction of left ventricular outlet in association with ventricular septal defect.' *Circulation* **22**, 110

McIntosh, M. D., Sealy, W. C., Whalen, R. E., Cohen, A. I. and Sumner, R. G. (1962). 'Obstruction to outflow tract of left ventricle.' *Archs intern. Med.* **110**, 312

Meerschwam, I. S. (1969). 'Electromyographic findings.' In *Hypertrophic Obstructive Cardiomyopathy*, p. 129. Amsterdam: Excerpta Medica Foundation

Molthan, M. E., Paul, M. H. and Lev, M. (1962). 'Common A-V orifice with pulmonary valvular and hypertrophic subaortic stenosis.' *Am. J. Cardiol.* **10**, 291

Neufeld, H. N., Ongley, P. A. and Edwards, J. E. (1960). 'Combined congenital sub-aortic stenosis and infundibular pulmonary stenosis.' *Br. Heart J.* **22**, 686

Olsen, E. G. J. (1971). 'Morbid anatomy and histology in hypertrophic obstructive cardiomyopathy.' In *Hypertrophic Obstructive Cardiomyopathy*. Ciba Foundation Study Group. Ed. by G. E. W. Wolstenholme and M. O'Connor, pp. 183–191. London: Churchill

Parker, D. P., Kaplan, M. A., and Connolly, J. E. (1969). 'Coexistent aortic valvular and functional hypertrophic subaortic stenosis. Clinical, physiologic and angiographic aspects.' *Am. J. Cardiol.* **24**, 307

Pearse, A. G. E. (1964). 'The histochemistry and electron microscopy of obstructive cardiomyopathy.' *Cardiomyopathies*. Ciba Foundation Symposium. Ed. by G. E. W. Wolstenholme and M. O'Connor, p. 132. London: Churchill

Sonnenblick, E. H. (1968). 'Correlation of myocardial ultra-structure and function.' *Circulation* **38**, 29

Teare, R. D. (1958). 'Asymmetrical hypertrophy of the heart in young adults.' *Br. Heart J.* **20**, 1

Turner, G. M., Oakley, C. M. and Dixon, H. G. (1968). 'Management of pregnancy complicated by hypertrophic obstructive cardiomyopathy.' *Br. med. J.* **4**, 281

Van Noorden, S., Olsen, E. G. J. and Pearse, A. G. E. (1971). 'Hypertrophic obstructive cardiomyopathy, a histological, histochemical and ultra-structural study of biopsy material.' *Cardiovasc. Res.* **5**, 118

Vecht, R. J. and Oakley, C. M. (1968). 'Infective endocarditis in three patients with hypertrophic obstructive cardiomyopathy.' *Br. med. J.* **2**, 455

Walther, R. J., Madoff, I. M. and Zinner, K. (1960). 'Cardiomegaly of unknown cause occurring in a family. Report of three siblings and review of the literature.' *New Engl. J. Med.* **263**, 1104

Wallooppillai, D. P., Atukorale, D. P., Jayasinghe, M. de S. and Kala-thungam, S. (1973). 'Familial hypertrophic cardiomyopathy in Ceylon.' *Br. Heart J.* **35**, 181

Wolstenholme, G. E. W. and O'Connor, M. (Eds) (1971) *Hypertrophic Obstructive Cardiomyopathy.* Ciba Foundation Study Group No. 17. London: Churchill

Five

Idiopathic familial cardiomyopathy

In 1949 Evans reported on a number of patients with a familial incidence of cardiomyopathy, with sudden death and cardiac arrhythmias as particularly prominent features and was the first person to use the term 'familial cardiomyopathies'.

Since this time, there have been numerous reports (Parsons, 1952; Gaunt and Lecutier, 1956; Vaishnava, 1957; Beasley, 1960) on this condition although only a few (Soulie *et al.*, 1957) have provided data on two or more patients passing through two generations (Campell and Turner Warwick, 1956; Whitfield, 1961; Pare *et al.*, 1961; Barry and Hall, 1962).

There may be a difference in pathological findings within the same family and these changes, therefore, indicate that considerable variations may exist in the same disease. It is also quite likely that some of the differences between families may be due to different defects which we are not, at present, able to distinguish.

CARDIAC APPEARANCES

The heart may show generalized ventricular hypertrophy and varying degrees of dilatation. It may sometimes show an asymmetrical hypertrophy, usually involving the interventricular septum and encroaching on the outflow tracts of the left ventricle and sometimes on that of the right ventricle. Encroachment on the outflow tract with obstruction and narrowing of the mitral valve have been reported (Cullhead, 1962). Pare *et al.* (1961) found that cases of symmetrical and generalized hypertrophy may occur in the same family. Myocardial hypertrophy is a constant finding.

MICROSCOPIC CHANGES

The amount of myocardial fibrosis found varies considerably from its absence in some cases to a gross scarring of the myocardium in others; Garrett, Hay and Richards (1959) have suggested that those cases without fibrosis are rarer than, and different from, those with fibrosis. However, this difference is probably one of degree. Evans (1949) and Gaunt and Lecutier (1956) found evidence of vacuolation and glycogen accumulation in the heart, whereas Battersby and Glenner (1961) and Barry and Hall (1962) found a non-metachromatic polysaccharide material deposited within some of the myocardial fibres.

In most cases no abnormal deposits are found in the myocardium on microscopic examination, a finding confirmed by the reports of many other workers on this disease. Although inflammatory cells are not usually present, in a few cases there is a large enough infiltrate to indicate myocarditis (Blanshard, 1953; Sommers, 1956).

Only a few reports mention vascular lesions. Some workers describe changes in the smaller coronary arteries with medial and intimal thickening and encroachment on the lumen (Blanshard, 1953; Bishop, Campbell and Jones, 1962; Treger and Blount, 1965).

The myocardial cells are hypertrophied and many of them contain abnormally-shaped or pyknotic nuclei.

References

Barry, M. and Hall, M. (1962). 'Familial cardiomegaly.' *Br. Heart J.* **24**, 613

Battersby, E. J. and Glenner, G. G. (1961). 'Familial cardiomyopathy.' *Am. J. Med.* **30**, 382

Beasley, J. C. (1960). 'Familial myocardial disease.' *Am. J. Med.* **29**, 476

Bishop, J. M., Campbell, M. and Jones, E. W. (1962). 'Cardiomyopathy in fair members of a family.' *Br. Heart J.* **24**, 715

Blanshard, H. P. (1953). 'Isolated diffuse myocarditis.' *Br. Heart J.* **15**, 453

Campbell, M. and Turner Warwick, Margaret (1956). 'Two more families with cardiomegaly.' *Br. Heart J.* **18**, 393

Cullhead, I. (1962). 'Familial cardiomyopathy.' *Folia clin. int.* **12**, 235

Davies, L. G. (1952). 'A familial heart disease.' *Br. Heart J.* **14**, 206

Evans, W. (1949). 'Familial cardiomegaly.' *Br. Heart J.* **11**, 68

Garrett, G., Hay, W. S. and Richards, A. G. (1959). 'Familial cardiomegaly.' *J. clin. Path.* **12**, 335

Gaunt, R. T. and Lecutier, M. A. (1956). 'Familial cardiomegaly.' *Br. Heart J.* **18**, 251

Pare, J. A. P., Fraser, R. E., Pirozymski, J. J., Shankgh, J. A. and Stubington, D. (1961). 'Hereditary cardiovascular dysphasia.' *Am. J. Med.* **31**, 37

Parsons, F. J. (1952). 'Familial cardiac enlargement—report of two cases.' *Med. J. Aust.* **2**, 435

Sommers, B. (1956). 'Problems in the clinical diagnosis and identification of ventricular hypertrophy in adults.' *Minn. Med.* **39**, 153

Soulié, P., Di Mathéo, J., Abaza, A., Nouaille, J. and Thibert, M. (1957). 'Cardiomegalie familiale.' *Arch. mal. coeur.* **50**, 22

Treger, A. and Blount, S. G. (Jnr) (1965). 'Familial cardiomyopathy.' *Am. Heart J.* **70**, 40

Vaishnava, H. P. (1957). 'Familial cardiomegaly.' *J. Ind. med. Ass.* **28**, 312

Whitfield, A. G. (1961). 'Familial cardiomyopathy.' *Q. Jl Med.* **30**, 119

METABOLIC STORAGE DISEASE

OXALOSIS

The deposit of oxalate is usually much more massive in endogenous oxalosis than is that usually found in the acquired conditions.

It used to be thought that oxalosis, being the result of an inborn error of metabolism, would lead to death at an early age. Only about 20 of the 60 or so cases described in the literature have been adults (Largiader and Zollinger, 1960).

In view of the relatively rare occurrence of oxalosis of endogenous origin, it is important to exclude any secondary causes of oxalosis such as ethylene glycol poisoning (Friedman *et al.*, 1962).

AGE INCIDENCE

The maximum age reported has been 66 (Koten *et al.*, 1965) but in a larger series the oldest patient studied was aged only 54. The patients most commonly present with renal failure.

IDENTIFICATION OF CRYSTALS

Numerous birefringent crystals arranged mostly in the form of rosettes or sheeves are seen. The average size of the crystals is about 25 μm and they are yellow. If appropriately stained, periodic acid Schiff (PAS)-positive material may be seen at the surface of these crystals and sometimes in concentric rings around them.

CARDIAC PATHOLOGY

In most cases of primary oxalosis the heart is often found to be moderately enlarged. Sometimes the surface of the epicardium shows greyish patches or evidence of a pericarditis.

Microscopically the myocardium may show diffuse fibrosis and the epicardial patches are seen to consist largely of fibrous tissue. Much oxalate is present both in the muscle fibres and in the connective tissue. Many of the blood vessels contain oxalate crystals situated between the lamina elastica and the tunica media; these may protrude like a mushroom into the lumen.

The interstitial tissue often contains inflammatory cells and sometimes crystalline material can be seen, especially in the fibrotic areas.

References

Friedman, E. A., Greenberg, J. B., Merrill, J. P. and Damonin, G. J. (1962). 'Consequences of ethylene glycol poisoning. Report of four cases and review of the literature.' *Am. J. Med.* **32**, 891

Koten, J. W., van Gastel, C., Dorhout Mees, E. J., Holleman, L. W. J. and Schuling, R. D. (1965). 'Two cases of primary oxalosis.' *J. clin. Path.* **18**, 223

Largiader, F. and Zollinger, H. U. (1960). 'Oxalosis. Part II: Experimental studies on the rat.' *Virchows Arch. path. Anat. Physiol.* **333**, 390

HAEMOCHROMATOSIS

The familial iron storage disease haemochromatosis is discussed in Chapter 14 because the cardiac lesions found are identical with those found in acquired disease.

POMPE'S DISEASE (GLYCOGEN STORAGE DISEASE)

The variety of glycogen storage disease which mainly involves the heart, and also the skeletal and smooth muscle, is the second (type II) of the six types of defective glycogenosis first described by Cori (1954). A large amount of an abnormal glycogen may be found in the heart. In type III a deficiency of the normally formed debrancher enzyme limits the accumulation of glycogen in the tissue but does not cause the conspicuous cardiac enlargement seen in the type II disease.

This disease was first described in 1932 by Pompe. The 54 cases described up to 1952 have been collected and reviewed by Ehlers *et al.* (1962), and since then a further 28 cases have been described in the English literature (Caddell and Whittemore, 1962; Huijing, Van Creveld and Losekoot, 1963; Crome, Cumings and Duckett, 1963; Kahana *et al.*, 1964; Rosenstein, 1964; Hohn *et al.*, 1965; Perez-Trevino *et al.*, 1965; Dincsoy *et al.*, 1965; Hernandez *et al.*, 1966; Cardiff, 1966; Hug *et al.*, 1966; Smith, Amick and Sidburg, 1966; Spach *et al.*, 1966; Nihill, Wilson and Hugh-Jones, 1970).

Infants with this disease are usually normal when born, but fail to thrive, and develop symptoms within some three to six months later (Ruttenberg *et al.*, 1964). A generalized muscular hypotonia then develops so that the child is often unable to sit up without support and becomes lethargic and flabby.

Clinical Signs

The child often adopts a typical frog-like position (*Figure 5.1*). Reflexes are diminished and there is often an excessive amount of sweating. The tongue usually becomes enlarged and protruberant, so

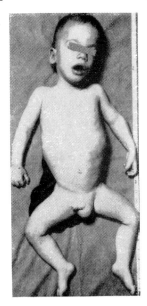

Figure 5.1.   Typical frog-like position exhibited by infants with Type II glycogenosis (Spach et al., 1966)

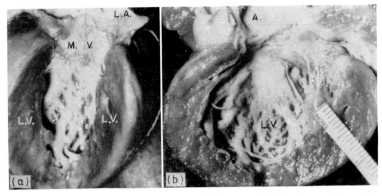

Figure 5.2.   A gross specimen of a heart. (a) Interior of left atrium and ventricle demonstrating a normal mitral valve (MV), a very thick left ventricular wall (LV) and milky-white thickening of the left ventricular and left atrial endocardium characteristic of endocardial sclerosis. (b) Left ventricular outflow tract and aorta (A). There is no evidence of sub-acute or valvular stenosis (picture taken before fixation) (Ruttenberg et al., 1964)

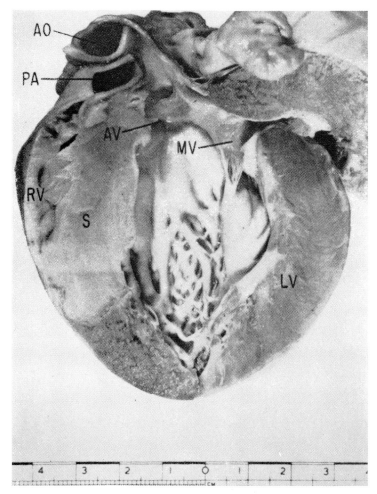

Figure 5.3. The heart from a case of Pompe's disease with left ventricle opened to show grossly thickened left ventricular wall (LV) and septum (S) with fibro-elastosis of the left ventricular septal wall. The right ventricular cavity (RV) is small and compressed by the thickened septum. (AO—aorta; PA—main pulmonary artery: AV—aortic valve: MV—mitral valve) (Nihill, Wilson and Hugh-Jones, 1970)

that the child often has the appearance of a case of Down's syndrome; consequently feeding may become difficult. The child, however, may first be noticed to be ill when it presents with either congestive heart failure or pneumonia. The average time of survival of these children is about six months; the longest so far described being 34 months.

At autopsy the heart is pale in colour and considerably enlarged, usually four or five times the weight found in a normal infant of similar age and weight. Cardiac enlargement of this degree may often so completely compress the lung in the left side of the chest that there is a serious loss of respiratory function. The cardiac enlargement is found to be predominantly left-sided to origin, but all chambers are usually dilated, the most marked thickening being that of the wall of the left ventricle, which may be up to 1·2–1·5 cm in thickness (*Figure 5.2*). The endocardial surface of the left ventricle is usually found to be opaque and thickened due to the development of endo-cardial fibro-elastosis, especially where the endocardium is overlying the base of the interventricular septum. The mitral and aortic valves may be mildly involved and thickened. The left ventricular cavity is often reduced in size due to an enlargement of the interventricular septum, which then bulges into the right ventricle, and reduces its cavity size to an even greater degree (*Figure 5.3*). These cardiac changes also, on occasions, give rise to obstruction of the ventricular outflow (Ehlers and Engle, 1963).

Histological Examination

The myocardium shows the presence of a great deal of glycogen—the greatest quantity being immediately beneath the endocardium. The myocardium shows a typical 'lacework' pattern in longitudinal section and a 'honeycombed' appearance on transverse section (*Figure 5.4*). There is often marked vacuole formation in the central portion of the muscle fibres and around the nucleus which, however, may be forced to one side, although the nuclei themselves appear normal. Therefore, in the muscle cells there may only be a small rim of cytoplasm around the cell wall, while the remainder of the cell consists of an open space which originally contained glycogen in the paraffin-fixed specimen. The glycogen is best demonstrated by the PAS stain or by Best's carmine stain for glycogen; provided the material has originally been fixed and stored in absolute alcohol, although more specific reactions may be obtained by exposing sections of fresh, unfixed material to diastase digestion, when large clear spaces will be left in the cytoplasm where the glycogen has been digested away. These glycogen stains will show diffuse deposits of glycogen within the vacuoles as well as in the fibrillar portions of the cells, and these changes in the myofibres are present throughout the myocardium. A marked degree of endocardial fibro-elastosis is also

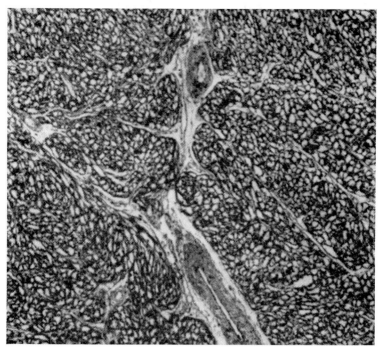

Figure 5.4. Section of myocardium showing lacework pattern caused by accumulation of intracellular glycogen granules (haematoxylin and eosin × 55) (Nihill, Wilson and Hugh-Jones 1970)

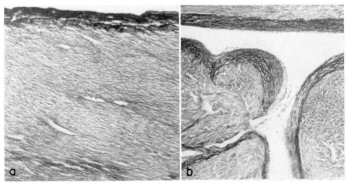

Figure 5.5. (a) Photomicrograph of the left ventricle demonstrates the lace-like appearance of the myocardium in cardiac glycogenosis. Endocardial sclerosis is also present. The thickened endocardium of the left ventricle forms a dark zone above the myocardium (elastic tissue stain × 125, reduced to 8/10). (b) Junction of left ventricular sinusoid and ventricular cavity. Marked thickening of the endocardium and of the sinusoidal lining (elastic tissue stain × 75, reduced to 8/10) (Ruttenberg et al., 1964)

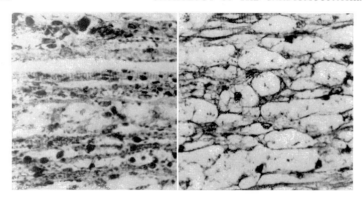

Figure 5.6.   Skeletal muscle in a case of Pompe's disease (cardiac glyco-genosis) showing cyst-like spaces which in fact are areas where glycogen has been present but has not stained (haematoxylin and eosin × 250 reduced to 8/10) (Ruttenberg et al., 1954)

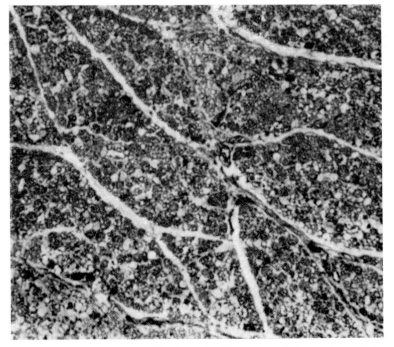

Figure 5.7.   Cross-section of deltoid muscle showing vacuolation and granulation of the cytoplasm (haematoxylin and eosin × 55) (Nihill, Wilson and Hugh-Jones, 1970)

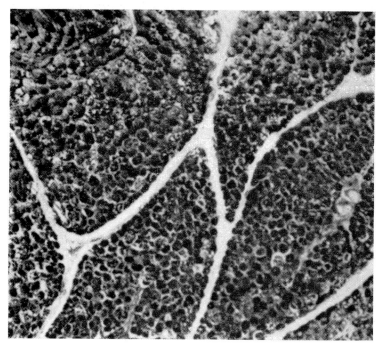

Figure 5.8.   Deltoid muscle showing darkly-staining glycogen granules (PAS × 55) (Nihill, Wilson and Hugh-Jones, 1970)

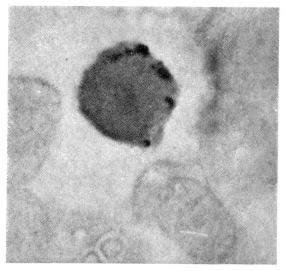

Figure 5.9.   Lymphocyte from peripheral blood showing large glycogen granules (PAS × 1,200) (Nihill, Wilson and Hugh-Jones, 1970)

usually found (*Figure 5.5*). The mechanism for this is suggested to be a predisposition for the deposition of fibrin on the endocardial surface. The amount of fibro-elastosis present seems to be directly related to the length of time of survival of the patient.

Diagnosis

Glycogen is also found in all the other somatic tissues. Muscle biopsy should always be used to confirm the presence of glycogen storage disease. It shows the presence of many vacuoles in the cytoplasm of muscle cells in haematoxylin and eosin-stained sections. Most of these cells, however, contain darkly-staining deposits, which represent glycogen when stained with Best's carmine stain. Most of the skeletal muscle fibres are vacuolated and appear cyst-like. When the skeletal muscle is exposed to diastase digestion before staining, the cyst-like areas in the muscle fibres are more clearly seen (*Figure 5.6*). A similar finding is noted when hepatic tissue is examined (Cori, 1958).

Glycogen may also be demonstrated in skeletal muscle by the PAS stain (*Figures 5.7* and *5.8*).

When the peripheral blood is examined, it is found to contain lymphocytes with small vacuoles and granules in their cytoplasm, which prove to be glycogen when stained by the PAS stain (*Figure 5.9*). This is a useful and simple diagnostic test but is not as diagnostically accurate as muscle biopsy.

Inheritance

Pompe's disease is inherited as an autosomal recessive with an equal sex distribution (Spach *et al.*, 1966). Studies of heterozygotes have been few (Nitowsky and Grunfeld, 1967). This disease has sometimes been described in sibs (Lewis and Sutherland, 1964).

Aetiology

Illingworth, Cori and Cori (1956) demonstrated amylo 1–6 glucosidase in muscle tissue in glycogen storage disease. Hers (1963) has shown that the accumulation of intercellular glycogen in all the tissues of the body in type II glycogenosis is due to an inherited deficiency of alpha-1-4 glucosidase (acid maltase). Recent work by Bauduin, Hers and Loeb (1964) have shown that much of the accumulated hepatic glycogen is found within membrane-lined vacuoles which they refer to as 'lysosomes'. Structurally the glycogen appears to be the same as that found elsewhere in the cytoplasm. Glycogen contained in the vacuoles, as well as the free cytoplasmic glycogen, is digested *in vivo* by amylase. It appears that the lysosomes

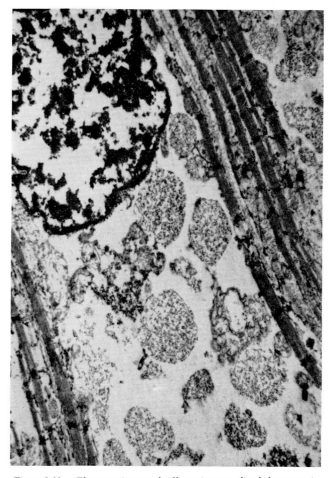

Figure 5.10.   Electronmicrograph of heart in generalized glycogenosis. There are several vascular masses near the nucleus which are composed of fine granular material and partially surrounded by a membrane. There is preservation of the normal myofibrillar pattern (phosphotungstic acid × 10,000, reduced to 8/10) (Spach et al., 1966)

have accumulated glycogen, and that they have then been unable to use normal glycogenic processes, and have thus been unable to utilize this glycogen. It is believed, therefore, that this accumulation is due to the absence of alpha-1-4 glucosidase or other enzymes from the lysosomes, and thus the hydrolysis of glycogen is prevented. Similar electron microscopic studies have been carried out on cardiac

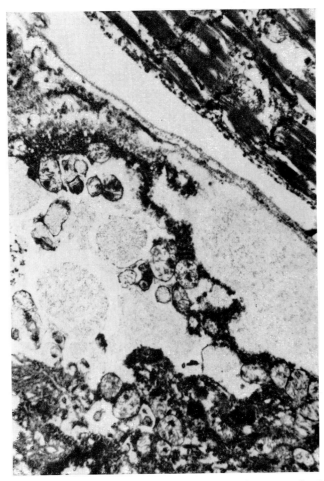

Figure 5.11. Electronmicrograph of skeletal muscle in generalized glycogenosis. There are several vacuoles containing fine granular material and partially surrounded by a membrane. There is also a conglomerate of granular material and mitochondria and absence of normal myofibrillar pattern. A portion of a more normal myofibre appears in the upper right-hand corner (phosphotungstic acid × 10,000, reduced to 8/10) (Spach et al., 1966)

muscle from patients with type II glycogen storage disease (Spach *et al.*, 1966).

It is demonstrated in the electron microgram shown in a representative section of heart muscle (*Figure 5.10*) that glycogen in these cases is only present inside lysosomes. This is a longitudinal section and above the nucleus there are several vacuoles of granular material resembling glycogen. These masses of material are incompletely surrounded by a membrane. It can be assumed that these masses of glycogen were originally completely surrounded by a membrane and were thus within lysosomes.

Aside from the pathological changes described so far, the most striking changes—at least histologically—are seen in skeletal muscle. In most cases of glycogenosis these muscles are grossly unremarkable. However, microscopically there is widespread vacuolar dilatation and degeneration of long segments of myofibres with clumps of basophilic material at the periphery of the fibre. Frequently, webs of this material extend across the damaged fibres and the nuclei in these areas appear to by pyknotic. Much glycogen can be detected in the damaged cells by histochemical means as well as in the adjacent, more normal fibres. *Figure 5.11* shows the electron microscopic features of skeletal muscle in the disease. In the upper right-hand corner is a portion of a normal fibre with good fibrillary structure. In the adjacent damaged fibre (lower left-hand portion of the picture) there are masses of granular material adjacent to the sarcolemma membrane. Occasionally, this material extends in strands or masses across the muscle fibre and coincides with the position of acid mucopolysaccharide shown by light microscopy.

These changes are not unlike those seen in early necrosis of muscle, and it seems that, pathologically, skeletal muscle damages much more than cardiac muscle, although the reverse is clinically true. It has been postulated that other glycolitic enzymes are absent from Pompe's disease (Brown and Zellweger, 1966).

References

Bauduin, P., Hers, A. G. and Loeb, H. (1964). 'An electron microscopic and biochemical study of type II glycogenosis.' *Lab. Invest.* **13**, 1139

Brown, B. I. and Zellweger, H. (1966). 'Alpha-1,4-glucosidase activity in leucocytes from the family of two brothers who lack this enzyme in muscle.' *Biochem. J.* **101**, 16c

Caddell, J. and Whittemore, R. (1962). 'Observations on generalised glycogenosis with emphasis on electrocardiographic changes.' *Paediatrics* **29**, 743

Cardiff, R. D. (1966). 'A histochemical and electron microscopic study of skeletal muscle in a case of Pompe's disease (glycogenosis II).' *Pediatrics, Springfield* **28**, 743

Cori, G. T. (1954). 'Glycogen structure and enzyme deficiencies in glycogen storage disease.' *Harvey Lect.* **48**, 145

Cori, G. T. (1958). 'Biochemical aspects of glycogen deposition disease.' *Med. Prob. Paediat.* **3**, 344

Crome, L., Cumings, J. N. and Duckett, S. (1963). 'Neuropathological and neurochemical aspects of generalized glycogen storage disease.' *J. Neurol. Neurosurg. Psychiat.* **26**, 422

Dincsoy, M. Y., Dincsoy, H. P., Kessler, A. D., Jackson, M. A. and Sidburg, J. B. Jnr (1965). 'Generalised glycogenosis and associated endocardial fibro-elastosis. Report of 3 cases with biochemical studies.' *J. Pediat.* **67**, 728

Ehlers, Katherine H. and Engle, Mary A. (1963). 'Glycogen storage disease of myocardium.' *Am. Heart J.* **65**, 145

— Hogstran, J. W. C., Lukas, D. S., Redo, S. F. and Engle, M. A. (1962). 'Glycogen storage disease of the myocardium with obstruction to the ventricular out-flow.' *Circulation* **25**, 96

Hernandez, A. Jnr, Marchesi, V., Goldring, D., Dissane, J. and Hartman, A. F. Jnr (1966). 'Cardiac glycogenosis. Haemodynamic, angiocardiographic, and electron microscopic findings. Report of a case.' *J. Pediat.* **68**, 400

Hers, H. G. (1963). 'α-Glucosidase deficiency in generalised glycogenstorage disease (Pompe's disease).' *Biochem. J.* **86**, 11

Hohn, A. R., Lowe, C. V., Sokal, J. E. and Lambert, E. C. (1965). 'Cardiac problems in the glycogenose—with special reference to Pompe's disease.' *Pediatrics, Springfield* **35**, 313

Hug, G., Garancis, J. C., Schubert, W. K. and Kuplan, S. (1966). 'Glycogen storage disease, types 2, 3, 8 and 9. A biochemical and electron microscopic analysis.' *Am. J. Dis. Child.* **111**, 457

Huijing, F., Van Creveld, S. and Losekoot, G. (1963). 'Diagnosis of generalised glycogen storage disease (Pompe's disease).' *J. Pediat.* **63**, 984

Illingworth, Barbara, Cori, Gerty, T. and Cori, C. F. (1956). 'Amylo 1–6 glucosidase in muscle tissue in generalised glycogen storage disease.' *J. biol. Chem.* **218**, 213

Kahana, D., Telem, C., Steinitz, K. and Solomon, M. (1964). 'Generalized glycogenosis. Report of a case with deficiency of alpha glucosidase.' *J. Pediat.* **65**, 243

Lewis, G. M. and Sutherland, T. W. (1964). 'Sibs with cardiac glycogenosis.' *Archs. Dis. Child.* **39**, 523

Nihill, M. R., Wilson, D. S. and Hugh-Jones, K. (1970). 'Generalised glycogenosis type II (Pompe's disease).' *Archs Dis. Childh.* **45**, 122

Nitowsky, H. M. and Grunfeld, A. (1967). 'Lysomal alpha-glucosidase in type II glycogenosis activity in leucocytes and cell cultures in relation to genotype.' *J. Lab. clin. Med.* **69**, 472

Perez-Trevino, C., Milino-Zapala, B., Guzman-Gercia, C., Merizalde, A. and Ricalde, A. (1965). 'Glycogen storage disease of the heart.' *Am. J. Cardiol.* **16**, 137

Pompe, J. C. (1932). 'Over idiopatische hypertrophy van het hart.' *Ned. Tijdschr. Geneesk.* **76**, 304

Rosenstein, B. J. (1964). 'Glycogen storage disease of the heart in a newborn infant.' *J. Pediat.* **65**, 126

Ruttenburg, H. D., Steil, R. M., Carey, L. C. and Edwards, J. E. (1964). 'Glycogen storage disease of the heart. Haemodynamic, angiocardio-graphic features of the disease.' *Am. Heart J.* **67**, 469

Spach, M. S., Martin, A. M., Sidburg, J. B., Hacker, D. B. and Canewt, R. V. (1966). 'Clinico-pathologic conference in a case of Pompe's disease (type II glycogen).' *Am. Heart J.* **72**, 265

Smith, H. C., Amick, L. D. and Sidburg, J. B. Jnr (1966). 'Type III glyco-genosis. "Report of a Case with Four Years' Survival and Absence of Acid Maltase Associated with Abnormal Glycogen".' *Am. J. Dis. Child.* **111**, 475

REFSUM'S DISEASE

Refsum's disease is rare and familial with a recessive inheritance. The clinical presentation is comprised of hemianopia, retinitis pigmentosa, cerebellar ataxia, nerve deafness and icthyotic skin changes.

Laboratory Findings

There is a marked rise in albumen and globulin in the cerebro-spinal fluid (but not cells). Electroencephalogram changes are usually present.

Cardiac Changes

Cardiac changes have been reported in a paper by Gordan and Hudson (1959). The heart weighed between 500 and 600 g; it was not possible to obtain an exact cardiac weight as part had been removed before the specimen was received. The right ventricle was 1 cm thick and the left venticle 2·2 cm thick. The cut surface of the left ventricle showed streaky fibrosis but the coronary arteries showed only minimal atherosclerotic changes.

Microscopically there were widespread, non-specific changes affecting all the chambers, and in quite large areas the muscle fibres had lost their identity in a kind of syncitium appearing empty and somewhat atrophic (no focal amyloid or glycogen deposits were found). There was no inflammation. The process in the ventricles was most marked in the subendocardial muscle; endocardial fibro-elastosis was also present and there was haemorrhage in the atrio-ventricular sulcus. The autonomic nerves in the epicardium and within the myocardium seemed unduly prominent; the sino-atrial node and the bundle of His were larger than normal.

References

Gordan, E. and Hudson, R. E. B. (1959). 'Refsum's syndrome heredo-pathic atactica polyneuritis fermie. A report of three cases including a study of cardiac pathology.' *Brain* **82**, 41

FABRY'S DISEASE

Fabry's disease (angiokeratoma corporis diffusum universale) originally considered to be a cutaneous manifestation of an inherited disease. The disease is due to the presence of an abnormal sphingo-lipid and glycolipid in the walls of small blood vessels (Sweeley and Klionsky, 1963).

Clinical signs develop during childhood and initially consist of dark-purple keratotic lesions in the skin, bouts of fever, proteinuria and abdominal pain. These manifestations may persist without aggravation for a considerable period of time (Pompen, Ruiter and Wyers, 1967). In male patients oedema, cardiac dysfunction, renal failure and uraemia develop during the third or fourth decades of life (Sweeley and Klionsky, 1966; Kahlke, 1967).

Hypertension is frequently encountered but is seldom of great severity.

Inheritance

The disease is transmitted by a sex-linked gene that is variably and incompletely recessive. Homozygous male patients exhibit the full spectrum of the disease; most heterozygous female patients show only a typical corneal dystrophy and some degree of renal involvement (Opitz *et al.*, 1965).

Cardiac Involvement

Cardiac involvement may result in anginal chest pain, myocardial infarction, congestive heart failure and cardiac dilatation and hypertrophy (Kahlke, 1967).

Their true incidence cannot be estimated because of the lack of complete data in many of the reported cases. Cardiac involvement, however, is a constant feature. At autopsy the heart is enlarged—often considerably so—i.e., weighing 600–800 g. It is dilated in all chambers and shows well-marked ventricular hypertrophy. Several young patients with Fabry's disease have been shown to have a myocardial infarction (Falck and Weicksel, 1957; Parkinson and Sunshine, 1961; Wise, Wallace and Jellinek, 1962). This infarction has been attributed to the deposit of glycolipid in the coronary vasculature. Death related to valvular involvement has been reported in three patients with Fabry's disease (Hofmann and Hauser, 1962; Leder and Bosworth, 1965; Ferrans, Hibbs and Burda, 1969).

Microscopic Changes

Hypertrophy of the muscle fibres with extensive cytoplasmic vacuolation and birefringent lipid deposits have been observed in all the cases studied. A neutral glycolipid can be demonstrated in the muscle cells, connective tissue elements and vascular smooth muscle of the heart. It seemed evident that the accumulation of glycolipid in these sites leads to progressive cardiac enlargement and failure.

The histological alterations of the cardiac muscle cells in Fabry's disease, that is the central vacuolization and peripheral displacement of the myofibres, is not specific for this disease. Practically identical changes are seen in types II and III glycogenosis, in which they are caused by the accumulation of glycogen. In all these disorders the vacuoles of the muscle fibres contain various PAS-positive staining substances and often show some degree of basophilia in haematoxylin and eosin stained preparations. Therefore, the disease must be differentiated from Fabry's disease clinically, and on the basis of biochemical, histochemical, polariscopic and electron microscopic studies.

Electron Microscopy

The lamellar intrastructure of the glycolipid deposits in the heart muscle are in the form of lamellar bodies with a periodicity of 40–50 Å. These probably represent non-specific degenerative changes.

Similar lamellar structures have been seen in other types of lipidoses, but they have a different chemical composition. The possibility that the lamellar bodies found in Fabry's disease are of lysosomal origin has been proposed by Hashimoto, Gross and Lever (1965), and it is now thought that the lamellar bodies in Fabry's disease appear to be a form of lysosome-derived residual bodies that retain very little of their original complement of hydrolytic enzymes.

The development of such changes in the blood vessels of smooth muscle is thought to account for the ischaemic type of pain experienced on exercise by some patients with Fabry's disease.

References

Ferrans, V. J., Hibbs, R. G. and Burda, C. D. (1969). 'The heart in Fabry's disease. A histochemical and electron microscopic study.' *Am. J. Cardiol.* **24**, 95

Flack, I. and Weicksel, A. (1957). 'Angiokeratoma corporis diffusum Fabry mit vasorenalen Symptomen Komplex.' *Samml. selt. klin. Fälle* **13**, 20

Hashimoto, K., Gross, B. G. and Lever, W. F. (1965). 'Angiokeratoma corposis diffusum (Fabry). Histochemical and electron microscopic studies of the skin.' *J. invest. Derm.* **44**, 119

Hofmann, A. and Hauser, W. (1962). 'Angiokeratoma corporis diffusum (Fabry) mit cerebralen Manifestationen.' *Dt. Z. Nerv. Heilk.* **183**, 351

Kahlke, W. (1967). 'Angiokeratoma corporis diffusum universale (Fabry's disease).' In *Lipids and Lipidoses*. Ed. by G. Schettler, p. 332. Berlin: Springer

Leder, A. A. and Bosworth, W. C. (1965). 'Angiokeratoma corporis diffusum universale (Fabry's disease) with mitral stenosis.' *Am. J. Med.* **38**, 814

Opitz, J. H., Stiles, F. C., Wise, D., Race, R. R., Sanger, R., Von Gemminge, G. R., Kickland, R. R., Cross, E. G. and Degroot, W. P. (1965). 'The genetics of angiokeratoma corporis diffusum (Fabry's disease) and its linkage relations with the Xg locus.' *Am. J. hum. Genet.* **17**, 325

Parkinson, J. E. and Sunshine, A. (1961). 'Angiokeratoma corporis diffusum universale (Fabry). Presenting as suspected myocardial infarction and pulmonary infarcts.' *Am. J. Med.* **31**, 951

Pompen, A. W. N., Ruiter, M. and Wijers, H. J. G. (1947). 'Angiokeratoma corporis diffusum universale (Fabry), as a sign of unknown internal disease; two autopsy reports.' *Acta med. scand.* **128**, 234

Sweeley, C. C. and Klionsky, B. (1963). 'Fabry's disease: classification as a sphingolipidosis and partial characterisation of a novel glycolipid.' *J. biol. Chem.* **238**, 3148

— — (1966). 'Glycolipid lipidosis Fabry's disease.' In *The Metabolic Basis of Inherited Disease*. Ed. by J. B. Stanbury, J. B. Wyngaarden and D. S. Fredrickson, p. 618. New York: McGraw Hill

Wise, D., Wallace, H. T. and Jellinek, E. H. (1962). 'Angiokeratoma corporis diffusum. A clinical study of eight affected families.' *Q. Jl. Med.* (NS) **31**, 177

GARGOYLISM (HURLER'S SYNDROME)

Gargoylism is a generalized disease in which there is widespread deposition of an acid mucopolysaccharide substance in various tissues, including the heart. Storage of the polysaccharide material occurs in fibroblasts and parenchymal cells.

This disease, with its peculiar skeletal and other abnormalities, was first described by Hunter (1916). The name 'gargoylism' was first used by Ellis, Sheldon and Capon (1936) because of the ugliness of the child's features. The head is large with coarse hair and a thick skull; the ears large and low-set and deafness is often present. The nasal bridge is depressed, and the face rather flat. The eyebrows are heavy and the eyes wide-set; the lips are thick, the teeth widely spaced, and the tongue enlarged—often filling the mouth. The hands are stubby, wide and clawed. The skeletal changes in the trunk cause shortness of the neck and dorsolumbar kyphosis; there is broadening of the rib spaces and widening of the anterioposterior diameter of the chest. The eye changes, when present, are pathognomonic; the cornea becomes clouded with yellowish-white deposits in the middle and deeper layers. Mental deficiency is also common, and there is hepatosplenomegaly with prominence of the abdomen, and often umbilical hernia.

'Forme fruste' of gargoylism may occur when one or more features of the disease are absent (De Lange *et al.*, 1943–44); Jervis (1950) described a type which affects males only, but in which there is no corneal involvement, and is due to a sex-linked recessive gene (Millman and Whittick, 1952); Jackson (1951) described a typical case in a girl, skeletal changes in a mentally normal brother and an intermediate grade of this disease in another sister. The heart is involved in the majority of cases.

Incidence

Gargoylism may affect either sex and several members of one family; parental consanguinity is not usually concerned. The usual form of the disease is due to a single autosomal recessive gene (Halperin and Curtis, 1942). Most patients die young; the age range in the patients reviewed by Lindsay (1950) being 1–29 years of age. Fourteen of nineteen cases died of cardiac failure.

Dawson (1954) suggested that the primary disturbance was one of polysaccharide or mucopolysaccharide metabolism, and that there is a combination between polysaccharides and the lipoid substance, phosphatides or cerebrosides, occurring in neurones and in other tissues producing a substance of variable solubility. Dawson considered that the skeletal changes in the disease were dystrophic; the result of metabolic changes in skeletal muscle.

In recent years the various disturbances of mucopolysaccharide metabolism have been classified into five types (McKusick, 1964), types IV–V have aortic regurgitation as a manifestation.

Cardiovascular Changes

Lindsay (1950) found that of 25 autopsy cases in the literature, 17 had gross or microscopic involvement of the heart, and that cardiac failure was the cause of death in 14. Emmanuel (1954) estimated that 85 per cent of 32 reported autopsy cases showed heart involvement; it was enlarged in 73 per cent and its valves deformed in 77 per cent, endocardial thickening was present in 7 cases, and epicardial thickening in 3 cases. Lindsay considered that the cardiac disease was aggravated by the thoracic deformity and the common occurrence of bronchopneumonia, and by anaemia.

Pericardial effusion is commonly found at autopsy. The heart is usually enlarged and the left ventricle often hypertrophied: passive pulmonary hypertension from mitral stenosis may also cause right heart enlargement.

In the myocardium the muscle fibres may show vacuolation. The material in the vacuoles is water soluble and it is difficult to demonstrate the contents.

The intercellular connective tissue is increased (*Figure 5.12*) and

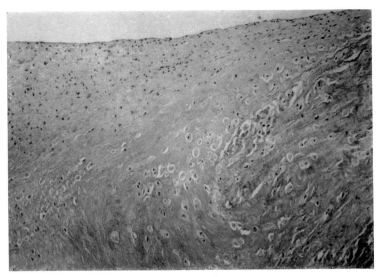

Figure 5.12. Hurler's syndrome showing the thickened ventricular endocardium while this, and the interstitial tissue of the underlying myocardium, is infiltrated with a large amount of mucopolysaccharides (PAS × 150, reduced to 2/3) (Reproduced by courtesy of Dr Ariela Pomerance)

shows hyaline or mucoid changes, the fibres being swollen and oedematous with clear vacuolated or granular cytoplasm and often with loss of its fibrillary character. This gives a pseudocartilanenous appearance.

The valves are thickened and show glistening translucent nodules, 1–3 mm in diameter, and the chordae tendinae may be thickened and shortened. The mitral valve orifice may be stenosed, and the edges of the aortic and pulmonary valves may be 'rolled'.

The endocardium (*Figure 5.13*) and especially the valves, may be thickened and sometimes small nodules (1–3 mm in diameter) are present in the cusps. Occasionally, in both the endocardium and valves a little calcium may be deposited and chronic inflammatory cells may appear.

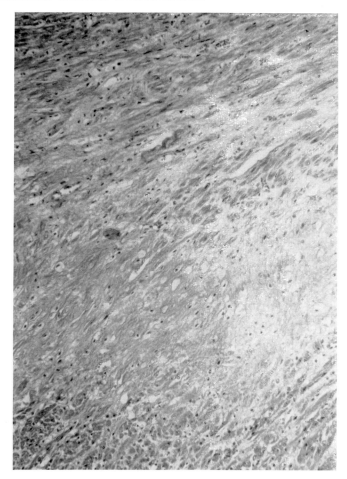

Figure 5.13. The myocardium showing that the interstitial tissue is diffusely infiltrated with mucopolysaccharides while the myocardial cells sometimes contain vacuoles, which are filled with clear material while others show perinuclear vacuolation (PAS × 150, reduced to 2/3) (Reproduced by courtesy of Dr Ariela Pomerance)

The epicardium may be thickened generally or in patches with fibrous tissue containing vacuolated cells and adipose tissues with a few mononuclear cells around the coronary artery branches.

The coronary arteries may show remarkable intimal proliferation with stenosis of the lumen which may cause myocardial ischaemia.

Vanace, Friedman and Wagner (1960) reviewed the condition and reported the case of an intelligent boy of 5 years of age in whom mitral stenosis was first diagnosed only four months before his death. Strauss and Platt (1957) reported a case associated with endocardial fibro-elastosis. In their case they were able to demonstrate granular material by Hale's dialysed iron method.

Laboratory Findings

Mild anaemia is common and the serum cholesterol may be raised. Reilly (1941) drew attention to the presence of abnormal dark violet granules in the leucocytes, seen especially well in neutrophils in blood films when stained with Wright's stain.

It is important to remember that all children with gargoylism have abnormal urinary polysaccharides, although they may have no symptoms; as in four of the six cases with gargoylism described by Scheibler et al. (1962).

The urine may contain an excess of two sulphated mucopolysaccharides, chondroitin sulphate and heparin sulphate, both of which contain uronic acid and are over-produced by the body in this disease; normal production is up to 30 mg/hr (Muir, Mittwoch and Bitter, 1963). These uronic acid compounds may be detected and assessed by the carbazole reaction; a simple method, using dialysed urine, was described by Segni, Romano and Tortorolo (1964).

References

Dawson, I. M. P. (1954). 'Histology and histochemistry of gargoylism.' J. Path. Bact. 67, 587

De Lange, C., Gerlings, P. G., De Kleyn, A. and Lettinga, T. W. (1943–44). 'Some remarks on gargoylism.' Acta Paediat. 31, 398

Ellis, R. W. B., Sheldon, W. and Capon, N. B. (1936). 'Gargoylism (Chondro- osteo- dystrophy, corneal opacities, hepato-splenomegaly and mental deficiency).' Q. Jl. Med. (NS) 5, 119

Emmanuel, R. W. (1954). 'Gargoylism with cardiovascular involvement in two brothers.' Br. Heart J. 16, 417

Halperin, S. L. and Curtis, G. M. (1942). 'Genetics of gargoylism.' Am. J. ment. Def. 46, 298

Hunter, C. (1916). 'A rare disease in two brothers. Elevation of scapula, limitation of movements of joints and other skeletal abnormalities.' Proc. R. Soc. Med. 10, 104

Jackson, W. P. U. (1951). 'Clinical features, diagnosis and osseous lesions of gargoylism exemplified in 3 siblings.' Archs Dis. Childh. 26, 549

Jervis, G. A. (1950). 'Gargoylism (Lipochondrodystrophy). A study of 10 cases, with emphasis on formes fruste of disease.' Archs Neurol. Psychiat. Chicago 63, 681

Lindsay, S. (1950). 'Cardio-vascular system in gargoylism.' *Br. Heart J.* **12**, 17

McKusick, V. A. (1964). 'A genetical view of cardiovascular disease. (The Lewis A. Conner Memorial Lecture.)' *Circulation* **30**, 326

Millman, C. G. and Whittick, J. W. (1952). 'A sex-linked variant of gargoylism.' *J. Neurol. Neurosurg. Psychiat.* **15**, 253

Muir, H., Mittwoch, Ursula, and Bitter, T. (1963). 'The diagnostic value of isolated urinary mucopolysaccharides and of lymphocyte inclusions in gargoylism.' *Archs Dis. Childh.* **38**, 358

Reilly, W. A. (1941). 'The granules in the leucocytes in gargoylism.' *Am. J. Dis. Childh.* **62**, 489

Scheibler, G. L., Lorincz, A. E., Brogdon, B. G., Shanklin, D. R., Bartley, T. D. and Krovetz, L. J. (1962). 'Cardio-vascular manifestations of Hurler's syndrome.' *Circulation* **26**, Suppl. 782

Segni, G., Romano, C. and Tortorolo, G. (1964). 'Diagnostic test for gargoylism.' *Lancet* **2**, 420

Strauss, L. and Platt, R. (1957). 'Endocardial sclerosis in infancy associated with abnormal storage (gargoylism); report of a case in an infant, aged 5 months and review of the literature.' *J. Mt Sinai Hosp.* **24**, 1258

Vanace, P. W., Friedman, S. and Wagner, B. M. (1960). 'Mitral stenosis in an atypical case of gargoylism; a case report with pathologic and histochemical studies of the cardiac tissues.' *Circulation* **21**, 80

PSEUDOXANTHOMA ELASTICUM

Pseudoxanthoma elasticum is a heritable disease of connective tissue characterized by morphological and functional alterations of the elastic fibres (McKusick, 1956).

The primary cardiac abnormalities in this condition are mentioned rarely in the literature but may be the mode of presentation and, indeed, the cause of death. The clinical symptoms are arrhythmias, cardiomegaly and congestive cardiac failure.

Usually, however, few symptoms of cardiovascular disease are noted in association with pseudoxanthoma elasticum.

Eddy and Farber (1962) in their clinical study of 200 cases, noted that 19 had angina pectoris.

The heart is usually enlarged and all the chambers are dilated especially the left ventricle. The myocardium is of normal thickness but usually flabby. The valves are normal, but may be thickened as more usually are the chordae tendineae. The endocardium of both atria and ventricles may exhibit a diffuse pearly-white thickening but localized areas of endocardial thickening, particularly below the atrioventricular valves, are more commonly seen.

The endocardium usually shows nodules and plaque-like thickenings microscopically; this is due to an increase of collagen and elastic tissue fibres. The elastic tissue fibres although staining positively are covered usually with a heavy deposition of calcium and are associated with a large amount of acid mucopolysaccharides in the surrounding connective tissue ground substance. In some places the thickened endocardium consists of fibrous tissue only.

The coronary arteries are unremarkable macroscopically, but microscopically areas of fragmentation and calcification of the internal lamina elastica are often seen.

Only nine cases with cardiac involvement have been reported, although the first was that of Balzer in 1884. This is difficult to explain and one must conclude that cardiac lesions have rarely been looked for.

References

Balzer, F. (1884). 'Recherches sur les caractères anatomiques du xanthelasma.' *J. Physiol. Path. gén.* **4**, 65

Eddy, D. D. and Farber, E. M. (1962). 'Pseudoxanthoma elasticum. Internal manifestations: a report of cases and a statistical review of the literature.' *Archs Derm.* **86**, 729

McKusick, V. A. (1956). 'Heritable disorders of connective tissue; pseudoxanthoma elasticum.' *J. Chron. Dis.* **3**, 263

PROGRESSIVE MUSCULAR DYSTROPHY

The non-myotonic muscular dystrophies are classified into four groups.

(1)   The pseudohypertrophic dystrophy of Duchenne (Duchenne, 1868; Gowers, 1879).

(2)   The limb girdle type of Erb (1884).

(3)   The fascioscapulohumeral dystrophy of Landouzy and Dejerine (1884).

(4)   'Benign Duchenne' limb girdle dystrophy with pseudohypertrophy (Morton, Chung and Peters, 1963; Pearson, 1963).

Published data describing cardiomyopathies in muscular dystrophies are numerous, but this relationship is not widely appreciated.

Table 5.1 illustrates the principal differences between the various types of muscular dystrophy. The first to describe progressive muscular atrophy in detail was Meryon (1852) but no mention of cardiac changes was made in this report. Ross (1863) was the first to describe myocardial atrophy in a muscular dystrophy occurring in a boy with pseudohypertrophic paralysis. Meerwein (1904), in reviewing the 480 cases of progressive muscular dystrophy reported prior to 1904, found that approximately 18 per cent had cardiovascular abnormalities.

Globus (1923) in an examination of the material published up to 1922, further suggested that the pathological findings in the heart were cardiac manifestation of the accompanying dystrophy.

Zatuchni et al. (1951) reviewed the literature from 1922–51 and discussed the cardiovascular data in 94 cases (out of 292), in which the findings were considered abnormal (Weisenfeld and Messinger, 1952; Rubin and Buchberg, 1952; Walton and Natrass, 1954; Demang and Zimmerman, 1969); and the detailed review of Perloff, de Leon and O'Doherty (1966). Manifestations of heart disease include arrhythmias (Ruben and Buchberg, 1952); cardiomegaly (Weisenfeld and Messinger, 1952); chest pain (Bert and Báráti, 1942); and sudden death (Goodhart, 1942). A detailed review of this subject was carried out by Berenbaum and Horowitz (1956).

PSEUDOHYPERTROPHIC DYSTROPHY OF DUCHENNE

The sex-linked recessive form occurs almost exclusively in males and characteristically begins during the first five years of life. Pseudohypertrophy of the calf muscles is especially marked in the early years of this disease and later there is a spread of the dystrophy to the shoulder girdle. Progression is usually constant and often rapid (Kiloh and Nevin, 1951). This disease may, however, present clinically as a cardiomegaly. Patients usually succumb to inanition or infections, especially pulmonary (Gilroy et al., 1963), but dystrophic cardiomyopathy may be an important cause of death (Weisenfeld and Messinger, 1952; Gilroy et al., 1963).

Skeletal muscle enzymes may enter the plasma as a result of myopathic disease. The demonstration of many enzymes, such as glutamic pyruvate transaminase, lactic and malic dehydrogenases and creatine phosphokinase has represented a major advance in the clinical study of muscular dystrophies. It has generally been accepted that the source of elevated enzymes is skeletal muscle, Sundermeyer et al. (1961) have detected the myocardial release of malic dehydrogenase and aldolase in several patients by comparing coronary sinus to systemic concentrations.

At Autopsy

At autopsy the heart is usually dilated and flabby while the endocardium is slightly thickened with elongation of chordae tendineae and papillary muscles. The circumference of the mitral annular ring may be markedly increased and the left atrium enlarged. A section of the myocardium shows marked interstitial fibrosis and extensive replacement of the myocardial fibres by connective tissue. Some parts of the myocardium, however, may show no significant increase in fibrous tissue. Histologically the myocardium shows replacement of myocardial fibres with connective tissue in addition to extensive interstitial fibrosis.

LIMB-GIRDLE DYSTROPHY OF ERB

Inheritance is usually by an autosomal recessive gene, although many cases occur sporadically.

The onset may be from childhood to middle age, but is generally in the second decade and the sexes are equally affected. The rate of progression is variable and cardiac involvement is not considered to occur in many cases (Walton, 1963). This finding is probably not correct as these cases often have some ECG changes and many show abnormal changes in serum enzyme levels. Perloff, de Leon and O'Doherty (1965) found abnormal concentrations of aldolase in 5 of 6; lactic dehydrogenase (LDH) in 5 of 9; serum glutamic oxaloacetic transaminase (SGOT) in 3 of 8; and serum glutamic pyruvic transaminase (SGPT) in 1 of 4 patients studied. In another two of these patients, coronary sinus levels of LDH, aldolase, SGOT and SGPT were not elevated when compared with systemic arterial concentrations and with that found in non-dystrophic subjects.

FASCIOSCAPULOHUMERAL DYSTROPHY

Inheritance is commonly by an autosomal dominant gene with equal expression in male and female.

Symptoms may begin from early childhood to middle life, although the onset is usually in adolescence and progression is characteristically insidious. Death is usually unrelated to the basic myopathic disease.

Cardiac involvement in fascioscapulohumeral dystrophy is also considered rare. In a few reports, where a definite diagnosis of this type of dystrophy has been made, abnormal electrocardiograms have been found (Gallini, Danowski and Fisher, 1958; Lisan, Ambriglia and Lickoff, 1959). No changes in cardiac enzymes have been reported in any of the patients studied.

'BENIGN DUCHENNE'

Some patients with limb-girdle dystrophy have pseudohypertrophy of the calves. Other patients (male but occasionally female) with an autosomal recessive form of Duchenne dystrophy experience a relatively slower progression of the disease than patients with the

TABLE 5.1
Points of Difference Between Dystrophies (1-4)

	Pseudohypertrophic dystrophy of Duchenne	Limb-girdle dystrophy of Erb	Fascioscapulohumeral dystrophy	Benign Duchenne
Sex affected	All male	More cases found in female	Both sexes equally affected	All male
Age at onset	5 years	2nd decade	Adolescence	Probably early 2nd decade
Mode of inheritance	X-linked recessive	Autosomal recessive	Autosomal dominant	Autosomal or X-linked recessive
Pseudohypertrophy of calf muscles	Marked	Mild	Rare	Moderate
Rate of progression	Rapid	Moderately rapid but may be variable	Insidious	Moderately rapid
Duration of disease	1-20	1-40	1-30	1-30
Serum enzyme changes	—	Moderate increase	Mild to moderate increase	Moderate increase
Cardiomyopathy overt	Common	Uncommon	Rare	May be common
Cardiomyopathy occult	Very common	May be common	Uncommon	May be common
Electrocardiogram abnormalities	Very common	Uncommon	Rare	May be common

classical aggressive, sex-linked form, but it is substantially later in onset and runs a slower course. It is difficult to find reported cases of cardiac involvement in such patients because the classification of the disease is unclear. However, in some patients there have been definite reports of cardiac failure and abnormal electrocardiograms, and we are probably dealing with a cardiomyopathy (Storstein and Kinge, 1961; James, 1962), although in none of these reports have any post-mortem details been given.

In conclusion Table 5.1 gives a summary of the differences between these various types of dystrophy.

References

Berenbaum, A. A. and Horowitz, W. (1956). 'Heart involvement in progressive muscular dystrophy.' *Am. Heart J.* **51**, 622

Bert, J. M. and Báráti, N. (1942). 'Le coeur dans les myopathics.' *Montpelier Med.* **21**, 13

Duchenne, G. B. (1868). 'Recherches sur la paralysie musculaire pseudo-hypertrophique, on paralysie myosclerosique.' *Archs gén. Méd.* Series **6**, 11: pp. 5, 179, 305, 421 and 522

Erb, W. (1884). 'Ueber die "juvenile form" der progressiven Muskelatrophie und ihre Beziehungen zur sogenannten pseudohypertrophie der Muskeln.' *Dt. Arch. klin. Med.* **34**, 467

Gallini, S., Danowski, T. S. and Fisher, D. S. (1958). 'Muscular dystrophy.' *Circulation* **17**, 583

Gilroy, J., Cahalan, J. L., Berman, R. and Newman, M. (1963). 'Cardiac and pulmonary complications in Duchenne's progressive muscular dystrophy.' *Circulation* **27**, 484

Globus, J. H. (1923). 'Pathologic findings in the heart muscle in progressive muscular dystrophy.' *Archs Neurol. Psychiat., Chicago* **9**, 59

Goodhart, S. P. (1942). 'Progressive muscular dystrophies; necropsy studies in four cases.' *J. Mt Sinai Hosp.* **9**, 514

Gowers, W. R. (1879). Clinical lecture on *pseudohypertrophic muscular paralysis. Lancet* **2**, 37

James, T. N. (1962). 'Observations on the cardiovascular involvement including the cardiac conduction system, in progressive muscular dystrophy.' *Am. Heart J.* **63**, 48

Kiloh, L. G. and Nevin, S. (1951). 'Pseudohypertrophic muscular dystrophy with cardiomegaly.' *Proc. Soc. Med.* **441**, 694

Landouzy, L. and Dejerine, J. (1884). 'De la myopathie atrophique progressive.' *Proc. R. Acad. Sci.* **1**, 53

Lisan, P., Ambriglia, J. and Lickoff, W. (1959). 'Myocardial diseases associated with progressive muscular dystrophy.' *Am. Heart J.* **57**, 913

Meerwein (1904). 'Verhältnisse von Herz und Zunge bei den primaren Myopathien.' Basel: Dissert

Meryon, E. (1852). 'On granular and fatty degeneration of the voluntary muscles.' *Med.-chir. Trans.* **35**, 73

Morton, N. E., Chung, C. S. and Peters, H. (1963). 'Genetics of muscular dystrophy.' In *Muscular Dystrophy in Man and Animals*. Ed. by G. H. Bourne and M. N. Golarz, p. 324. Basel: Karger

Pearson, C. M. (1963). 'Muscular dystrophy.' *Am. J. Med.* **35**, 632

Perloff, J. K., de Leon, A. E. and O'Doherty, D. (1966). 'The cardiomyopathy of progressive muscular dystrophy.' *Circulation* **33**, 625

Ross, J. (1863). 'On a case of pseudohypertrophic paralysis.' *Br. med. J.* **1**, 200

Rubin, I. C. and Buchberg, A. S. (1952). 'Heart in progressive muscular dystrophy.' *Am. Heart J.* **43**, 161

Storstein, O. and Kinge, F. O. (1961). 'Heart involvement in progressive muscular dystrophy.' *Acta psychiat. scand.* **36**, 489

Sundermeyer, J. F., Gudrjarnason, S., Wendt, V. E., den Bakker, P. B. and Bing, R. J. (1961). 'Myocardial metabolism in progressive muscular dystrophy.' *Circulation* **24**, 1348

Walton, J. N. (1963). 'Clinical aspects of human muscular dystrophy.' In *Muscular Dystrophy in Man and Animals*. Ed. by G. H. Bourne and M. N. Golarz, p. 264. Basel: Karger

— and Nattrass, F. S. (1954). 'On classification, natural history and treatment of myopathies.' *Brain* **77**, 169

Weisenfeld, S. and Messinger, W. J. (1952). 'Cardiac involvement in progressive muscular dystrophy.' *Am. Heart J.* **43**, 170

Zatuchni, J., Aegerter, E. E., Molthan, L. and Schuman, C. R. (1951). 'The heart in progressive muscular dystrophy.' *Circulation* **3**, 846

MYOTONIA CONGENITA

Few pathological studies on the heart muscle in myotonia congenita have been reported.

In 1933, Keschner and Davison described one patient and this was later followed by the paper of Fisch and Evans (1954), when they reported the cardiac findings in a man of 41 with myotonia congenita, who died suddenly. This patient had no cardiac symptoms or signs of cardiomegaly, although the presence of AV block and auricular flutters had been observed. Lesions of the conduction system have also been reported by Thompson (1968).

Black and Ravin (1947) described the pathological changes in the hearts of five cases detailing many of the findings listed below.

The only paper so far published, which deals with the cardiac findings in detail, is that of Cannon (1962).

The heart, at post-mortem, is seen to be soft and flabby while the walls of both ventricles may be slightly thickened. The endocardium contains a few grey areas, due to slight endocardial thickening and an occasional petechial haemorrhage may be seen. On section the myocardium is usually normal except that it may contain an

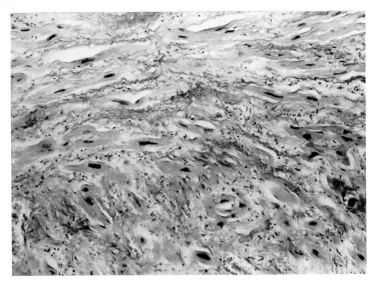

Figure 5.14. Myocardial fibrosis with splitting of muscle fibres and variation in size of nuclei (van Gieson × 100, reduced to 7/10) (Arnason et al., 1964)

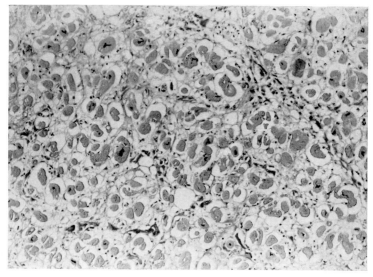

Figure 5.15. Transverse section of myocardium showing muscle fibres of varying thickness (van Gieson × 40, reduced to 7/10) (Arnason et al., 1964)

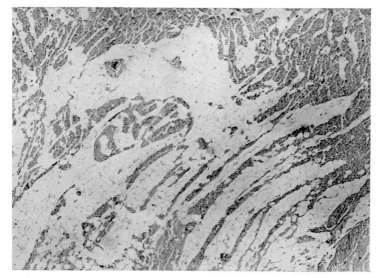

Figure 5.16. Fatty infiltration of the myocardium (van Gieson × 10, reduced to 7/10) (Arnason et al., 1964)

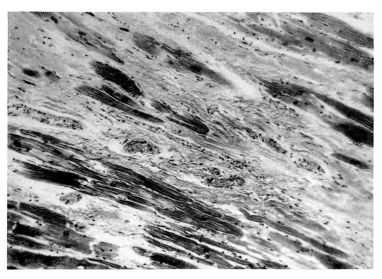

Figure 5.17. Microscopic section of the left ventricular myocardium from a case of myotonia congenita. A distinct cardiomyopathy analogous to the degeneration of skeletal muscle which occurs in myotonic muscular dystrophy (haematoxylin and eosin × 186, reduced to 2/3). (Reproduced from Cannon (1970) by courtesy of the author and Editor of the American Journal of Medicine)

increased amount of fibrous tissue and a moderate amount of fatty tissue.

Microscopic examination of the cardiac tissue shows a marked variation in the size of the muscle fibres, many of which are hypertrophied. Many of these cells have large rectangular nuclei, others being pyknotic, or of irregular shape (*Figure 5.14*).

In other places many of the cells have disappeared, leaving only a few nuclear remnants. There is often a great increase in the amount of fibrous tissue present, particularly in that the interstitial fibrous tissue in all parts of the myocardium is increased. This gross variation in nuclear cell size is best seen in a transverse section (*Figure 5.15*).

In many places there is also a marked infiltration of both the myocardial cells and the interstitial tissues with fat (*Figure 5.16*).

In the later stages of the disease, atrophy of muscle fibres is commonly seen with rows and clusters of nuclear remnants scattered throughout the surrounding connective tissue and lying between scattered fat cells (*Figure 5.17*).

In conclusion, it can be stated that the changes found in cardiac muscle in myotonia are similar to, but less severe than, those found in the skeletal muscle of an affected individual.

References

Arnason, G., Berge, Th. and Dahlbergh, L. (1964). 'Myocardial changes in dystophia myotonica.' *Acta med. scand.* **176**, 535

Black, W. C. and Ravin, A. (1947). 'Studies in dystrophia myotonica; autopsy observations in five cases.' *Archs Path.* **44**, 176

Cannon, P. J. (1962). 'The heart and lungs in myotonic muscular dystrophy.' *Am. J. Med.* **32**, 765

Fisch, C. and Evans, P. V. (1954). 'Heart in dystrophia myotonica; report of autopsied case.' *New Engl. J. Med.* **251**, 527

Keschner, M. and Davison, C. (1933). 'Dystrophia myotonica; clinico-pathologic study.' *Archs Neurol. Psychiat., Lond.* **30**, 1260

Thomson, A. M. P. (1968). 'Dystrophia corotic myotonica studied by serial histology of the pacemaker and cardiatry systems.' *J. Path. Bact.* **96** 285

FRIEDREICH'S ATAXIA

It has been known for many years that the heart is frequently abnormal in Friedreich's ataxia—Friedreich, himself, noted cardiac disturbances in his original cases in 1863.

A recent study (Hewer, 1973) has shown that 56 of 82 fatal cases of Friedreich's ataxia died of heart failure and another 17 cases had

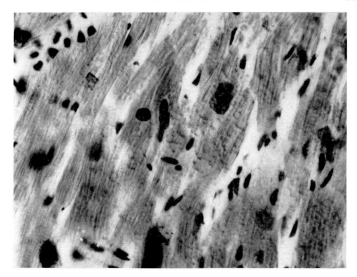

Figure 5.18. Large and bizarre muscle fibre nuclei (haematoxylin and eosin × 395, reduced to 9/10) (Hewer, 1969)

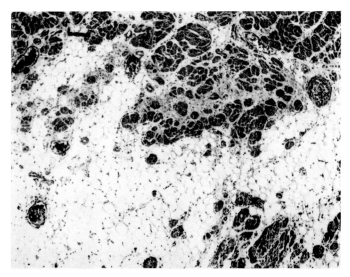

Figure 5.19. Extensive fatty infiltration (haematoxylin and eosin × 40, reduced to 9/10) (Hewer, 1969)

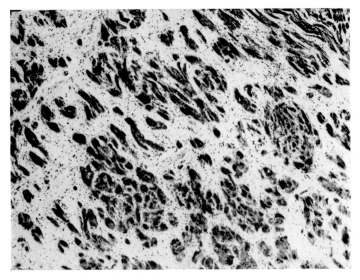

Figure 5.20. Myocardium showing severe interstitial fibrosis in Friedreich's ataxia (van Gieson × 40, reduced to 9/10) (Hewer, 1969)

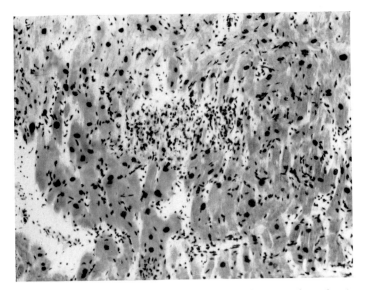

Figure 5.21. Single focus of muscle fibre necrosis (haematoxylin and eosin × 96, reduced to 9/10) (Hewer, 1969)

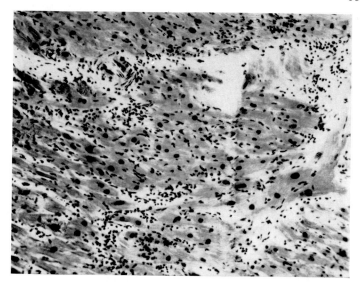

Figure 5.22. Several foci of inflamatmory cells and muscle fibre necrosis (haematoxylin and eosin × 96, reduced to 9/10) (Hewer, 1969)

cardiac symptoms before death. Thorén (1964) has noted that other studies show that 92 per cent of cases have abnormal electrocardiograms. Cardiac function is little impaired during the early years of life. Several authors (Thorén, 1964; Hewer, 1969) have reported that the electrocardiogram changes in adolescence and that heart failure in this disease when it occurs is rarely found in patients less than ten years old. It is interesting to speculate whether the heart in these cases of Friedreich's ataxia is normal in the early years of life or whether it is abnormal since birth.

It is only very recently that a detailed account of pathological changes in the heart has been reported (Hewer, 1969) and much of the description which follows is taken from his paper.

The heart is usually enlarged but the cardiac weight may vary from 250 to 750 g. Thickening of the left ventricle is seen in most hearts and these hearts are commonly found to contain ante-mortem thrombi when first opened.

MICROSCOPIC EXAMINATION

The cardiac muscle fibres are often markedly hypertrophied and irrespective of their size, contain many large and bizarre-shaped

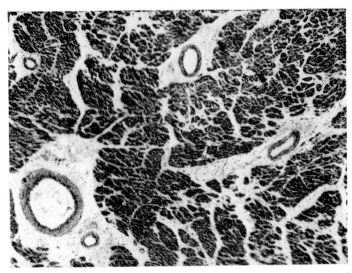

Figure 5.23. Several normal small cardiac arteries (haematoxylin and eosin × 40, reduced to 9/10) (Hewer, 1969)

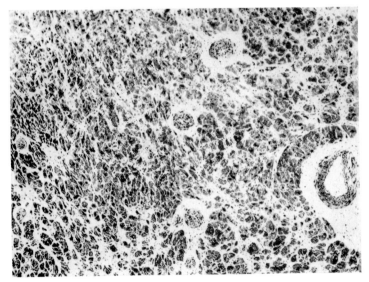

Figure 5.24. Several narrowed arteries (haematoxylin and eosin × 40, reduced to 9/10) (Hewer, 1969)

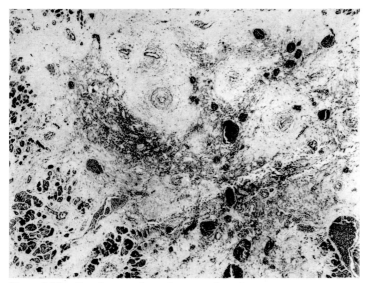

Figure 5.25. Grossly-scarred papillary muscle with many narrowed arteries (haematoxylin and eosin, × 40, reduced to 9/20) (Hewer, 1969)

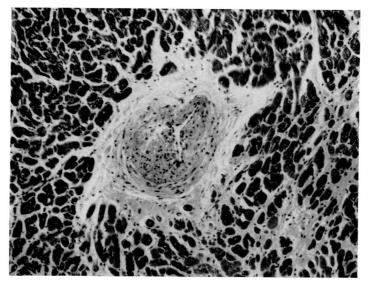

Figure 5.26. Single grossly-narrowed artery (haematoxylin and eosin × 96, reduced to 9/10) (Hewer, 1969)

nuclei, which are often square-ended and contain much darkly-staining material (*Figure 5.18*). Extensive fatty infiltration of the myocardium is uncommon but is sometimes seen (*Figure 5.19*).

In some parts of the myocardium there may be a severe degree of interstitial fibrosis, thin strands of fibrous tissue being seen between most of the muscle fibres (*Figure 5.20*), and in some cases it seems that the myocardial cells have disappeared and been replaced by fibrous tissue. In some areas these have united to form small scars.

Perivascular fibrosis is seen around some of the smaller blood vessels but much of this is not severe. In some parts of the myocardium small foci of muscle necrosis may be seen, usually alone and surrounded by lymphocytes (*Figure 5.21*), and they are usually not an important part of the histological picture. Numerous foci of active muscle necrosis together with numerous inflammatory cells may be present (*Figure 5.22*). The foci consist of disintegrating muscle fibres surrounded by collections of inflammatory cells which are mainly lymphocytes but may include a few polymorphs, mast cells and monocytes.

ARTERIAL CHANGES

All the main branches of the coronary arteries are normal although the internal elastic laminar frequently shows reduplication. The great majority of the small cardiac arteries are normal (*Figure 5.23*) but may be surrounded with small areas of perivascular fibrosis. In a few cases the lumen is narrowed—the decrease being due to hyperplasia of the medial musculature and not to endothelial proliferation (*Figure 5.24*). The narrowing is largely due to severe fibrosis and not so much to endothelial proliferation (*Figure 5.25*). In some vessels the endothepial proliferation has progressed to such a degree that the lumen is almost, or sometimes completely, obliterated (*Figure 5.26*).

Active foci of myocardial necrosis are sometimes seen in these cases, and this indicates that this disease process goes on for many years. It is not possible to say if the process ever completely 'burns itself out'.

Comparatively few of the small cardiac arteries are diseased (Hewer, 1969) and it seems certain that the cardiac lesions seen in the arteries are non-specific, and are a reaction to atrophy and involution of the surrounding cardiac muscle (Ivemark and Thorén, 1964).

References

Friedreich, N. (1863). 'Über degenerative Atrophie der spinalen Hinter-stränge.' *Virchows Arch. path. Anat. Physiol.* **26**, 391, 433

Hewer, R. L. (1969). 'The heart in Friedreich's ataxia.' *Br. Heart J.* **31**, 5

Hewer, R. L. (1973). To be published.

Ivemark, B. and Thorén, C. (1964). 'The pathology of the heart in Friedreich's ataxia. Changes in coronary arteries and myocardium.' *Acta med. scand.* **175**, 227

Thorén, C. (1964). 'Cardiomyopathy in Friedreich's ataxia. With studies of cardiovascular and respiratory function.' *Acta paediat., Stockh.* **53**, Suppl. 153

Six

Peri-partal cardiomyopathy

For more than a century (Ritchie, 1849a, b, 1850), physicians have been aware of a clinical syndrome of post-partal, non-valvular myocardial disease of unknown origin. Sporadically cases have been reported (Blacker, 1907; Campbell, 1923) and various aetiological theories have been proposed but the relative rarity of this disease and inconsistent, incomplete descriptions have rendered it difficult to understand. Hull and Hidden (1937) and Hull and Hafkesbring (1938) were the first to suggest its existence as a clinical entity and to stress the possible importance of 'peri-partal factors' in its aetiology. Not the least of the problems is the lack of a universally-accepted definition of the syndrome (Walsh and Burch, 1967). It is little wonder that its very existence is disputed (Bashour and Winchell, 1954; Benchimol, Carneiro and Schlesinger, 1959).

To make a diagnosis of this disease, attention must be paid to the following criteria which should be fulfilled.

(1)   The absence of a history of symptoms or physical signs of heart disease in the patient prior to the puerperium.

(2)   The appearance of signs and symptoms of heart disease between weeks 1 and 20 of the puerperium.

(3)   An inability to establish an aetiological basis for the heart disease from any other known cause.

The first week of the puerperium is purposely disregarded in order to eliminate patients who develop mild heart failure during delivery, and who may not be regarded as such until several days after delivery has taken place, in addition to those patients with possible pre-existing cardiac diseases which only become noticeable during pregnancy or after delivery.

RACIAL INCIDENCE

Although cases of this disease have been reported in Caucasian women (Hughes *et al.*, 1970) from England, France (Michon, Larcon and Renaud, 1959), Canada (MacKinnon and McKeen, 1949) and elsewhere, the majority of patients to be so affected are Negroes who come from many widely-separated places such as New Orleans (Walsh *et al.*, 1965), South Africa (Seftel and Susser, 1961) and Jamaica (Stuart, 1968). This disease has also been reported in Chinese (Chang, 1952) and Arabian women (Perrine, 1967).

AGE

This syndrome appears at an earlier age in female patients than does idiopathic myocardial disease in the male. The majority of these patients are housewives, but many have been working for brief periods as domestic servants.

CLINICAL HISTORY

About half of the patients reported the presence of a history of heart disease, which was most commonly either hypertensive or arteriosclerotic heart disease in one or both parents. The high incidence of familial heart disease in such relatively young patients raises the possibility of an hereditary susceptibility to cardiovascular disease. Some patients recall an uncomplicated respiratory infection prior to the onset of the congestive heart failure.

Although the possibility must be considered that this cardio-myopathy is of infectious origin, these findings are of only doubtful significance.

The majority of the patients who present with peri-partal cardio-myopathy come from a socio-economic group which, characteristic-ally, suffers from inadequate nutrition. Few patients give a history of adequate nutrition for any extended period of time: in the majority of cases, adequate nutrition occurs during brief periods of relative affluence only. As a rule the diet consists largely of carbohydrates, usually in the form of maize meal, while meat is only very rarely consumed and fish, eggs and milk are, for practical purposes, never eaten. This dietary history is not, however, found in all cases.

OBSTETRIC HISTORY

The majority of the patients described fall into the grand multipara class (i.e., they have had five or more pregnancies) although this disease may occur in women who have had only one or two preg-nancies. The majority of these patients also give a history of 'toxaemia' and 'pre-eclampsia' in the proceeding pregnancy, but it is not known what is actually described by these terms, and therefore this history is of little value.

Brown *et al.* (1967) also describes fifteen cases of heart failure manifesting in the last trimester of pregnancy or in the puerperium. The authors did not consider post-partum cardiomyopathy to be an entity, however, and only one of these fifteen cases qualified for such a title (although necropsy confirmation was not obtained).

CLINICAL PRESENTATION

Orthopnoea, paroxysmal nocturnal dyspnoea, oedema and cough are all experienced by practically all these patients during the evolution of their illnesses. Invariably the initial appearance of left heart failure is followed at various intervals by symptoms of right heart failure. The majority of the patients also complain of chest pain or haemoptysis and this is shown later, by clinical or autopsy evidence, to have been due to a pulmonary embolism. Sometimes, however, there may be central chest pain without any evidence of thrombo-emboli. Less frequently, but not uncommonly, some of these patients present with clinical evidence of cerebral infarction or obstruction of a major limb artery, or vessel supplying an abdominal viscus, and are proved at autopsy to have been embolic in origin. Prolonged bed rest does not seem to predispose these patients to thrombo-embolic phenomenon.

An interesting factor is the high incidence of colicky, severe, persistent abdominal pain. With the return of cardiac compensation and decrease in hepatomegaly these symptoms generally subside, although they tend to persist to a mild degree for many months without demonstrable heart failure or intrinsic gastro-intestinal changes. The frequency of palpitations and cough are greater than those normally seen in congestive heart failure.

LABORATORY INVESTIGATIONS

HAEMATOLOGY

Patients are found in all the normal blood groups. Some patients have abnormal haemaglobins, such as AC or AS haemaglobins, but taking into account the fact that abnormal haemaglobins are apparently more common in Negro populations, these findings seem to be of no significance. All have total and differential white cell counts within normal limits, but may often have a normochromic microcytic anaemia. The erythrocyte sedimentation rate is normal in most of the cases but, in a few, it is raised for no apparent reason or because of the presence of some underlying but unassociated disease. No other haematological tests reveal changes of any significance.

SERUM PROTEINS

These are within normal limits in the majority of cases seen but the albumin-globulin ratio may be reduced to 1 in a few cases. With bed rest the levels of serum albumin and total protein eventually increase to normal values. Re-examinations after several years of apparent good health may show a slight increase in serum albumin levels.

RENAL FUNCTION

There is initially a trace to one plus of protein in about half the patients, many of whom are in congestive heart failure. Some of these patients with abnormally low renal concentrating ability fail to exhibit decrease in heart size after treatment and about half of these eventually die of congestive heart failure.

ELECTROCARDIOGRAPHY

All these patients have electrocardiogram changes consistent with left ventricular hypertrophy. Rhythm disturbances are transitory and usually limited to premature ventricular contractions.

COMPLICATIONS

Thrombo-embolism

The most frequently encountered complication in this disease is pulmonary thrombo-embolism. About one-third of the emboli arise from thrombo-embolism in the lower limbs but the majority of the emboli found arise initially in the heart.

Associated cerebral emboli and infarctions are seen less often but are still fairly frequent.

Bronchopneumonia

Bronchopneumonia is commonly found as the termination of intractable heart failure in many of these patients.

NATURAL COURSE OF THE DISEASE

The typical patient with post-partum heart disease is a young multiparous Negress with long-standing marginal or inadequate nutrition and a high probability of having had a history of 'toxaemia' related to her previous pregnancy, following which heart disease had appeared between weeks 1 and 20 after delivery. After 1–2 weeks the patient, who by now has developed symptoms and signs of right-sided ventricular heart failure, seeks medical advice. The initial response to treatment is good and rather prompt with the exception of a persisting cardiomegaly. A sizeable minority of these patients have thrombo-embolic episodes. Symptomatic response to treatment is so good that the patient usually insists on leaving hospital and returning to work.

Congestive heart failure may soon occur again when the patient has a further pregnancy and, almost certainly, will follow a full-term delivery. Intermittent pyelonephritis, discontinuation of digitalis and possibly resumption of poor dietary habits and undue physical exertion may cause another relapse.

The subsequent course is characterized by frequent exacerbations requiring hospital treatment and may be associated with thrombo-embolic episodes.

Cardiomegaly persists and eventually increases. The possibility of sudden cardiac death is extremely likely.

Further Pregnancies

About half of the patients with post-partum cardiomyopathy develop congestive heart failure in their next and subsequent pregnancies.

Post-mortem Findings

The lesions found at autopsy, apart from coincidental diseases, are limited either directly or indirectly to the cardiovascular system.

GROSS FINDINGS IN THE HEART

The heart is usually pale and flabby and the weight most commonly varies between 400 and 600 g, usually about 525 g, so that the heart is normally considerably enlarged.

A small pericardial effusion of clear straw-coloured fluid, or small fibrinous adhesion is often present. The coronary arteries are always dilatated and free from atheromatous changes, except occasionally, from minor scattered lesions. Maximal left ventricular wall thickness varies from 0·5–2·5 cm, the median width usually being between 1 and 1·5 cm.

The valves appear normal, their size being within the upper limit of normal. In most hearts the endocardium is normal but in some other cases there are numerous grey-white scattered patches of endocardial thickening which are most commonly seen in the left ventricle, but also, although to a much lesser extent, in the right ventricular wall when there are plaques in the left ventricle.

The plaques usually involve both the free and septal walls of the ventricles and are prominent at the apices, 2–3 mm in thickness, and do not involve the myocardium. Patches may vary from 0·5–4 cm in diameter and are usually associated with minimal thickening of the chordae tendineae, apparently by the same process.

The large plaques may contain areas of calcification which are often extensive and mural thrombi may be found to be present overlying the thickened endocardial patches in the ventricles. The lungs may be subjected to recurrent embolization and when these emboli are not large, the patient develops pulmonary heart disease due to the emboli becoming incorporated into the walls of the small pulmonary arteries and arterioles.

MICROSCOPIC FINDINGS

Myocardium

Microscopically the principal feature is degeneration of myocardial fibres.

(1) Interstitial oedema and scattered areas of interstitial infiltration with inflammatory cells are found in the myocardium of all the hearts. This cellular infiltrate consists mainly of lymphocytes, but histiocytes and plasma cells are sometimes seen. The inflammatory cells, chiefly lymphocytes, are usually scattered diffusely throughout areas where there are necrotic muscle fibres (*Figure 6.1*). Small discrete foci of lymphocytes are only rarely seen. Dispersed throughout the myocardium are often areas of acellular fibrosis (*Figure 6.2*). Many fibres are atrophic with loss of the normal staining properties of the cytoplasm and, often with hyperchromatic or abnormally-shaped nuclei (*Figure 6.3*). Some other cells may have lost their cross striations or nuclei and degeneration of myocardial fibres may have occurred (*Figure 6.4*). There is much variation in muscle fibre size in different parts of the myocardium. These fibres may be oedematous and sometimes undergoing hyaline degeneration (*Figure 6.5*).

(2) The amount of lipofuscin present is within the normal limits accepted for the age of these patients.

(3) No increase in mast cells can be demonstrated by the cresyl violet stain and no areas of metachromasia are present.

(4) No accumulations of amyloid or other PAS-positive material can be seen in the myocardial fibres—as has been reported by Evans (1949) in familial cardiomyopathies.

(5) Sometimes small vacuoles of fat are seen within the sarcoplasm of degenerating myocardial fibres (*Figure 6.6*). These small

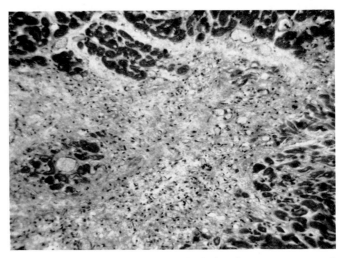

Figure 6.1.   The inflammatory cells, chiefly lymphocytes, are scattered among remnants of degenerating myocardial fibres (haematoxylin and eosin × 180, to 2/3) (Johnson et al., 1968)

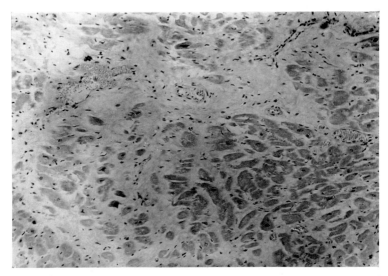

Figure 6.2.   Dispersed throughout the myocardium are often cellular areas of fibrosis (haematoxylin and eosin × 120, reduced to 2/3)

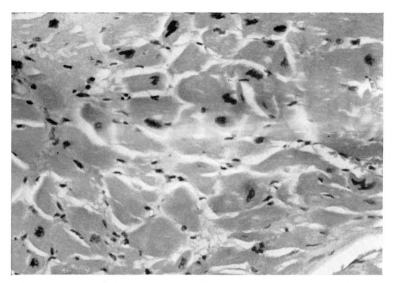

Figure 6.3. Puerperal cardiomyopathy showing many abnormally-shaped nuclei, some of which show perinuclear vacuolation while in other areas myocardial cells have become completely replaced by pale staining areas of necrotic tissue. There is also a generalized infiltrate with small round cells (haematoxylin and eosin × 625, reduced to 2/3). (Reproduced by courtesy of Dr Hughes)

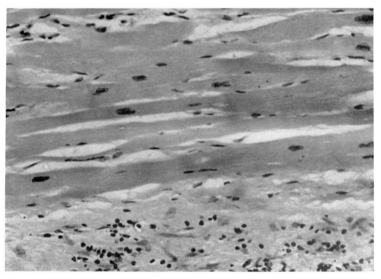

Figure 6.4. Myocardium showing numerous myocardial cells which have lost their usual striated appearance. Some of the nuclei are abnormally shaped. In some, even the myocardium has been replaced by fibrous tissues and contains many small lymphocytes (haematoxylin and eosin × 625, reduced to 2/3). (Reproduced by courtesy of Dr Hughes)

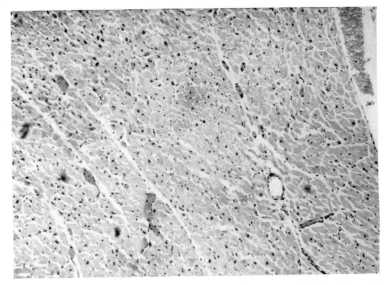

Figure 6.5. Peri-partal cardiomyopathy showing variation in both nuclear cell size and intensity of staining. Also note variation in intensity of staining of the myocardial cells, the dilated blood vessels and the diffuse infiltration with chronic inflammatory cells—lymphocytes (haematoxylin and eosin × 80, reduced to 2/3). (Reproduced by courtesy of Dr Hughes)

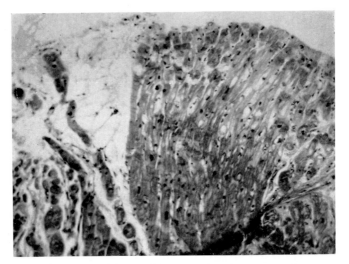

Figure 6.6. Surgical biopsy of heart revealing degeneration of myocardial fibres within the sarcoplasm and pyknosis of many of the nuclei (haematoxylin and eosin × 240, reduced to 2/3). (Johnson et al., 1968)

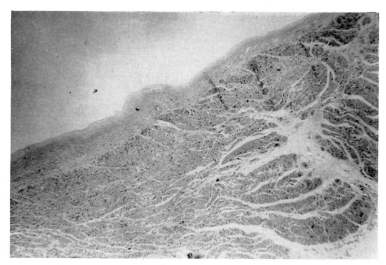

Figure 6.7. The endocardium may be slightly thickened (haematoxylin and eosin × 125, reduced to 2/3). (Reproduced by courtesy of Dr Hughes)

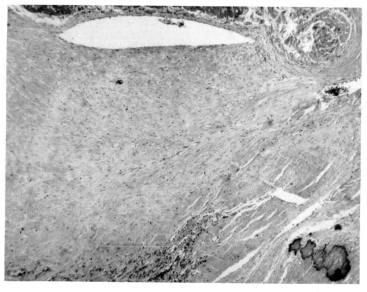

Figure 6.8. Section through attached mural thrombus. A papillary muscle is enmeshed in the thrombus at the upper right. Focal calcification is seen at lower right (haematoxylin and eosin × 60, reduced to 2/3). (Reproduced by courtesy of Dr Hughes)

lipid deposits, due to their size are best stained by benzopyrene and demonstrated fluorescently by ultraviolet light.

These changes can be interpreted as evidence of mitochondrial damage with resultant impairment of oxidation of lipids which, therefore, accumulate.

The lipid in the droplets has been identified as triglycerides (Walsh *et al.*, 1965). Occasional lipid-laden macrophages are also seen in these areas.

(6)   Plasmal reactions are localized to the mitochondria between myofibrils and at the poles of nuclei, in interfibrilliary spaces and intercalary discs. Fat droplets, myofibrils and lipofuscin granules are negative for these substances while areas of fatty change in the myocardium show a moderate to marked decrease in the intensity of their plasmal reactions.

(7)   Succinic dehydrogenase and cytochrone oxidase reactions are localized to the mitochondria of muscle fibres. A faint reaction can sometimes be observed in some inflammatory cells. The sharpness of localization of these enzyme changes is very variable due to post-mortem changes, which affect the mitochondria rapidly so that only limited credence may be drawn from these findings. In general, intensity of reaction is somewhat decreased when compared with the findings in a normal heart in similar post-mortem autopsies. There are spotty zones of varying degrees of lessened activity within some fibres while others are almost completely negative.

In this respect, the succinic dehydrogenase reaction seems to be a more sensitive indicator of cell damage than the reaction used to demonstrate cytochrome oxidase.

Endocardium

The endocardium may be found to be slightly thickened (*Figure 6·7*) and if present the thickening is usually in the wall of the ventricle or at the apex. Small foci of fibrin may be present within the thickened endocardium.

In the thickened endocardium, the elastic tissue content is not increased. Sometimes the endocardial thickening is caused by the organization and incorporation of an overlying thrombus (*Figure 6.8*).

DISCUSSION

The clinical presentation of this disease may vary from a symptom-less cardiac enlargement, without, or with little evidence of, cardiac failure to a rapidly fatal illness. The clinical features noted in many reports have usually been of the latter type and the selection of these cases may, therefore, account for the uniformity of descriptions of this condition. That the histological changes found in this disease are essentially similar, when cases reported from different centres are compared, has been clearly illustrated by Meadows (1960) (*Figure 6.9*).

The myocardial changes discussed in this disease are in contrast to the findings in the hearts of patients with alcoholic cardiomyopathy, which show many minute fat droplets widely distributed throughout the myocardium, along with more marked focal areas of fatty metamorphosis.

It is important to remember that the aetiology of this disease is frequently not associated with pregnancy, because of the long period that may divide the illness from a previous pregnancy. It is, therefore, very difficult to assess the true incidence of this disease, but it is probably much higher than is at present thought. When examining the heart of a patient who is thought to be suffering from peri-partal cardiomyopathy, the lesions of some other cardiac disease may be found, as in the case described by Hudson (1970) where the underlying disease was, very probably, rhabdomyomatosis and not peri-partal cardiomyopathy as he stated.

It is, therefore, important to take account of the possible association of pregnancy, especially when repeated in rapid succession, with cardiac disease. Pregnancy, however, may only unmask and precipitate a cardiac disease already present. On statistical grounds this is likely to occur from time to time, especially in those tropical areas, such as South Africa or the West Indies, where primary myocardial diseases are common.

However, this observation does not explain one of the most striking features of the peri-partal cardiomyopathies—their common occurrences weeks or even months after delivery, where the haemodynamic stresses of pregnancy have passed.

If pregnancy were a non-specific precipitant of this disease one would expect to see cases of unexplained cardiomegaly and congestive cardiac failure developing in men of the same age range, who had been exposed to heavy manual labour or similar environmental stresses.

It can, therefore, be concluded that pregnancy plays a more precise role in the development of cardiac disease, rather than merely a non-specific precipitant for cardiac enlargement and failure.

It is thought that pregnancies, particularly when occurring in rapid succession, have an adverse effect on myocardial function, probably by impairing myocardial metabolism, and that this effect is maximal in the post-partal period.

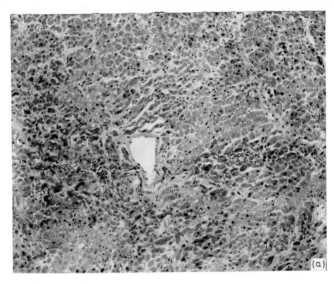

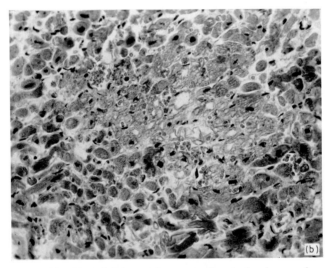

Figure 6.9.   Foci of disintegrating myocardium in the absence of an inflammatory reaction and progressing to fibrosis as noted in the myocardium in cases of peri-partal cardiomyopathy (haematoxylin and eosin) (a) and (b), original magnification × 120, reduced to 3/4. (b) and (c), original magnification × 300, reduced to 3/4. (Reproduced by courtesy of Dr Meadows)

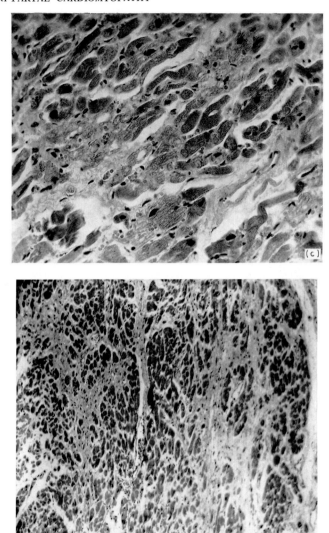

For caption see facing page

The aetiology of this disease is unknown, although it has recently been suggested that it may be viral in origin. This view is largely based on the fact that the post-partal state may, in some patients, be favourable for the initiation of viral disease.

At least four patients with post-partal heart disease, secondary to Coxsackie virus infection, have been described (Sainani, Krompotic and Slodki, 1968). The concept that the pregnant and post-partal states may be more conducive to the development of viral heart disease is supported by the observation that pregnant mice are more susceptible to the encephalomyocarditis virus than non-pregnant mice (Farber and Glasgow, 1970).

This view is, however, extremely speculative and it is difficult to see how it could be proved.

References

Bashour, F. and Winchell, P. (1954). ' "Post-Partal" heart disease—a syndrome?' *Ann. intern. Med.* **40**, 803

Becker, F. F. and Taube, H. (1962). 'Myocarditis of obscure etiology associated with pregnancy.' *New Engl. J. Med.* **266**, 62

Benchimol, A. B., Carneiro, R. D. and Schlesinger, P. (1959). 'Post-partum heart disease.' *Br. Heart J.* **21**, 89

Blacker, G. F. (1907). 'A clinical lecture on heart disease in relation to pregnancy and labour.' *Br. Med. J.* **1**, 1225

Brown, A. K., Doukas, N., Riding, W. D. and Jones, E. W. (1967). 'Cardiomyopathy and pregnancy.' *Br. Heart J.* **29**, 387

Campbell, D. G. (1923). 'Pregnancy and heart disease.' *Can. med. Ass. J.* **13**, 244

Chang, Y. H. (1952). 'Post-partal heart disease: Report of a case.' *Chin. med. J.* **70**, 227

Evans, W. (1949). 'Familial cardiomegaly.' *Br. Heart J.* **11**, 68

Farber, P. A. and Glasgow, L. A. (1970). 'Viral myocarditis during pregnancy; encephalomyocarditis virus infection in mice.' *Am. Heart J.* **80**, 96

Hudson, R. E. B. (1970). 'Cardiomyopathy in late pregnancy and the puerperium.' In *Cardiovascular Pathology*, Vol. 3, p. 536. London: Edward Arnold

Hughes, R A. C., Kapur, P., Sutton, G. C. and Honey, M. (1970). 'A case of fatal peri-partum cardiomyopathy.' *Br. Heart J.* **32**, 272

Hull, E. and Hafkesbring, E. (1937). ' "Toxic" post-partal heart disease.' *New Orl. med. surg. J.* **89**, 550

— and Hidden, E. (1938). 'Post-partal heart failure.' *Sth med. J.* **31**, 265

Johnson, J. B., Hussain, G., Flores, P. and Mann, M. (1968). 'Idiopathic heart disease associated with pregnancy and the puerperium.' *Am. Heart J.* **72**, 809

MacKinnon, H. H. and McKeen, R. A. H. (1949). 'Post-partum heart disease (case reports).' *Can. med. Ass. J.* **61**, 308

Meadows, W. R. (1960). 'Post-partum heart disease.' *Am. J. Cardiol.* **6**, 788

Michon, P., Larcan, A. and Renaud, J. (1959). 'Myocardie et état gravido puerpéral. Contribution à l'étude de la cardiopathie du post-partum de Meadows.' *Gynéc. Obstét.* **58**, 269

Perrine, R. P. (1967). 'An obscure myocardiopathy in post-partum Saudi Arabs.' *Trans. R. Soc. trop. Med. Hyg.* **61**, 834

Ritchie, C. (1849a). 'Clinical contributions to the pathology and treatment of certain chronic diseases of the heart.' *Edinburgh med. surg. J.* **1**, 7, 14, 21 and 29

— (1849b). 'Clinical contributions to the pathology and treatment of certain chronic diseases of the heart.' *Edinburgh med. surg. J.* **2**, 333

— (1850). 'Clinical contributions to the pathology and treatment of certain chronic diseases of the heart.' *Edinburgh med. Surg. J.* **2**, 2, 8, 29 and 256

Sainani, G. S., Krompotic, E. and Slodki, S. J. (1968). 'Adult heart disease due to the Coxsackie virus B infection.' *Medicine, Baltimore* **47**, 133

Seftel, H. and Susser, M. (1961). 'Maternity and myocardial failure in African women.' *Br. Heart J.* **23**, 43

Stuart, K. L. (1968). 'Cardiomyopathy of pregnancy and the puerperium.' *Q. Jl. Med.* **37**, 463

Walsh, J. J. and Burch, G. E. (1967). 'Post partal heart disease.' *Arch. intern. Med.* **108**, 817

— — Black, W. C., Ferrans, V. J. and Hibbs, R. G. (1965). 'Idiopathic myocardiopathy of the puerperium (postpartal heart disease).' *Circulation* **32**, 19

Part Two

Secondary Cardiomyopathies

Seven

Tropical cardiomyopathy

Endomyocardial fibrosis and cardiomegaly of unknown origin are two idiopathic cardiomyopathies commonly found in tropical and sub-tropical areas but normally affect only the indigenous inhabitants. However, there are also descriptions of endomyocardial fibrosis from temperate areas but usually in people who are either natives of the tropics, or who have lived there for many years.

Whether these are, in fact, two different diseases—a view held by the WHO study group on cardiomyopathies (WHO Bulletin, 1965)—or are both one disease presenting in different ways when modified by associated factors, a view held by other workers such as Thomson (1961) and McKinney (1970a) is still in dispute. It seems possible that the first description of these tropical cardiomyopathies was made by Gelfand (1944) when he described cases, of what he termed 'beriberi heart disease' which were resistant to thiamine. No autopsies, unfortunately, were done on these patients.

These diseases will, therefore, be described separately and only brought together when aetiology and classification are discussed.

ENDOMYOCARDIAL FIBROSIS

Endomyocardial fibrosis was first reported by Bedford and Konstam (1946) when describing cases of congestive heart failure occurring in West African (Nigerian) troops in the Middle East, towards the end of World War II. Probably this report also included cases of cardiomegaly of unknown origin and rheumatic heart disease.

Recognition of this disease as a distinct entity first came when Davies (1948) described the cardiac lesions, although when he first wrote about this disease, which he incorporated in an M.D. thesis to the University of Bristol, he used the term *endomyocardial necrosis* and not endomyocardial fibrosis as he later called it. Since this time, much of the work on this disease has come from Uganda from Davies and later from Connor *et al.* (1967, 1968).

TABLE 7.1
Distribution of Tropical Cardiomyopathies

Country	Year reported	No. of cases		
		Non-class	EMF	CUO
Australia	1965	–	1	–
Brazil	1962	–	–	5
North	1964	–	4	–
South	1963	–	3	–
Cameroun	1962	–	1	–
	1965	–	1	–
Central African Republic	1961	–	1	–
Central Pacific	1951	–	1	–
Ceylon	1956	–	1	–
	1959	–	3	–
Colombia	1963	28	–	–
Congo: Brazzaville	1964	–	1	–
	1964	–	1	–
	1966	–	1	–
Kinshasha	1962	–	1	–
	1966	–	1	–
	1967	–	1	–
Dominica	1964	1	–	1
England	1957	1	–	1
	1957	4	–	–
	1963	2	–	–
	1965	4	–	–
Gabon	1961	–	1	–
Gold Coast	1954	–	7	3
Hawaii	1957	–	1	–
India: Bombay	1970	–	3	–
Delhi	1965	–	2	–
South India	1960	–	3	–
	1964	–	1	–
	1965	–	1	–
Ivory Coast	1956	–	1	–
Jamaica	1963	–	–	29
	1967	–	–	8
	1971	–	–	16
Kenya	1960	–	3	–
Malaya	1957	–	2	–
	1957	–	2	–
Nigeria	1951	–	1	1
	1954	–	1	–
	1955	7	2	5
	1959	53	–	–
	1963	43	–	–
	1965	1	–	–
	1965	–	100	–
	1967	–	1	–
Rhodesia	1959	–	–	14
	1961	–	–	25
	1961	–	–	25
	1971	–	–	16
South Africa	1951	30	–	–

TABLE 7.1 (contd.)

Country	Year reported	No. of cases		
		Non-class	EMF	CUO
South Africa (*contd*).	1952	–	–	12
	1953	–	–	30
	1961	–	–	1
	1963	–	–	90
	1972	–	2	–
Sudan	1954	25	–	–
Tanzania	1960	–	1	–
	1969	–	16	–
Turkey	1960	1	–	–
Uganda	1948	–	36	–
	1954	–	20	–
	1955	–	32	–
	1964	–	48	78
	1967	–	15	12
United States of America	1936	–	2	–
	1941	5	–	–
	1952	1	1	–
	1952	1	–	–
	1953	–	2	–
	1953	2	–	–
	1955	–	1	–
	1962	–	1	–
West Africa	1946	40	–	–
	1946	–	1	–

DISTRIBUTION

Endomyocardial fibrosis has an extremely extensive distribution (Table 7.1) in tropical and sub-tropical areas. Although this disease was originally described in the Sudan (O'Brien, 1954) and Uganda (Davies and Ball, 1955), it has also been commonly found in Nigeria (Edington and Jackson, 1963); Kenya and Tanganyika [Tanzania] (Turner and Manson-Bahr, 1960); Ghana (McKinney, 1968); Brazil (Andrade and Guimãraes, 1964); the Congo [Brazzaville] (Peuchot, Latour and Puech, 1960), [Leopoldville] (Cochlo and Pymental, 1963) and other parts of tropical Africa; from Malaya (La Brooy, 1957); Ceylon (Nagaratnam and Dissanayake, 1959); and India (Reddy, Parvathi and Rao, 1970). Scattered reports of this condition in other parts of the world have come from such countries as Britain or the USA (Ishak and Tschumy, 1962), but they largely consist of cases occurring in migrants from the tropics, or of people who have spent a large part of their lives in these places. Some cases, however, do occur in temperate zones (Black and Fowler, 1965) probably much more frequently than is commonly thought.

Many case reports seem, however, to be based on incorrect interpretations of the cardiac pathology as, for example, the case of endomyocardial fibrosis reported by Ogan (1960) from Turkey and those cases reported from Australia (Brown and Burnell, 1965) and Japan (Yoshida *et al.*, 1964); in all of which the diagnosis seems actually to be that of endocardial fibro-elastosis.

RACIAL INCIDENCE

Endomyocardial fibrosis is most commonly found in the Negro races but cases have been reported in Europeans living in these areas (Brockington, Olsen and Goodwin, 1967), or in Europeans who have spent long periods of time in tropical Africa (Gray, 1951). Some others have spent shorter periods under prolonged conditions of dietary privation as, for example, in subjects who spent long periods of time as prisoners of war in the Far East or in concentration camps (Lynch and Watt, 1957) during the last war. The disease is found equally in both sexes.

AGE

This is principally a disease of young adults. Most of the cases occur in patients aged between 15 and 35, although all ages have been affected and cases have been reported in subjects varying from 4 to 74 years of age.

CLINICAL PRESENTATION

This disease usually presents as congestive heart failure but it less commonly presents as *constrictive pericarditis* or as thrombo-embolic episodes which are commonly pulmonary, due to an embolus which has arisen in the right atrium or ventricle.

On clinical examination the heart is usually of normal size but it sometimes may be increased in size, or much less commonly diminished. Very commonly there is a pericardial effusion which may be massive and, on tapping, is found to contain fluid under considerable pressure; but is in fact normally under no pressure and consists of clear yellow fluid and contains only a few cells and little protein or fibrin. A haemopericardium is only found when the paracentesis has been attempted and carried out incorrectly.

Signs of congestive heart failure may be well marked and the patient may complain of an enlarged tender liver, upper abdominal or thoracic pain or dyspnoea, or sometimes swelling of the feet, liver or limbs—due to dependent cardiac oedema.

Thrombo-embolism may involve any organ and occurs most usually to the limbs or lungs, although cerebral embolism is fairly frequently seen. Myocardial infarction, due to embolic obstruction of a coronary artery, may also sometimes occur.

The patients who develop this disease usually come from the lower socio-economic classes. In Uganda, for instance, the commonly-affected subjects are the Banyaruanda who are poorly-paid, itinerant labourers. This disease may, however, affect people who are well-off economically.

No specific diagnosis of endomyocardial fibrosis can be made from the electrocardiogram but low voltage QRS complexes and other non-specific changes are common (Williams and Somers, 1960).

These patients are often found to be anaemic, but this is thought to be due to their general state of malnutrition. The white cell count is normal both in number and distribution except for the fact that there may sometimes be an eosinophilia.

The ESR may be raised but this is due to anaemia or other associated diseases where plasma proteins are low and often the albumin/globulin ratio is reversed. Few enzyme studies have been carried out in this disease, and apart from cases where the patients have associated liver damage or very rarely a myocardial infarction, are non-specific.

PATHOLOGY

The pericardium is usually found to contain a small amount of clear yellow fluid which is usually not blood stained, nor under any increased pressure while the pericardium is not thickened.

The heart (*Figure 7.1*) itself is of variable size, although it is usually small. The most marked feature of the heart to be seen externally is the almost invariable gross atrial enlargement, due to ventricular back pressure because of cardiac failure; and, at the junction of the left and right ventricles an indentation (notch), due to the pulling apart of the two ventricles, because of their loss of elasticity and the shrinkage in size of the ventricles when they become lined with a thickened and fibrotic endocardium.

On opening the heart the endocardium lining, the auricles and the inflow tracts of both ventricles are seen to be massively thickened, especially the apical region of both the ventricles, which are very often entirely filled by plugs of thickened endocardium.

The ventricular cavities are very markedly decreased in size, while the atria are usually massively distended. The atrioventricular valves may be distorted by an extension of the fibrous process from the endocardium to the valve cusps and they may become adherent to the underlying ventricular wall. This change is most commonly seen in

the involvement of the posterior cusp of the mitral valve which may
be tightly bound down to the posterior ventricular wall.

The endocardium of the outflow tract is quite normal in appearance, there being a ridge about half way up the wall of the ventricle,

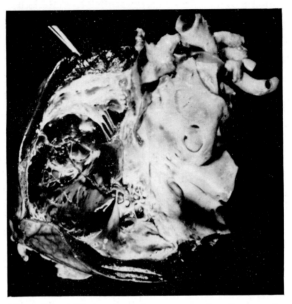

*Figure 7.1. This specimen demonstrates that the posterior
cusp of the mitral valve is tightly bound down to the ventricular
wall and also the endocardium of the outflow tract is normal.
(Reproduced from Connor et al. (1967) by courtesy of the
author and Editor of the* American Heart Journal)

where the thickened endocardium ends. The pulmonary and aortic
valves are also normal.

Ante-mortem thrombi are commonly seen to be present in one or
more of the cardiac cavities; these thrombi are most often found at or
towards the apices of one or both ventricles, and on the lateral aspects
of the ventricular walls or the septum. They are normally firm but
may fragment easily when touched.

When cut, the myocardium is found to be firm and often contains a
considerable amount of fibrous tissue which appears to have extended
in fine strands from the overlying endocardium.

The endocardium itself usually appears of normal thickness in the
outflow tracts of the ventricles but in other parts of the ventricles it is

thickened, often to a considerable degree, so that it may consist of a layer of fibrous tissue 1–2 cm or more in thickness. The endocardium lining the atria is not as thick as in the ventricles but, because of the much thinner muscular wall thickness, the thickness is proportionately much more marked. At the apex the amount of fibrous thickening of the endocardium may be very marked; the whole apex

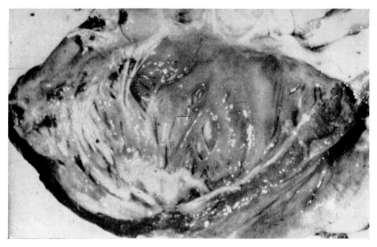

Figure 7.2. The heart has been opened to show that the fibrosis in the ventricles is limited to the apex and the ventricular inflow tract while the outflow tract is normal. Note that the posterior cusp of the mitral valve is firmly-bound down to the ventricular wall. (Reproduced by courtesy of Professor M. S. B. Hutt, Makerere University, Uganda)

being replaced by a plug of fibrous tissue which may extend completely or almost completely to the pericardium at this point.

In some places the thickened endocardium, particularly in the thickened parts of the endocardium adjacent to atrioventricular valves, may contain foci of calcification which may be up to 1–2 cm in diameter, or even larger. At the base of this thickened endocardium in the region where it meets the underlying myocardium, some small dilated blood vessels may be present but they can usually only be seen as small bleeding points against the uniform white background of the thickened endocardium, when the adjacent endocardium and myocardium are compressed.

The coronary arteries are usually normal and dilated and are not seriously affected by atherosclerosis or any other disease process. No obstruction in the lumina of these vessels can be found at any point.

The coronary sinus and other cardiac veins are normal in appearance.

Histologically the endocardium is seen to consist of a single layer of endothelial cells in the region of the outflow tracts of the ventricles.

In the other portions of the ventricles, the endocardium is usually markedly thickened and, with haematoxylin and eosin stains, is seen to consist of a thick layer of fibrous tissue (*Figure 7.2*).

Here the underlying muscle may have been reduced to a few cells in the centre of a column of fibrous tissue. Often thin strands of fibrous tissue which appear to have arisen *de novo*, perhaps from old thrombi, may be seen passing from one portion of the endocardial surface to another through the ventricular cavity. In some parts of the endocardium mural thrombi are to be found, and in some cases, these thrombi are undergoing re-organization and becoming incorporated in the underlying endocardium by strands of fibrous tissue passing from the overlying, organizing thrombus into the underlying myocardium (*Figure 7.3*). Some strands of fibrosis pass from the thickened endocardium into the myocardium. In some places the endocardium contains small foci of inflammatory cells. Towards the junction between the endocardium (*Figure 7.4*) and the myocardium there are often numerous small capillaries which are normal, except that they are congested and dilated, a few may have ruptured and be associated with small groups of inflammatory cells which are usually large lymphocytes.

In the underlying myocardium many of the cell nuclei are distorted in shape and pyknotic, especially in the myocardium immediately beneath the endocardium (*Figure 7.5*). Here, and in other parts of the myocardium, the cytoplasm may have become hyaline in appearance having lost its normal fibrillary appearance, while elsewhere only outlines of cell walls may remain, the nuclei and cytoplasm being lost. Whether this loss of cell contents has happened during life, or during the preparation of the specimen and is artefactual, is not known.

The myocardial cells are often hypertrophied although this conclusion may not be gained after a cursory inspection of some sections, while in others it appears that the cells are hypoplastic. The cells may also be abnormally shaped (*Figure 7.6*). Detailed comparative studies have shown that the cells are often enlarged (McKinney, 1972) but this is not always so.

There is a diffused infiltration in many areas of the myocardium, with foci of lymphocytes (*Figure 7.7*) and other chronic inflammatory cells, while a few eosinophils are often also present throughout the myocardium and endocardium.

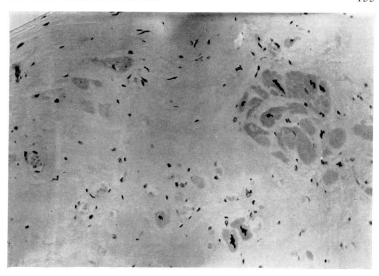

Figure 7.3. This illustration shows a gross thickening of the endocardium with, towards its base, a few small muscle cells, many of which contain abnormally-shaped nuclei (haematoxylin and eosin × 120, reduced to 2/3)

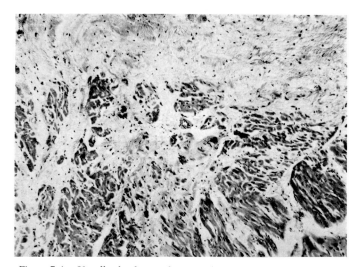

Figure 7.4. Usually the division between the thickened endocardium and the underlying myocardium is clearly marked but sometimes, as shown here, strands of fibrous tissue may pass into the underlying myocardium (haematoxylin and eosin × 90, reduced to 2/3)

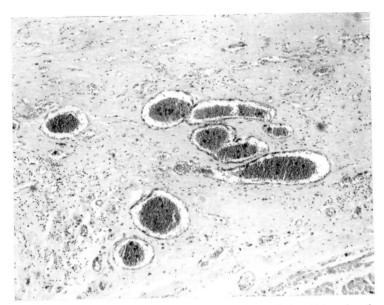

Figure 7.5. Small dilated blood vessels at the base of the thickened endo-myocardium associated with a diffuse infiltration with chronic inflammatory cells—lymphocytes (haematoxylin and eosin × 200, reduced to 2/3)

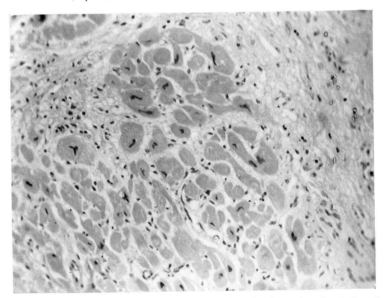

Figure 7.6. Myocardium showing myocardial cells with pyknotic 'staghorn'-shaped nuclei surrounded by fibrous tissue and lymphocytes (haematoxylin and eosin × 200, reduced to 2/3)

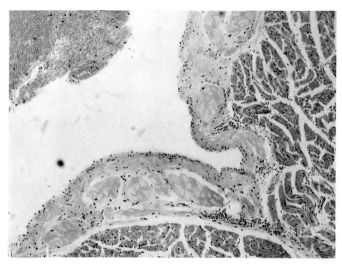

Figure 7.7. This photograph shows small foci of inflammatory cells (lymphocytes) in thickened endocardium and myocardium (haematoxylin and eosin × 200, reduced to 6/10)

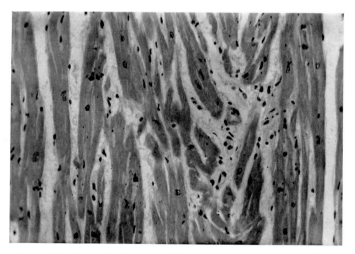

Figure 7.8. A small intramyocardial arteriole is seen surrounded by a small zone of perivascular fibrous tissue in which are a small number of chronic inflammatory cells—lymphocytes (haematoxylin and eosin × 260, reduced to 6/10)

The small intracardiac arteries and arterioles are usually normal, and in most places are surrounded by small zones of peri-vascular fibrosis (*Figure 7.8*) containing small collections of lymphocytes. All parts of the myocardium usually show signs of chronic venous congestion. As a long-standing pericardial effusion is usually present in these cases, the myocardium immediately adjacent to the pericardium may show a considerable lymphocytic infiltrate.

The pericardium itself may show an increase in thickness, perhaps two or three layers of cells instead of one, but usually it is normal as is any pericardial adipose tissue which may be present in the sections examined, except that the small blood vessels contained in it may be congested and dilated. A few may have ruptured and, in many places, the cells are separated by small pools of oedema fluid.

Any coronary arteries found in the section will be dilated but otherwise normal except, perhaps, for minimal atherosclerotic changes.

Similar histological changes are usually seen in the atria but the endocardial thickness is usually much less than in the ventricles. The number of strands of fibrous tissue passing into the underlying myocardial cells is, however, greater and, in places, the myocardium is practically replaced by areas of fibrosis. There is usually some slight infiltration with lymphocytes and a few eosinophils are also present in the myocardium, and a few foci of lymphocytes are seen in the endocardium. No foci of calcification are usually seen in the atria or auricular endocardium.

A thin layer of fibrin is commonly found overlying most of the endocardium (*Figure 7.9*). The layer is very thin but in the ventricles may have become appreciably thicker (*Figure 7.10*).

Foci of fibrin, some fairly large, are often found in the thickened endocardium, sometimes considerably below the endocardial surface and often adjacent to the zone of dilated blood vessels found immediately above the myocardium. In other parts of the thickened endocardium no fibrin is present or is found in the form of many small particles perhaps 3–5 μm in diameter, and usually surrounded by areas of fibrous tissue. Apart from some of the fibrin which is present on the endocardial surface, and is shown to be red in colour by Lendrum's picro-mallory stain or by using the Martius' scarlet blue technique, much of the fibrin deposits are blue and therefore have been present in the endocardium for a considerable time. Probably the large deposits have not yet undergone organization, although in some cases this appears to be happening.

Elastic tissue stains show that, usually, the thickened endocardium does not contain any elastic tissue except for a thin layer at the base of the thickened endocardium, and this appears to be part of the elastic

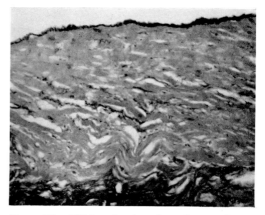

Figure 7.9. Thickened endocardium showing absence of elastic tissue fibres (*Verhoeff and van Gieson* × 240, reduced to 6/10)

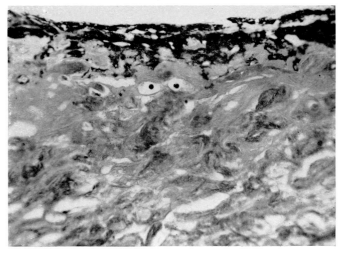

Figure 7.10. This shows a thick layer of fibrin covering the outer surface of the thickened endocardium (*Martius' scarlet blue* × 275, reduced to 6/10)

tissue layer of the original endocardium (*Figure 7.11*). In some places, particularly near the atrioventricular valve, the thickened endocardium may contain a considerable number of elastic tissue fibres which may consist of long, straight and unfragmented strands (*Figure 7.12*); in other parts of the thickened endocardium where elastic tissue

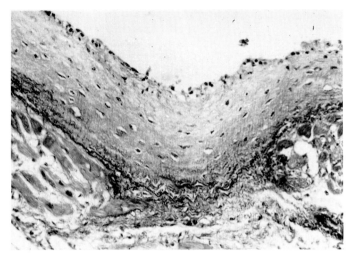

Figure 7.11.   This shows an area of thickened endocardium which contains no elastic tissues except for the normal basement layer (Verhoeff and van Gieson × 50, reduced to 6/10)

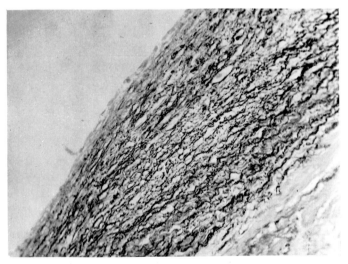

Figure 7.12.   This section shows that the thickened endocardium sometimes contains many elastic tissue fibres (Orcein and van Gieson × 180, reduced to 6/10)

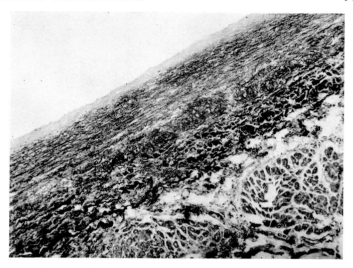

Figure 7.13. In this section the thickened endocardium is seen to contain much elastic tissue except for a thin zone at its outer edge (Orcein × 80, reduced to 6/10)

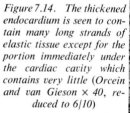

Figure 7.14. The thickened endocardium is seen to contain many long strands of elastic tissue except for the portion immediately under the cardiac cavity which contains very little (Orcein and van Gieson × 40, reduced to 6/10)

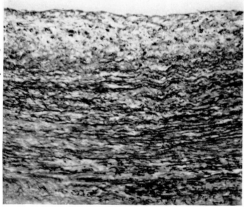

fibres are present they are usually thin, disorganized and fragmented into many small pieces. A few of these elastic tissue fibres may pass together with the fibrotic tissue into the underlying myocardium, but not to any great extent. No deposits of fibrin can be seen in the myocardium. Sometimes the more superficial part of the endocardium contains no elastic tissue (*Figure 7.13*), or the elastic tissue present in the more superficial parts of the thickened endocardium consists only of scanty fragments (*Figure 7.14*).

The alcian blue stain usually shows a great deal of acid mucopolysaccharides on the surface of the endocardium and also within it, but acid mucopolysaccharides are also seen to be present in the fibrous tissue and the interstitial spaces between myocardial cells.

CARDIOMEGALY OF UNKNOWN ORIGIN

The heart disease 'cardiomegaly of unknown origin'—having been given this name by the WHO Study Group on cardiomyopathies—was first described in South Africa by Becker, Chetgidakis and Van Lingen (1953) under the name 'cardiovascular collagenosis'; and by Gillanders (1951) with the name 'nutritional heart disease', although these workers now recognize that they were describing the same disease process. The disease has also been reported from Nigeria (Edington and Jackson, 1963) under the name of heart muscle disease; Jamaica (Stuart and Hayes, 1963; Hill, Still and McKinney, 1967); Brazil (Guimãraes and Andrade, 1956); Uganda (Hutt, 1970); Rhodesia (McKinney and Ashworth, 1973); Ceylon (Nagaratnam and Dissanayake, 1959); India (Gopi, 1968; Reddy, Parvathi and Rao, 1970); while isolated cases usually among immigrant people from areas where the disease normally occurs are now commonly being seen in hospitals in England (McKinney, 1970b), or reported as a chance finding at autopsy (Davies and Hollman, 1965).

CLINICAL PRESENTATION

This form of heart disease commonly presents as congestive heart failure, as in the case of endomyocardial fibrosis—the patient usually saying that he has been well until shortly before coming to hospital, although he may have complained, for some time previously, of dyspnoea, palpitations or liver tenderness.

These patients very commonly present with an arrhythmia, which is most commonly auricular fibrillation, an infarction, usually to the lung, liver or limb, which has been due to a thrombus, or with congestive heart failure. Although, as in the case of endomyocardial fibrosis, patients of all ages may be affected from young children (Seftel and Susser, 1961) to old people, the characteristic age group to be affected is that of early middle-aged adults characteristically 35–45 years of age. These patients are not usually found only in the very poor or indigenous classes, although they are usually Africans or people who eat or have eaten African diets for long periods.

On clinical examination, the heart is found to be grossly enlarged and when the patient presents with congestive heart failure, there is usually an associated pericardial infusion, which is sometimes of considerable size but which, on aspiration, is usually found to contain clear yellow fluid with few white and no red blood cells.

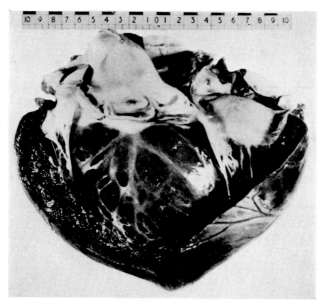

Figure 7.15. This is the heart of a 30 year old African male. Note thickening of the aortic valve cusps and only slight thickening of the ventricular endocardium, although some of the papillary muscles are largely replaced by fibrous tissue and a few patches of endocardial thickening are present in the ventricles. (Reproduced by courtesy of Dr T. G. Ashworth)

The electrocardiogram is usually of low voltage, the QRS complexes may be diminished in size and there may be ectopic beats, flutter or fibrillation or heart block, but no diagnostic changes can be found.

Examination of the blood reveals little of importance except perhaps an eosinophilia. The aorta and its branches may show marked atherosclerosis but the coronary arteries, sinuses and cardiac veins are all normal.

Macroscopically, the heart is found to be greatly enlarged, the ventricular walls in particular. When opened the endocardium is not usually found to be greatly thickened, although some parts of the endocardium may show white patches, where the endocardial thickening is slightly increased (*Figure 7.15*).

Microscopically, the endocardium appears to be only very slightly thickened over most parts of the atria and ventricles (*Figure 7.16*), but is often much more thickened in the region of the ventricular apices and around the atrioventricular valves. The endocardial thickening is usually also seen to be more marked over papillary muscles but, in most places, is seen to be only a few cells thick. Strands of fibrous tissue do not usually pass down from the endocardium into the underlying myocardium, in those areas where the endocardial thickening is only very slight, but usually do so where the endocardial thickening is greater (as in the region of the apices of the ventricles). In the region of the atrioventricular valves and in the atria where the endocardial thickening is, proportionately, much more marked and the underlying myocardium often appears to have been replaced, or almost completely replaced, by strands of fibrous tissue passing down from the overlying endocardium. The myocardium, in many places, has many abnormally-shaped, distorted and pyknotic nuclei, which are most easily seen in the myocardial cells immediately below the endocardium but are found in all parts of the myocardium (*Figure 7.17*). The cytoplasm of many of the myocardial cells has lost its normal striations and appears to have undergone a hyaline change, while other cells show evidence of cloudy swelling only. Some of the cells also contain small vacuoles in their cytoplasm but these vacuoles cannot be made to take up any stain and, therefore, what their contents are cannot be known. In other parts of the myocardium only myocardial cell walls remain, the cytoplasm and nuclei apparently appearing to have fallen out. This finding is not as commonly seen as in endomyocardial fibrosis. Many workers have said that the myocardial cells in cardiomegaly of unknown origin show evidence of hypertrophy and some workers in fact make it a diagnostic point when distinguising histologically cardiomegaly of unknown origin from endomyocardial fibrosis. Studies of the diameter of muscle fibres seen in cardiomegaly of unknown origin (Reid, 1966; McKinney, 1973) show that they are not hypertrophied, at least in their transverse diameter, although they may be elongated when compared with normal myocardial cells.

The fibrous tissue, when it extends into the underlying myocardium from the endocardium, may in some areas completely surround either small groups of myocardial cells or separate myo-

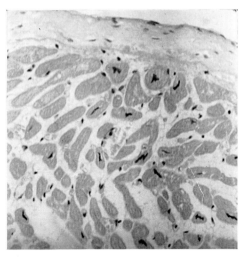

Figure 7.16. The endocardium is only slightly thickened. The underlying myocardial cells show considerable variation in size while many of their nuclei are pyknotic and distorted in shape— 'staghorn' (haematoxylin and eosin × 295, reduced to 6/10)

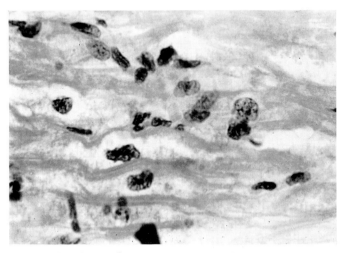

Figure 7.17. Myocardium containing many abnormally shaped and distorted nuclei (haematoxylin and eosin × 200, reduced to 6/10)

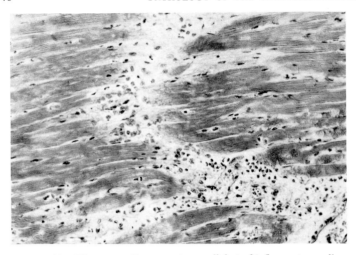

Figure 7.18.   The myocardium contains small foci of inflammatory cells—largely lymphocytes but a few plasma cells and eosinophils are present. Some parts of the muscle fibres have lost their striations and, in some, perinuclear vacuolation can be seen (haematoxylin and eosin × 60, reduced to 6/10)

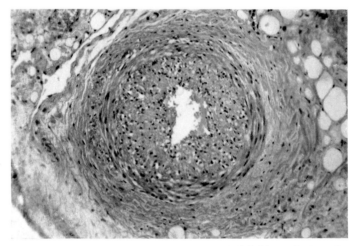

Figure 7.19.   Small artery showing marked endothelial hyperplasia so that the lumen is almost completely occluded (haematoxylin and eosin × 50, reduced to 6/10)

cardial cells completely. The small intracardiac arteries and arterioles also show well-marked perivascular fibrosis. There is also a diffuse infiltration of some areas of the myocardium with lymphocytes (*Figure 7.18*), less commonly with eosinophils and sometimes a few plasma cells. In these cases which have a pericardial effusion this lymphocytic infiltration is most marked in the myocardium immediately below the pericardium. This lymphocytic infiltrate may also extend into any deposits of pericardial adipose tissue and there may be a few small foci of lymphocytes in the visceral pericardium. The myocardium usually shows the changes of prolonged congestive cardiac failure—the myocardial cells appear to be more unduly separated than those seen in normal tissue; the separation being due to infiltration with oedema fluid. Many of the small blood vessels also show marked congestion and dilatation while some have apparently ruptured and the red blood cells are found to be lying freely in the myocardium. In some of these hearts, usually a marked minority, some of the small arteries show endothelial proliferation (*Figure 7.19*). The lumen may be almost completely blocked so that very few erythrocytes may pass along the course of the vessels, or they may be completely blocked. This change is known as 'endothelial vasculosis' and when present is best seen in some of the small vessels of the pericardial fat, although it may also be present in the myocardium. A change, which is more commonly seen, is the presence of marked thickening of the walls of many of the small intramyocardial arteries, so that the vessels' lumen may be greatly reduced (*Figure 7.20*). The thickening consists mainly of fibrous tissue where an increased number of elastic tissue fibres are seen. The coronary arteries are normal or show only very slight atherosclerotic changes while the intramyocardial and cardiac veins are normal in appearance.

In the myocardium itself the small blood vessels are often surrounded by much perivascular fibrosis (*Figure 7.21*). Sometimes relatively large areas of fibrosis are found (*Figure 7.22*), although sometimes particular muscle fibres are surrounded by fibrous tissue and oedema fluid (*Figure 7.23*). Sometimes a thrombus overlying the endocardium is seen to be undergoing a process of organization and incorporation (*Figure 7.24*).

Fibrin stains usually show a thin layer of fibrin covering the surface of the endocardium (*Figure 7.25*). In those places where the endocardium has become thick, small foci of fibrin may be seen in the deeper parts of the endocardium while thrombi are present on the overlying endocardium and are undergoing a process of organization. The result of this is that the fibrin layer becomes incorporated with

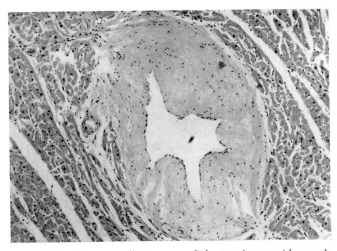

Figure 7.20. Here a small intramyocardial artery is seen with a markedly thickened wall: the thickening consists of fibrous tissue which has also replaced most of the medial muscle (haematoxylin and eosin × 80, reduced to 6/10)

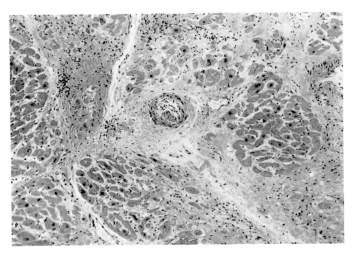

Figure 7.21. This shows a small intramyocardial artery which is surrounded by a zone of perivascular fibrosis. A considerable number of lymphocytes are also present in association with the zones of fibrous tissue (haematoxylin and eosin × 80, reduced to 6/10)

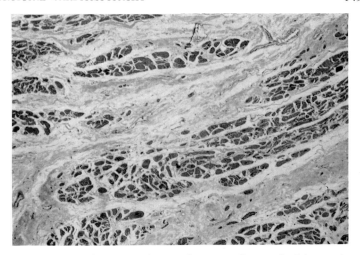

Figure 7.22. In this section of ventricular myocardium much of the muscle has been replaced by fibrous tissue (haematoxylin and eosin × 60, reduced to 6/10)

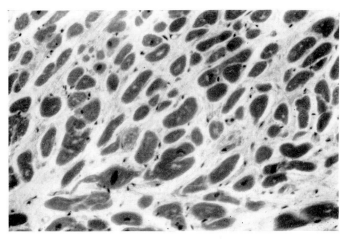

Figure 7.23. In some areas the myocardial fibres may be separated by numerous strands of connective tissue and oedema fluid (haematoxylin and eosin × 50, reduced to 6/10)

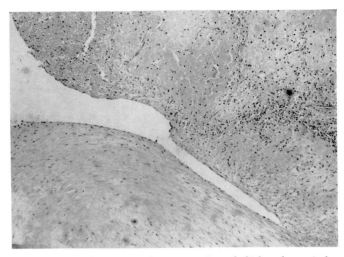

Figure 7.24. This section shows a portion of thickened ventricular endocardium—overlying which is a thrombus which is in the process of becoming organized—it is at the bottom right hand corner (haematoxylin and eosin × 50, reduced to 6/10)

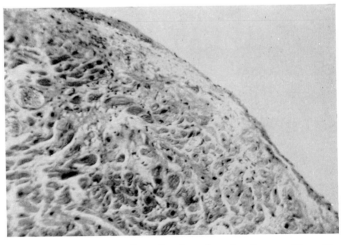

Figure 7.25. This section shows that the endocardium is covered by a thin layer of fibrin (Martius' scarlet blue × 50, reduced to 6/10)

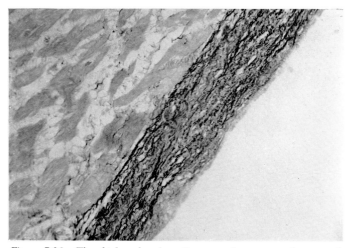

Figure 7.26. The thickened endocardium contains many unfragmented elastic tissue fibres (Verhoeff and van Gieson × 90, reduced to 6/10)

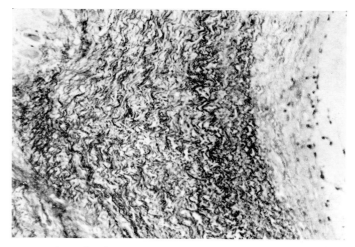

Figure 7.27. The deeper parts of the endocardium in this photograph contain many thickened endocardial elastic tissue fibres but the more superficial layer of endocardium contains none (Verhoeff and van Gieson × 50, reduced to 6/10)

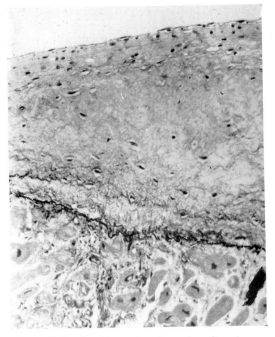

Figure 7.28. In this section the endocardium is considerably thickened but contains only scanty elastic tissue fibres apart from a basal layer (Verhoeff and van Gieson × 295, reduced to 2/3)

the underlying endocardium. No fibrin deposits can be seen in the myocardium or can be associated with any foci of inflammatory cells or blood vessels.

Elastic tissue stains usually show a good deal of elastic tissue in the thickened endocardium (*Figure 7.26*) which consists of long, thin and largely unfragmented strands. Often, however, the parts of the endocardium immediately below the cardiac cavity do not contain any elastic tissue (*Figure 7.27*), as this is the area where overlying thrombus has recently been incorporated in the thickened endocardium.

In a few places, especially in the area of the atrioventricular valves, or at a ventricular apex, the thickened endocardium can be seen to contain no elastic tissue fibres (*Figure 7.28*) or only a few scattered and fragmented strands.

The alcian blue stain shows the presence of much acid mucopolysaccharides in the endocardium most particularly in those areas where the endocardium is considerably thickened and in small foci within the endocardium. Alcian blue is also found to stain much of the fibrous tissue placed more deeply within the myocardium, particularly that in the areas of perivascular fibrosis around the small blood vessels and small scattered foci of inflammatory cells.

Toluidine blue has been used by some workers to demonstrate metachromasia of the endocardium (Becker, 1963) but in my hands has shown very inconsistant results and cannot be regarded as showing any definite specificity for this disease by its staining of the endocardium.

The amount of alcian blue staining seems to be roughly similar to that found in endomyocardial fibrosis.

CLASSIFICATION

It will be seen from these results that there is no clear line of demarcation between endomyocardial fibrosis and cardiomegaly of unknown origin—pathologically or histologically. Although the distinction between typical cases can be made, there are many other cases where this distinction cannot be made. It is, therefore, of importance to the pathologist to bear these facts in mind and, although he may often be able to classify a cardiomyopathy as either endomyocardial fibrosis or cardiomegaly of unknown origin, he should not be too anxious if he can only place it in the group which is regarded as being tropical cardiomyopathies.

Table 7.2 shows a list of the main points of difference and similarity in these two conditions.

AETIOLOGY

It has been suggested that endomyocardial fibrosis may be caused by an infectious agent (Parry and Abrahams, 1965); particularly as a report by Parry from West Africa stated that many of the patients with endomyocardial fibrosis gave a history of having had a febrile illness some months previously. In fact, they sometimes continued to have febrile episodes when presenting with this heart disease. These findings have not been confirmed by workers dealing with cases of endomyocardial fibrosis in other parts of Africa. The other suggestion put forward by this group of workers in Nigeria (Brockington, Olsen and Goodwin, 1967) that the disease is caused by filarial infection has not been supported by filarial antibody studies carried out in Uganda (Somers, 1967 personal communication). Here it has been shown that many cases of endomyocardial fibrosis have not had a previous filarial infection; in many other areas of Africa, infection with non-pathogenic strains of filariae such as *Filaria perstans*, is so common. If Filariae were the cause of this disease, one would expect

TABLE 7.2

	Endomyocardial fibrosis	Cardiomegaly of unknown origin
Age	15–25 but the disease may occur at any age	Most commonly 35–45
Sex	Equally affected	Equally affected
Heart weight	Usually small but may be enlarged to 450 or 500 g	Usually enlarged—400–600 g
Thrombo-embolism	Frequent	Frequent
Eosinophilia	Sometimes seen	Sometimes seen
Endocardium	Usually markedly thickened and the elastic tissue is usually absent except for the original basal layer but sometimes scattered fragments are seen	Usually slightly thickened except for the apex or near the atrioventricular valves. Elastic tissue is usually present and usually takes the form of long, thin strands. It may, however, be absent especially immediately below the cardiac cavity or completely so in the region of the atrioventricular valves; only small scattered fragments may be present
Myocardium	Cell hypertrophy. Abnormally-shaped nuclei. Hyaline change or vacuolation of cytoplasm is sometimes seen	No cell hypertrophy. Abnormally-shaped nuclei. Hyaline change or vacuolation of cytoplasm is sometimes seen

Cell infiltrates	This largely consists of lymphocytes found in scattered foci throughout the endocardium. Eosinophils are sometimes seen
Fibrin	Present in both diseases on the endocardial surface but the largest deposits are seen within the thickened endocardium; usually in endomyocardial fibrosis
Alcian blue	Equal staining of connective tissue for acid mucopolysaccharides in both conditions
Blood vessels	(1) 'Endothelial vasculosis'—i.e., marked endothelial hyperplasia in the smaller intracardiac arteries—is not found in endomyocardial fibrosis but is sometimes found in cardiomegaly of unknown origin but not essential for diagnosis
	(2) Thickening of the walls of small intramyocardial arteries is more commonly seen in cardiomegaly of unknown origin—the thickening being due to fibrous tissue and elastic fibres may be present
	(3) Hyaline thickening of the walls of small arteries and arterioles is sometimes seen in both endomyocardial fibrosis and cardiomegaly of unknown origin (*Figure 7.24*)

all the inhabitants of these areas to have endomyocardial fibrosis. The mechanisms by which this cardiac lesion may be produced has not been discovered, but it is thought that they work by producing obstruction of cardiac lymphatics and that endocardial thickening subsequently results through the sclerosing action of lymph. The mechanism of obstruction of cardiac lymphatics has been shown to produce endocardial thickening, although there is much more elastic tissue, similar to that found in fibro-elastosis by the experimental work of Miller, Pick and Katz (1963).

Viral infections such as those with certain strains of encephalomyo-carditis virus—meningo-encephalomyocarditis virus—have been supported by the fact that they have been isolated from animals in some places where endomyocardial fibrosis occurs. Also, it has been suggested that these viruses have not been isolated from any affected human beings nor have any specific antibodies to the viruses been found in affected patients as these viruses are specific species for man.

Infection with malaria has also been suggested as a cause for this disease but with little supporting evidence. Shaper (1966) postulated that endomyocardial fibrosis may be an atypical variant of rheumatic heart disease. This worker thinks that streptococcal infection, acting on a background of altered immunological status, may produce endomyocardial fibrosis. He goes on to say that this particular immunological status could be produced by parasitic diseases, such as malaria or possibly even filariasis. The febrile episodes described by patients could be due either to these infections or to the streptococcal invasion precipitating the rheumatic variant.

The idea that the disease may have an auto-immune aetiology has been put forward by some workers but cardiac antibodies have been estimated in the sera of some of these patients, and found to be normal or no more than is often found in normal controls.

Vitamin B_2 (thiamine) deficiency has also been suggested as a possible aetiological agent for endomyocardial fibrosis. This may be disregarded when one considers that endomyocardial fibrosis occurs very commonly in areas where vitamin B_2 deficiency is not found; the lesions of experimental B_2 deficiency are not found in the heart even after prolonged periods of time.

It has been suggested that both endomyocardial fibrosis and cardiomegaly of unknown origin may be due to malnutritional causes, as can be noted from the fact that one of the original names for the latter in South Africa was 'nutritional heart disease' (Gillanders, 1951); and that in Uganda the former is found to be most common among the most lowly-paid group of immigrant labourers the Banyaruanda. It has been shown that the diet of groups of patients who are likely to develop cardiomegaly of unknown origin are tryptophan deficient and that patients with this heart disease have low serum tryptophan levels (Reid and Berjak, 1967).

These findings have been extended by Reid and Berjak (1966) who have fed rats for long periods (1–2 years) on maize diets, similar to those usually eaten by the South African Bantu, and have produced lesions that appear to be identical with cardiomegaly of unknown origin in man. It has also been noted that endomyocardial fibrosis is found (most commonly) in those places where the dietary staples are plantains (Crawford, 1963), a food which contains a high concentration of 5-hydroxytryptamine but little tryptophan. Diet containing low tryptophan has previously been used to produce 'carcinoid'-like lesions when combined with injections of 5-hydroxytryptamine (Spatz, 1964). This work was extended by McKinney and Crawford (1965) when they produced some cardiac lesions in guinea-pigs fed on plantain diets for long periods—8–12 months. It is only recently, however, that this work has been extended; using the pure chemicals and deficiency diets in attempts to produce hearts showing the exact lesions of endomyocardial fibrosis, and appears to have been successful (Spatz, 1969). It is suggested that 5-hydroxytryptamine has a protective action on the myocardium and so tryptophan deficiency may be prevented from producing cardiomegaly of unknown origin. However, it does produce the lesions of endomyocardial fibrosis in the presence of high dietary intake of 5-hydroxytryptamine.

It is to be hoped that later work will repeat these findings when foods similar to those used by the indigeneous inhabitants of these areas, where the disease are found, are used.

The only way in which cases of both these diseases can be diagnosed with certainty is by stating that enlarged hearts—over 500 g and with little endocardial thickening—are cases of cardiomegaly of unknown origin, while those of under 500 g and with endocardial thickening are cases of endomyocardial fibrosis. This fact clearly demonstrates how artificial this pathological classification is, which separates both these diseases into two separate classes.

References

Andrade, Z. A. and Guimãraes, A. C. (1964). 'Endomyocardial fibrosis in Bahia, Brazil.' *Br. Heart J.* **26**, 813

Becker, B. J. P. (1963). 'Idiopathic mural endocardial disease in South Africa.' *Med. Proc.* **9**, 124

— Chetgidakis, C. G. and Van Lingen, B. (1953). 'Cardiovascular collagenosis with parietal endocardial thrombosis, clinicopathologic study of 40 cases.' *Circulation* **7**, 345

Bedford, D. E. and Konstam, G. L. S. (1946). 'Heart failure of unknown aetiology in Africans.' *Br. Heart J.* **8**, 236

Black, M. and Fowler, J. M. (1965). 'Endomyocardial fibrosis in Britain.' *Br. med. J.* **1**, 682

Brockington, I. F., Olsen, E. G. and Goodwin, J. F. (1967). 'Endomyocardial fibrosis in Europeans resident in Tropical Africa.' *Lancet* **1**, 583

Brown, J. M. and Burnell, R. H. (1965). 'A case of endomyocardial fibrosis.' *Med. J. Aust.* **1**, 973

Cochlo, E. and Pymental, J. C. (1963). 'Diffuse endomyocardial fibrosis.' *Am. J. Med.* **35**, 369

Connor, D. H., Somers, K., Hutt, M. S. R., Mannion, W. C. and D'Arbela, P. (1967). 'Endomyocardial fibrosis in Uganda (Davies disease). Part I: An epidemologic, clinical and pathologic study.' *Am. Heart J.* **74**, 687

— — — — — (1968). 'Endomyocardial fibrosis in Uganda (Davies disease). Part II: An epidemologic, clinical and pathologic study.' *Am. Heart J.* **75**, 107

Crawford, M. A. (1963). 'Endomyocardial fibrosis and carcinoidosis. A common denominator.' *Am. Heart J.* **66**, 273

Davies, J. N. P. (1948). 'Endocardial fibrosis in Africans.' *E. Afr. med. J.* **25**, 10,

— and Ball, J. D. (1955). 'Pathology of endomyocardial fibrosis in Uganda.' *Br. Heart J.* **17**, 337

— and Hollman, A. (1965). 'Becker type cardiomyopathy in a West Indian woman.' *Am. Heart J.* **70**, 225

Edington, G. M. and Jackson, J. G. (1963). 'The pathology of heart muscle disease and endomyocardial fibrosis in Nigeria.' *J. Path. Bact.* **86**, 333

Gelfand, M. (1944). 'Description of beri-beri heart disease.' In *The Sick African; a clinical study* 1st Edition, pp. 209–10. Capetown: Stewart Printing

Gillanders, H. D. (1951). 'Nutritional heart disease.' *Br. Heart J.* **13**, 177

Gopi, C. K. (1968). 'Idiopathic cardiomegaly.' *Bull. Wld Hlth Org.* **38**, 979

Gray, I. R. (1951). 'Endocardial fibrosis.' *Br. Heart J.* **13**, 387

Guimãraes, A. C. and Andrade, Z. A. (1962). 'Miocardiopatia de etiologia obscura (Relato anatomo-clinico de cinco casos).' *Hospital, Rio de J.* **62**, 1023

Hill, K. R., Still, W. J. S. and McKinney, B. (1967). 'Jamaican cardiomyopathy.' *Br. Heart J.* **29**, 594

Hutt, M. S. R. (1970). 'Pathology of African cardiomyopathies.' *Pathologica Microbiol.* **35**, 37

Ishak, K. G. and Tschumy, W. O. (1962). 'Endomyocardial fibrosis— report of a case in a 12 year old youth.' *Am. J. Med.* **32**, 645

La Brooy, E. B. (1957). 'Endomyocardial fibrosis.' *Proc. Alumni Ass. Malaya* **10**, 303

Lynch, J. B. and Watt, J. (1957). 'Diffuse endomyocardial sclerosis.' *Br. Heart J.* **19**, 173

McKinney, B. (1968). 'Endomyocardial fibrosis in Ghana.' Personal observation.

— (1970a). 'A comparative histological study of endomyocardial fibrosis and cardiomegaly of unknown origin.' *Pathologica Microbiol.* **35**, 70

— (1970b). 'Cardiomegaly of unknown origin in England.' Personal observation.

— (1970c). 'Rhodesian cardiomyopathy.' Personal observation.

McKinney, B. (1973). 'Muscle fibre size in cardiomyopathies in Africa.' *Am. Heart J.* (In press)

— and Ashworth, T. G. (1973). 'Spontaneous cardiomyopathies found in adult Africans in Rhodesia.' *Pathologica Microbiol.*

— and Crawford, M. A. (1965). 'Fibrosis in guinea pig heart produced by plantain diet.' *Lancet* **2**, 880

Miller, A. J., Dick, Ruth and Katz, L. N. (1963). 'Ventricular endomyocardial changes after impairment of cardiac lymph flow in dogs.' *Br. Heart J.* **25**, 182

Nagaratnam, N. and Dissanayake, R. V. (1959). 'Endomyocardial fibrosis in the Ceylonese.' *Br. Heart J.* **21**, 162

O'Brien, W. (1954). 'Endocardial fibrosis in Sudan.' *Br. med. J.* **2**, 899

Ogan, H. (1960). 'Diffuse endomyocardial sclerosis.' *Bull. Soc. Int. Chir.* **19**, 469

Parry, E. H. O. and Abrahams, D. G. (1965). 'The natural history of endomyocardial fibrosis. *Q. Jl. Med.* **34**, 383

Peuchot, G., Latour, H. and Puech, P. (1960). 'Anatomoclinical records of acquired retractile endomyocardial fibrosis.' *Archs Mal. Coeur* **53**, 1137

Reddy, C. R. M., Parvathi, G. and Rao, N. R. (1970). 'Pathology of cardiomyopathy from South India.' *Br. Heart J.* **32**, 2, 226

Reid, J. V. O. (1966). 'Muscle fiber content of the heart in African cardiomyopathy.' *Am. Heart J.* **71**, 352

— and Berjak, P. (1967). 'Tryptophan and serotonin levels in patients with, or susceptible to African cardiomyopathy.' *Am. Heart J.* **74**, 337

— — (1966). 'Dietary production of myocardial fibrosis in the rat.' *Am. Heart J.* **71**, 240

Seftel, H. and Susser, M. (1961). 'Maternity and myocardial failure in African women.' *Br. Heart J.* **23**, 43

Shaper, A. G. (1966). 'Endomyocardial fibrosis and rheumatic heart disease.' *Lancet* **1**, 639

Spatz, Maria (1964). 'Pathogenetic studies of experimentally induced heart lesions and their relation to the carcinoid syndrome.' *Lab. Invest.* **13**, 288

— (1969). 'Tryptophan metabolism and cardiac disease.' *Ann. N.Y. Acad. Sci.* **156** Article 1, 152

Stuart, K. L. and Hayes, J. A. (1963). 'A cardiac disorder of unknown aetiology in Jamaica.' *Q. Jl. Med.* **32**, 99

Thomson, J. G. (1961). 'Cardiopathy of unknown origin in Africa.' In Recent Advances in Human Nutrition. Ed. by J. F. Brock, pp. 389–394. London: Churchill

Turner, P. P. and Manson-Bahr, P. E. (1960). 'Endomyocardial fibrosis in Kenya and Tanganyika Africans.' *Br. Heart J.* **22**, 305

WHO (1965). 'Cardiomyopathies.' *Bull. Wld Hlth Org.* **33**, 257

Williams, A. W. and Somers, K. (1960). 'The electrocardiogram in endomyocardial fibrosis.' *Br. Heart J.* **22**, 311

Yoshida, T., Nimura, Y., Sakakibara, H., Metsutani, K., Nishizaki, K. and Nakata, T. (1964). 'A diffuse endocardial fibroelastosis with markedly dilated right atrium observed in an adult.' *Jap. Heart J.* **5**, 85

Eight

Viral myocarditis

GENERAL CONSIDERATIONS

In some patients myocarditis may be evident at the start of a viral illness but there is usually a latent period of several days, during which the patient is asymptomatic. This latent period may then be followed by obvious symptoms of myocarditis. However, because there are usually temporarily related phenomena, physicians often have difficulty in relating an infection, regardless of type, to the cardiac disease.

The electrocardiogram in viral myocarditis is usually non-specific with T wave inversion, ST segment abnormalities or various types of atrioventricular conduction disturbances. Sometimes the electrocardiogram changes of myocardial infarction, due to areas of electrical silence produced by fairly large isolated areas of myocardial damage, may be found.

It can, therefore, be seen that the diagnosis of viral myocarditis is usually entirely indirect, that is, obtained by clinical logic. The clinical findings, isolation of the virus from the stool, urine, pharyngeal washings, blood or cerebrospinal fluid and changes in specific viral antibody titre may all contribute to establishing a clinical diagnosis.

COXSACKIE AND ECHO VIRUS INFECTIONS

Coxsackie B virus, of which there are six types, causes spastic paralysis in experimental mice, with focal necrosis in muscle, pancreas, liver, brain and myocardium. In the human they can cause aseptic meningitis, myocarditis and pericarditis, epidemic myalgia and Bornholm disease. Grist and Bell (1969) of Glasgow mentioned that 22 cases of myocarditis and/or pericarditis had been diagnosed in the period 1959–68; viruses concerned and numbers of cases were A1 (1), A4 (3), A9 (1), B2 (2), B3 (3), B4 (5) and B5 (7). Eight cases were in the first decade, five in the second and third, and nine in the fourth to seventh decades. The incidence of cardiac involvement has been at least 5 per cent of most recorded outbreaks. Other types of Coxsackie A viruses, of which 23 types are known, can also involve the heart. Grist and Bell (1968) referred to cases of A1 pericarditis, A4 myocarditis and myopericarditis; A16 myocarditis; and A8 infections in an infant with atrial septal defect and in a two year old girl with paroxysmal tachycardia.

Infection with one of the above groups of viruses, commonly group B, produces a wide variety of clinical manifestations. These include pleurodynia, meningo-encephalitis (Rapmund et al., 1959) and benign pericarditis. These conditions are almost invariably associated with a favourable prognosis.

A Public Health Laboratory Report (1967) from Colindale, England stated that 1,160 notifications of Coxsackie B5 infection were made during 1967—mainly from London and the south-east of England, reaching a peak in July and August. Forty-one per cent of the infections were in children up to 9 years old and 19 per cent in those aged between 10 and 19; few adults over 50 years of age were affected. Of 900 cases the central nervous system was involved in 31 per cent (usually aseptic meningitis); 23 per cent had myalgia or Bornholm disease; 15 per cent had respiratory infection; 9 per cent had gastro-intestinal symptoms; and 5 per cent (45) had cardiac involvement (41 pericarditis and 4 myocarditis). There were six deaths: an infant of 11 days and an adult died of myocarditis, and two infants died of respiratory involvement. Respiratory, gastro-intestinal and central nervous system symptoms are dominant in the under 10s and muscular and central nervous system involvement in those above this age.

In neonatal infections, however, the organ most commonly involved is the heart, and a fatal outcome is frequent. In older children and adults myocarditis has been recorded only rarely (Null and Castle, 1959; Connolly, 1961), and only one fatal case, which was due to infection with Coxsackie virus group B, has been recorded so far (Sanyal et al., 1965).

ECHO viruses have a range of pathogencity in man somewhat similar to Coxsackie viruses, particularly where nervous tissue is concerned. They may occasionally be a cause of pleurodynia, but their relationship to cardiac disease is less well established. ECHO virus strains exceed thirty in number, and of these types 6, 9, and 14 seem to be related to cardiac disease (Bell and Grist, 1970). During an epidemic of 513 cases of ECHO virus infection in Holland in 1967, 0·8 per cent were classified as causing myocarditis or pericarditis.

ECHO virus type 9 has been reported to cause myocarditis with conduction defects and arrhythmias (Cherry, Juhn and Meyer, 1967), and similar findings were recorded for types 6 and 9 by Kibrick (1964).

Several virus types have been isolated from cases of acute pericarditis in man and Johnson *et al.* (1961) describe a series of 34 patients while Kavelman, Duncan and Lewis (1961) review others.

Only one case has been recorded in the literature so far of death from myocarditis in an adult, with recovery of the virus from myocardial tissue alone, and no lesions or virus elsewhere in the body (Monif, Lee and Hsiung, 1967). The interesting histopathology of this case will be referred to later. Lou and Werner (1962) found two strains of ECHO virus (types 2 and 14) which readily produce myocarditis in monkeys, but these types have not yet been reported to do so in man.

Most of the fatal cases of neonatal myocarditis described so far and due to Coxsackie virus infection have been associated with nursery epidemics. These outbreaks have been fully described by Montgomery *et al.* (1955) from Southern Rhodesia; by Javett *et al.* (1956) from Johannesburg; and by van Creveld and de Jager (1956) and Verlinde, van Tongeren and Kret (1956) from Amsterdam. Sporadic fatal cases have also been reported elsewhere, mostly from the USA (Kibrick and Benirschke, 1956; Hosier and Newton, 1958; Fechner, Smith and Middlekamp, 1963), but also elsewhere, as the case reported from England by Jennings (1966).

Coxsackie virus infection normally occurs soon after birth, but in some instances infection is intra-uterine and the infection is transplacental in origin (Kilbrick and Benirschke, 1956). Not uncommonly there is a history of an acute illness in the mother, either before or shortly after the birth of the sick child (Ronino *et al.*, 1962).

The affected infant usually presents with an acute fulminating illness together with evidence of circulatory failure and respiratory distress. The only clinical finding present may be an extremely rapid rate of respiration.

Most of the necropsy reports stress the generalized nature of the infection, and in addition to the myocarditis, necrotizing lesions may be found in the liver, adrenals, pancreas and bone marrow. A meningo-encephalitis has often been found to be present (van Creveld and de Jager, 1956; McLean *et al.*, 1961; Ronino *et al.*, 1962). Perhaps the most characteristic finding in Coxsackie viral myocarditis is the presence of cardiomegaly which has been found in most cases (Saphir and Cohen, 1957; Hosier and Newton, 1958;

Jennings, 1966), but is absent in others (Fechner, Smith and Middlekamp, 1963). A compensatory hypertrophy, presumably due to hypertrophy of the remaining muscle fibres with normal function, to replace the widespread necrotic foci of damaged muscle, is often found. The possibility of hyperplasia shortly before or after birth cannot be completely ruled out (Black-Schaffer and Turner, 1958).

Macroscopically at autopsy the heart is found to be enlarged, usually markedly so, due to thickening of the walls of both ventricles, while there is usually a small excess of slightly turbid pericardial fluid present. On section the myocardium is uniform in appearance, and normal in consistency but may be much browner than normal in colour.

Histological examination of the heart shows inflammatory foci consisting mainly of lymphocytes and mononuclear cells with some polymorphs together with associated areas of muscle necrosis which may be present throughout both ventricles, atria and auricular appendages (*Figure 8.1*). There may also be a slight pericarditis, but more frequently there are signs of endocarditis (Sanyal *et al.*, 1965), with thrombi overlying areas of subendocardial necrosis.

The virus has been isolated at necropsy from a variety of sites: including the myocardium (Montgomery *et al.*, 1955); spinal cord (Kibrick and Benirschke, 1956); liver and lungs (McLean *et al.*, 1961); and frequently from the intestine (Ronino *et al.*, 1962).

In the investigation of these cases the cardiac muscle itself is the organ of choice when attempting to isolate the virus. All of the group B viruses have been isolated, at one time or another, from cases of neonatal myocarditis, but no one serological type is predominant.

There is some evidence to suggest that Coxsackie virus infection during pregnancy has teratogenic effects, and this was first noted by Evans and Brown (1963).

Fruhling *et al.* (1962) carried out a survey on myocarditis in 81 newborn and young babies with fibro-elastosis. In 28 of the more recent cases virological investigations were done, and Coxsackie B virus was recovered from the myocardium in several instances.

Infection early in pregnancy was found to produce rigidity of the left side of the heart by endocardial sclerosis, sometimes involving also mitral valve and aorta. Where infection occurred later on in the first trimester a persistent inflammatory cell process was predominant. The authors considered the aetiology to be an infective pancarditis, and the direct cause of death in fibro-elastosis to be either from ventricular involution or from lesions of the conducting tissue.

Recent serological evidence by Evans and Brown (1967) provides further confirmation of a causal relationship between Coxsackie virus infection and congenital heart disease. In a six-year investigation they found that a greater number of mothers of infants with congenital abnormalities experienced Coxsackie virus infections than did a matched control series. Half of the infections were completely subclinical.

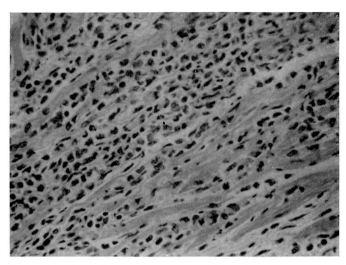

Figure 8.1. Coxsackie myocarditis in a child aged two years causing cardiomegaly. Note diffuse infiltration of the myocardium with small round cells, mainly lymphocytes and a few plasma cells. Some of the myocardial cells appear to be undergoing necrosis and replacement by areas of fibrosis (haematoxylin and eosin × 120, reduced to 8/10). (Reproduced from Jennings (1966) by courtesy of the author and Editor of the Journal of Clinical Pathology)

In adults Coxsackie virus infection is not thought by many physicians to have serious effect on the myocardium, and usually other signs of virus infection, such as pleurodynia, predominate. However, reports of fatal cases of Coxsackie virus myocarditis do exist, although they are rare. It is reasonable to suggest that this does not reflect the true frequency of the condition (Sainani, Krompotic and Slodki, 1968), and it may well be that many cases are missed and classified as idiopathic or Fiedler's myocarditis. Sometimes, however, cases of obscure heart failure have been shown to be the result of Coxsackie viral myocarditis (Burch *et al.*, 1967) and in some other cases evidence of viral valvulitis has been seen. It is noteworthy that Cossart, Burgess and Nash (1965) and

Friedberg (1966) have made similar comments concerning the electrocardiogram, and studies in monkeys (Lou, Werner and Kamitsuka, 1961) have shown that the electrocardiogram is commonly found to be normal in Coxsackie virus myocarditis.

Smith (1966) of Perth, Western Australia, reported a remarkable series of 10 adults (1 woman aged 30, and 9 men aged 27–56), with heart involvement, 6 also had symptomatic pericarditis, and all had leucocytosis, neutrophilia and a raised ESR. The virus type was B5 in 4 cases, B4 in 3, B2 in 3, and B1 in the remaining case. Seven patients recovered completely, although one had severe heart failure and nephritis, and another had persistent electrocardiogram changes. The 8th case had 4 recurrences of pericarditis in 2 years, the 9th had mitral regurgitation and the 10th, a doctor aged 45, died of coronary artery disease 5 weeks after leaving hospital. Smith noted that especially young men could be affected, and that other manifestations might present such as myalgia, septic meningitis and nephritis.

The myocarditis caused cardiac dilatation and was nearly always accompanied by acute benign, non-specific pericarditis. Most recovered completely, depending on the degree of cardiac involvement and underlying heart disease; haemopericardium was not seen. A few patients developed constrictive pericarditis or electrocardiogram abnormalities.

Some workers have succeeded in isolating the Coxsackie virus from the adult heart at necropsy (Sanyal et al., 1965; Cossart, Burgess and Nash, 1965) or by myocardial biopsy (Sutton et al., 1967), but these have not received the attention they have deserved.

Longson, Cole and Davies (1969) have reported a fatal case of myocarditis in an adolescent male—a boy aged 15—which was confirmed at necropsy by the isolation of Coxsackie B5 virus from the myocardium and bowel. At necropsy the heart was somewhat enlarged, 350 g in weight, while the pericardium contained a small amount of straw-coloured fluid, but showed no other evidence of pericarditis. At the apices of both ventricles there was recent mural thrombus and the left ventricle was dilated. The myocardium throughout was pale and soft. Macroscopically the endocardium showed no abnormality and the coronary arteries were normal. Identical microscopical changes were seen in all parts of the myocardium but were most severe in the ventricles. The predominant feature was extreme muscle fibre necrosis, but the necrotic fibres were often adjacent to fibres which appeared normal, while the sarcoplasm of the affected cells was eosinophilic and granular with loss of striations (*Figure 8.2*). Many fibres showed cytoplasmic vacuolation while nuclei were often grossly pyknotic or absent and there was active myocarditis. Throughout the heart muscle and, particularly in relation to necrotic areas, there was a diffuse lymphocyte cell infiltrate, with occasional plasma cells and neutrophils, while inflammatory oedema separated many of the muscle fibres.

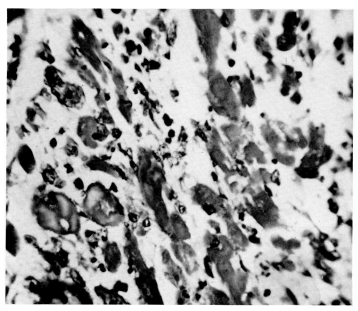

Figure 8.2. Focus of necrosis, showing myocarditis, loss of striations of myofibrils, macrophage activity, and round-cell infiltration (haematoxylin and eosin × 350, reduced to 9/10). (Reproduced from Longson, Cole and Davies (1969) by courtesy of the authors and Editor of the Journal of Clinical Pathology*)*

Some endocardial thickening was also noted in the atria and in fact consisted of endomyocardial fibrosis up to about 40 μ in thickness (*Figure 8.3*).

The fatal case of myocarditis due to ECHO virus reported by Monif, Lee and Hsiung (1967) occurred in a 34 year old male and was confirmed by recovery of ECHO type-9 virus solely from his tissue. On naked-eye examination numerous discrete greyish-white plaques measuring 0·2–0·7 cm were present throughout the entire myocardium and involved also the papillary muscles. A serious pericardial effusion was also present. The myocardium adjacent to the plaques was pale but firm in texture. Histopathological changes showed an extensive focal and diffuse inflammatory cell infiltration, with a massive focal necrosis of muscle fibres, and associated interstitial oedema. The cellular response consisted of lymphocytes, plasma cells, neutrophils and eosinophils, together with histiocytic cells with ovoid nuclei, all in varying proportions and at different sites. Occasional myofibres showed nuclear enlargement.

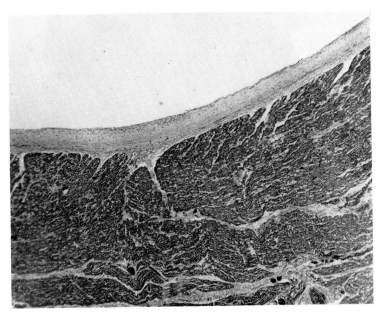

Figure 8.3. Myocardial wall showing endocardial thickening (haematoxylin and eosin × 90). (Reproduced from Longson, Cole and Davies (1969) by courtesy of the authors and Editor of the Journal of Clinical Pathology)

Smith (1966) has suggested that the Coxsackie virus may initiate an auto-immune reaction, as in traumatic carditis, or in the post-cardiac infarction and post-cardiotomy syndromes.

Perhaps the most interesting suggestion made in relation to Coxsackie virus infection is that this infection may be the primary aetiological cause of some forms of 'idiopathic' cardiomyopathy which are responsible for the production of some types of 'congestive cardiomyopathy' (Burch and de Pasquale, 1964), although this has not yet been conclusively established. It is perhaps interesting to note that experimental lesions have been produced in mice by Burch *et al.* (1966), who injected over 200 HAM/ICR strain with group B4 Coxsackie virus intraperitoneally. The animals were killed from 12 hours to 76 days later. Two-thirds showed lesions of the mitral valve and sometimes the aortic valve also. Early lesions were oedema and round-cell infiltration, later fibroblast proliferation, fibrosis and verruca formation occurred.

References

Bell, E. J. and Grist, N. R. (1970). 'Further studies on artero-virus infection in cardiac disease and pleurodynia.' *Scand. J. inf. Dis.* **2**, 1

Black-Schaffer, B. and Turner, M. E. (1958). 'Hyperplastic infantile cardiomegaly; a form of idiopathic hypertrophy with or without endocardial fibroelastosis, and a comment on cardiac atrophy.' *Am. J. Path.* **34**, 745

Burch, G. E. and De Pasquale, N. P. (1964). 'Noted that Coxsackie B endocarditis can occur in animals and may be the cause of unexplained acute and chronic endocarditis in man.' (Editorial) *Am. Heart J.* **67**, 721

— —, Sun, S. C., Mogabgab, W. J. and Hale, A. R. (1966). 'Endocarditis in mice infected with Coxsackie virus B4.' *Science, N.Y.* **151**, 447

— —, Colcolough, H. L., Sohal, R. S. and De Pasquale, N. P. (1967). 'Coxsackie B viral myocarditis and valvulitis identified in routine autopsy specimens by immunofluorescent techniques.' *Am. Heart J.* **74**, 13

Cherry, J. D., Juhn, C. L. and Meyer, T. C. (1967). 'Paroxysmal atrial tachycardia associated with E.C.H.O. 9 virus infection.' *Am. Heart J.* **73**, 681

Connolly, J. H. (1961). 'During Coxsackie B5 infection.' *Br. med. J.* **1**, 877

Cossart, Y. E., Burgess, J. A. and Nash, P. D. (1965). 'Fatal Coxsackie B myocarditis in an adult.' *Med. J. Aust.* **1**, 337

Evans, T. N. and Brown, G. C. (1963). 'Coxsackie virus infections in pregnancy.' *Am. J. Obstet. Gynec.* **87**, 749

— — (1967). 'Serologic evidence of Coxsackie virus etiology of congenital heart disease.' *J. Am. med. Ass.* **199**, 183

Fechner, R. E., Smith, M. G. and Middlekamp, J. N. (1963). 'Coxsackie B virus infections of the newborn.' *Am. J. Path.* **42**, 493

Friedberg, C. K. (1966). *Diseases of the Heart.* Philadelphia: Saunders

Fruhling, L., Korn, R., Lavillaureix, J., Surjus, A. and Foussereau, S. (1962). 'Chronic fibroelastic myoendocarditis of the newborn and the infant (fibroelastosis). New morphological, etiological and pathogenic data. Relation to certain cardiac abnormalities.' *Annls. Anat. Path.* **7**, 227

Grist, N. R. and Bell, E. J. (1969). 'Coxsackie viruses and the heart.' *Am. Heart J.* **77**, 295 (Editorial).

Hosier, D. M. and Newton, W. A. Jnr (1958). 'Serious Coxsackie virus infections in infants and children.' *Am. J. Dis. Child.* **96**, 251

Javett, S. N., Heymann, S., Mundel, B., Pepler, W. J., Lurie, H. I., Gear, J. H. S., Measroch, V. and Kirsch, Z. G. (1956). 'Myocarditis in the new born infant. A study of an outbreak associated with Coxsackie B Virus infection in a maternity home in Johannesburg.' *J. Pediat.* **48**, 1

Jennings, R. C. (1966). 'Coxsackie group B fatal neonatal myocarditis associated with cardiomegaly.' *J. clin. Path.* **19**, 325

Johnson, R. T., Portnoy, B., Rogers, N. G. and Buescher, E. L. (1961). 'Acute benign pericarditis: virologic study of 34 patients.' *Archs intern. Med.* **108**, 823

Kavelman, D. A., Duncan, I. B. and Lewis, J. A. (1961). 'Acute benign pericarditis.' *Can. med. Ass. J.* **85**, 1287

Kibrick, S. (1964). 'Current status of Coxsackie and E.C.H.O. viruses in human disease.' *Prog. med. Virol.* **6**, 27

— and Benirschke, K. (1956). 'Acute aseptic myocarditis and meningo-encephalitis in the newborn child infected with Coxsackie virus Group B, type 3.' *New Engl. J. Med.* **255**, 883

Longson, M., Cole, F. M. and Davies, D. (1969). 'Isolation of a Coxsackie virus group B, type 5 from the heart of a fatal case of myocarditis in an adult.' *J. clin. Path.* **22**, 654

Lou, T. Y. and Werner, H. A. (1962). 'Experimental infections with entro viruses. V. Studies on virulence and pathogenesis in cynomolgus monkeys.' *Arch. Virusforsch.* **12**, 303

— — and Kamitsuka, P. S. (1961). 'Experimental infections with Coxsackie viruses. II. Myocarditis in cynomolgus monkeys infected with B4 virus.' *Arch. Virusforsch.* **10**, 451

McLean, D. M., Donohue, W. L., Snelling, C. E. and Wyllie, J. C. (1961). 'Coxsackie B5 virus as a cause of neonatal encephalitis and myocarditis.' *Can. med. Ass. J.* **85**, 1046

Monif, G. R. G., Lee, C. W. and Hsiung, G. D. (1967). 'Isolated myocarditis with recovery of E.C.H.O. type 9 virus from the myocardium.' *New Engl. J. Med.* **277**, 1353

Montgomery, J., Prinsloo, F. R., Khan, M. and Kirsch, Z. G. (1955). 'Myocarditis in the newborn. An outbreak in a maternity home in Southern Rhodesia associated with Coxsackie Group B virus infection.' *S. Afr. med. J.* **29**, 608

Null, F. C., Jnr. and Castle, C. H. (1959). 'Adult pericarditis and myocarditis due to Coxsackie group B, type 5.' *New Engl. J. Med.* **261**, 937

Public Health Laboratory Service (1967). 'Report to the director from various laboratories in the United Kingdom: Coxsackie B5 virus infection in the United Kingdom during 1965.' *Br. med. J.* **4**, 675

Rapmund, G., Gauld, J. R., Rogers, N. G. and Holmes, G. E. (1959). 'Neonatal myocarditis and meningo encephalitis due to Coxsackie virus group B, type 4.' *New Engl. J. Med.* **260**, 819

Ronino, G., Periman, A., Togo, Y. and Reback, J. (1962). 'Coxsackie myocarditis and meningo encephalitis.' *J. Pediat.* **61**, 911

Sainani, G. S., Krompotic, E. and Slodki, S. J. (1968). 'Adult heart disease due to Coxsackie virus B infection.' *Medicine, Baltimore* **47**, 133

Sanyal, S. K., Mahdavy, M., Gabrielson, M. O., Vidone, R. A. and Browne, M. J. (1965). 'Myocarditis in an adolescent caused by Coxsackie virus, group B.' *Pediatrics, Springfield* **35**, 36

Saphir, O. and Cohen, N. A. (1957). 'Cardiomegaly in Coxsackie myocarditis,' *Archs Path.* **64**, 446

Smith, W. G. (1966). 'Adult heart disease due to the Coxsackie virus group B.' *Br. Heart J.* **28**, 204

Sutton, G. C., Harding, H. B., Truehart, R. P. and Clark, H. P. (1967). 'Coxsackie B4 myocarditis in an adult: successful isolation of virus from ventricular myocardium.' *Aerospace Med.* **38**, 66

Van Creveld, S. and de Jager, H. (1956). 'Myocarditis in newborns caused by Coxsackie virus.' *Annls paediat.* **187**, 100

Verlinde, J. D., van Tongeren, H. A. E. and Kret, A. (1956). 'Myocarditis in the newborn due to group B Coxsackie virus,' *Annls paediat.* **187**, 113

MUMPS MYOCARDITIS

There have been in the past two decades several papers describing electrocardiographic changes in many patients with mumps (Wendkos and Noll, 1944; Rosenberg, 1945; Irvin, Bacharach and Pullen, 1951; Bengtsson and Orndahl, 1954), as well as some dealing with the clinical signs and symptoms of myocarditis in patients with mumps (Felknor and Pullen, 1946; Bland, 1949; Horton, 1958).

There have, however, been only three recorded cases of autopsies on patients who died during mumps infection from what appears to be myocarditis (Manca, 1932; Krakower and Roberg, 1962; and Roberts and Fox, 1965).

These patients, whose ages ranged from 4 to 22 years, all presented with the typical signs of severe attack of mumps: tachycardia, cardiomegaly, and ventricular premature contractions were noted initially. All these cases subsequently developed congestive cardiac failure, which responded at first to digitalis and diuretic therapy, but all eventually succumbed to severe congestive heart failure. At autopsy the hearts were hypertrophied in every case, and all the chambers were dilated while the myocardium was soft. Recent and organizing thrombus was present in the apex of each ventricle and sometimes in the atria. The tricuspid and mitral valves and chordae were normal, but the valve rings were dilated. The endocardium was in some places markedly thickened while all the coronary arteries were normal both at their origin and in their distribution, and were free from diseases of the lumen, such as atherosclerosis.

Microscopically these hearts revealed diffuse interstitial myocardial

fibrosis, small focal areas of myocardial lysis, and a few mononuclear cells in the interstitial fibrous tissue and in the focal areas
of necrosis. Most myocardial fibres were hypertrophied but some
were atrophic. Staining of the myocardium for fat, glycogen,
amyloid and iron have all been found to be negative.

In Manca's case, the patient lived only 14 days, the heart was
neither dilated nor hypertrophied. Histologically this patient had
a fibrinous and leucocytic infiltrate in the interstitial tissues of the
myocardium, and the myocardial fibres showed various degenerative
changes. Roberts and Fox's (1965) patient had no significant
cellular infiltrate in the heart at autopsy, but the cellular response
would be expected to have disappeared long before death. Had the
myocardial inflammatory reaction persisted, a beneficial effect would
probably have resulted from the subsequent administration of
prednisolone, but this was not the case. The autopsy findings are,
however, similar to those of Krakower and Roberg's case (1962). In
all these cases the histology is consistent with a viral aetiology.

In viral myocarditis degeneration and actual muscle necrosis of
isolated, or groups of, myocardial fibres invariably occur and this
has been a prominent feature in all these cases.

The course and radiographical features in the patient of Roberts
and Fox (1965) are not unlike those described by Levy and Von
Glahn (1944) in patients with cardiac hypertrophy of unknown
origin, and these workers suggest that some cases of idiopathic
hypertrophy may have, as their aetiology, a clinically inapparent
infection by mumps virus.

A few years ago Noren, Adams and Anderson (1963) made the
interesting observation that children with endocardial fibro-elastosis
showed delayed-type skin hypersensitivity to mumps virus antigen.
Similar observations were made by St Geme, Noren and Adams
(1966) on children aged 2 months to 2 years, and the interesting
suggestion has been made that this disease may be related to intra-
uterine infection with mumps.

Reports by Sellers, Keith and Manning (1968) and Shone et al.
(1966) add weight to the above findings, although Gersony, Katz
and Nadas (1966) from the Childrens Hospital, Boston, failed to
establish a clear relationship between endocardial fibro-elastosis and
skin reactivity on exposure to mumps during pregnancy.

The significance of the findings is still in some doubt, and mumps
virus has so far not been recovered from the myocardium of fatal
cases. It could well be, however, that endocardial fibro-elastosis has a
multiple causation. In the section on Coxsackie viruses more definite
evidence of a viral aetiology of this condition is put forward.

References

Bengtsson, E. and Orndahl, G. (1954). 'Complications of mumps with special reference to the incidence of myocarditis.' *Acta med. scand.* **149**, 381

Bland, J. H. (1949). 'Mumps complicated by myocarditis, meningoencephalitis and pancreatitis. Review of the literature and report of a case.' *New Engl. J. Med.* **240**, 417

Felknor, G. E. and Pullen, R. L. (1946). 'Mumps myocarditis: Review of literature and report of case.' *Am. Heart J.* **31**, 238

Gersony, W. M., Katz, S. L. and Nadas, A. S. (1966). 'Endocardial fibroelastosis and the mumps virus.' *Pediatrics, Springfield* **37**, 430

Horton, G. E. (1958). 'Mumps myocarditis: Case report with review of literature.' *Ann. intern. Med.* **49**, 1228

Irvin, M. Z., Bacharach, T. H. and Pullen, R. L. (1951). 'Mumps Myocarditis.' *NW. Med., Seattle* **50**, 583

Krakower, C. A. and Roberg, N. B. (1962). 'Clinical pathologic conference.' *Am. Heart J.* **63**, 276

Levy, R. L. and Von Glahn, W. C. (1944). 'Cardiac hypertrophy of unknown cause. A study of the clinical and pathologic features in 10 adults.' *Am. Heart J.* **28**, 714

Manca, C. (1932). 'Miocardite da parotite epidemica.' *Archo ital. Anat. Istol. patol.* **3**, 707

Noren, G. R., Adams, P. and Anderson, R. C. (1963). 'Positive skin reactivity to mumps virus antigen in endocardial fibroelastosis.' *J. Pediat.* **62**, 604

Roberts, W. C. and Fox, S. M. (1965). 'Mumps of the heart. Clinical and pathologic features.' *Circulation* **32**, 342

Rosenberg, D. H. (1945). 'Electrocardiographic changes in epidemic parolitis (Mumps).' *Proc. Soc. exp. Biol. Med.* **58**, 9

Saphir, O. and Cohen, N. A. (1957). 'Myocarditis in infancy.' *Archs Path.* **64**, 446

Sellers, F. J., Keith, J. D. and Manning, J. A. (1964). 'The diagnosis of primary endocardial fibroelastosis.' *Circulation* **29**, 49

Shone, J. D., Muñoz Armas, S., Manning, J. A. and Keith, J. D. (1966). 'The mumps antigen skin test in endocardial fibroelastosis.' *Pediatrics, Springfield* **37**, 423

St Geme, J. W., Noren, G. R. and Adams, P., Jnr (1966). 'Proposed embryopathic relation between mumps virus and primary endocardial fibroelastosis.' *New Engl. J. Med.* **275**, 339

Wendkos, M. H. and Noll, J., Jnr (1944). 'Myocarditis caused by epidemic parotitis.' *Am. Heart J.* **27**, 414

INFLUENZA

The heart is involved in a proportion of cases of influenza but there is conflicting evidence as to the extent of involvement clinically and pathologically. Clinical manifestations include dyspnoea, palpitations, anginoid pain, arrhythmia and heart block.

Cardiac involvement rarely occurs during the acute phase of the disease but may follow a week or two later. Hamburger (1938) regarded the conduction system as especially vulnerable. Lucke, Wright and Kime (1919) in a series of 125 fatal cases of influenza found cloudy swelling, and vacuolation of fibres with oedema of the interstitial tissue, but did not describe an actual myocarditis. In two cases reported by Finland *et al.* (1945) the lesions consisted of interstitial infiltrations of plasma cells, lymphocytes and occasionally large mononuclears with neutrophils and eosinophils. Foci of muscle necrosis were noted and some fibres were invaded with mononuclear cells. Influenza A virus was isolated from the lungs of these cases.

Of 8 cases of viral myopericarditis reported by Adams (1959) 5 were associated with influenza B, 2 with both influenza A and B and 1 with influenza A. Coltman (1962) noted persistent elevation of serum transaminase and a strongly positive complement-fixation test for influenza A (titre 1:1024) in a patient with acute respiratory disease, tachycardia, an enlarged heart, atrial fibrillation and inverted T waves. Two weeks later these changes disappeared, and two months later a coronary anteriogram showed no abnormalities. In a study of 13 fatal cases of Asian influenza during the 1957 epidemic, Oseasohn, Adelson and Kaji (1959), found in 3 cases segmented or circumferential fibrinoid necrosis of myocardial arterioles, with secondary atrial thrombi, and in other 10, myocarditis ranging in severity from slight oedema with scattered foci of pleomorphic cells, to diffuse infiltrates of lymphocytes, monocytes and scanty neutrophils. In the vicinity of the exudate the muscle fibres were shrunken and intensely eosinophilic, the striations being lose while many of the nuclei were pyknotic. Eight of the patients were less than 40 years old and the duration of illness varied from 2 to 8 days.

Similar changes have been described in one of 46 cases of Asian flu reported by Giles and Shuttleworth (1957). It is not possible to determine the role of the myocardial lesions as a cause of death.

References

Adams, C. W. (1959). 'Post viral myopericarditis associated with the influenzae virus.' *Am. J. Cardiol.* **4**, 56

Coltman, C. A., Jnr. (1962). 'Influenza myocarditis.' *J. Am. med. Ass.* **180**, 204

Finland, M., Parker, F., Jnr, Barnes, M. W. and Jolliffe, L. S. (1945). 'Acute myocarditis in influenza A infections.' *Am. J. med. Sci.* **209**, 455

Giles, C. and Shuttleworth, E. M. (1957). 'Post mortem findings in 46 influenza deaths.' *Lancet* **2**, 1224

Hamburger, W. W. (1938). 'The heart in influenza.' *Med. Clins N. Am.* **22**, 111

Lucke, B., Wright, T. and Kime, E. (1919). 'Pathologic anatomy and bacteriology of influenza.' *Archs intern. Med.* **24**, 154

Oseasohn, R., Adelson, L. and Kaji, M. (1959). 'Clinico-pathologic study of 33 fatal cases of Asian influenza.' *New Engl. J. Med.* **260**, 509

PSITTACOSIS AND ORNITHOSIS

Humans may contract *psittacosis* from psittacine birds, such as parrots or budgerigars and from canaries, whilst the similar but milder condition *ornithosis* (Anderson, 1969) is contracted from non-psittacine birds, such as wild fowl. The agents responsible belong to the *Chlamydia bedsonia* group, which are larger than true viruses, smaller than rickettsiae and are sensitive to antibiotics. The symptoms of these diseases are cough with sputum, fever, sore throat, headache, aching muscles, chest pain, dyspnoea and sometimes haemoptysis. The ESR is raised and the x-ray of the lungs shows varying homogeneous ground-glass appearances. The disease often takes several weeks to clear up or may sometimes prove fatal. Adamy (1930) commented on the development of post-infectious myocardial degeneration in psittacosis. In the case reported by Walton (1954) there were only oedema and a few areas of mononuclear cell exudate in the interstitial tissue.

The occurrence of myocarditis, presumably caused by the psittacosis agent was reported by Vosti and Roffwarg (1961) in a 48 year old woman with pneumonia who developed gallop rhythm and hypotension, and died from ensuing encephalitis one month later; of six parakeets which she had kept in her home, one had died and another was found to harbour psittacosis virus. Her psittacosis complement-fixation test was positive to a dilution of 1:64. The heart showed thrombi attached to the posterior wall of the left ventricle, scattered foci of fibrosis, and soft areas in which there was a loss of muscle associated with recent granulation tissue. No coronary artery disease was present. Microemboli were observed in the brain, which also showed peri-vascular cuffing with lymphocytes, and in many other viscera.

Jannach (1958) reported psittacosis in an 18 month old girl. The myocardium contained foci of monocytes, macrophages and lymphocytes, interspersed between isolated necrotic muscle fibres. Subsequent to the child's death, the virus was isolated from a parakeet to which she had been exposed. Spherical intracytoplasmic (Levinthal–Coles–Lillie) inclusion bodies, 280–800 μm in diameter were observed within macrophages in the lungs. When treated with Giemsa's stain the aggregations were purple, with Macchiavello's stain red and blue, and with Castãneda's stain deep blue; virus particles were visualized using dark field, ultraviolet, phase contrast and electron microscopy.

Coll and Horner (1967) described myocarditis in a youth of 18 years who had headache, fever, leg pains with extremely tender calf muscles and retrosternal pain, possibly due to pericarditis. Psittacosis complement-fixation titres rose to 1 in 480 within the first month of the disease (1 in 16 being diagnostic).

MacLennan, Dymmock and Ross (1967) in the same year reported the case of a boy aged 13 who kept budgerigars; he developed a purulent cough and then later blood-stained sputum, with heart failure and pleural effusion. Necropsy revealed myocarditis and pulmonary embolism. Serum obtained three and a half weeks after the onset gave a titre of 1 in 1024 to the psittacosis group.

Sutton et al. (1967) in Chicago examined 599 sera from patients with suspected pericarditis or myocarditis, and found 3 (Group I) who had inflammatory heart disease (men of 33 and 45 years and a woman of 65) and 6 (Group II) who possibly had myocardial disease (3 men and 3 women aged 35–52 years). Group I had been exposed to parakeets, had radiological pulmonary infiltrates, showed a 4-fold rise of complement fixing-antibodies to psittacosis antigen, responded favourably to antibiotics and made a complete recovery. One patient had a pericardial effusion, 2 had fever, precardial pain or cardiomegaly, and 3 had ST changes in the electrocardiogram.

Diagnosis is confirmed by culture of the sputum, throat washings or blood for virus (if no antibiotics have been given) and the complement-fixation test for psittacosis should give a four-fold rise in titre for firm diagnosis. As the virus is quite sensitive to the tetracycline group, recovery of virus from specimens is often un-successful soon after the commencement of specific therapy.

From necropsies, spleen and lung tissue should be taken for culture of the virus in mia and eggs. The frequency of the disease in bird fanciers is well established and in the home, women seem particularly liable to infection, probably because they usually look after household pets, and children are somewhat more susceptible to the virus.

References

Adamy, G. (1930). 'Klinische studie über die Psittakose.' *Dt. Arch. klin.*, *Med.* **169**, 301

Anderson, J. P. (1969). 'Ornithosis—some current views.' *Med. News*, April 11, p. 9

Coll, R. and Horner, I. (1967). 'Cardiac involvement in psittacosis.' *Br. med. J.* **4**, 35

Jannach, J. R. (1958). 'Myocarditis in infancy with inclusions characteristic of psittacosis.' *Am. J. Dis. Child.* **96**, 734

MacLennan, W. J., Dymmock, I. W. and Ross, Constance (1967). 'Cardiac involvement in psittacosis.' *Br. med. J.* **4**, 620

Sutton, G. C., Marrissey, R. A., Tobin, J. R., Jnr and Anderson, T. O. (1967). 'Pericardial and myocardial disease associated with serological evidence of infection by agents of the psittacosis-group.' *Circulation* **36**, 830

Vosti, G. J. and Roffwarg, H. (1961). 'Myocarditis and encephalitis in a case of suspected psittacosis.' *Ann. intern. Med.* **54**, 764

Walton, K. W. (1954). 'The pathology of a fatal case of psittacosis showing intracytoplasmic inclusions in the meninges.' *J. Path. Bact.* **68**, 565

MEASLES

RUBELLA

Rubella, contracted by the mother during the first trimester of pregnancy, frequently results in congenital heart lesions (usually septal defects or patient ductus arteriosus) in the baby. At the time of infection the developing foetal heart is miniscule, and its capacity to produce a significant inflammatory response is questionable. It is not astonishing therefore, to observe no trace of the infection in the hearts of the afflicted neonatals.

In postnatal rubella, cardiac complications are infrequent. Logue and Hanson (1945) observed complete heart block, and Goldfinger, Schreiber and Wosika (1947) described permanent 2:1 AV block following rubella. Autopsy confirmation of active myocarditis following German measles, however, is lacking.

References

Goldfinger, D., Schreiber, W. and Wosika, P. H. (1947). 'Permanent heart block following German measles.' *Am. J. Med.* **2**, 320

Logue, R. B. and Hanson, J. F. (1945). 'Complete heart block in German measles.' *Am. Heart J.* **30**, 205

MORBILLI

Myocarditis is a relatively infrequent complication of measles. However, Giustra and Nilson (1950) observed tachycardia, 2:1 heart block and notched T waves in a young boy 13 days after the onset of measles. During the subsequent three years the child experienced recurrent episodes of acute arrhythmia, during one of which he died. At autopsy the heart exhibited diffuse subendocardial sclerosis and focal fibrosis involving the left bundle branch. Degan (1937) in reviewing 100 fatal cases of measles found lymphocytic infiltration, chiefly perivascular, in four of the hearts.

In a study of an epidemic of over 1600 measles patients in South Greenland, Christensen *et al.* (1953) found heart failure to have been a serious complication, accounting for 2·2 per cent of the deaths.

Ross (1952) studied 125 electrocardiograms from 71 children and found 30 per cent with prolonged PR intervals and 29 per cent with altered QT complexes.

Goldfield, Bayer and Weinstein (1955), in a series of cases studied intensively, found electrocardiographic abnormalities occurred in nearly 20 per cent.

Myocarditis has also been seen in the prodromal stage of measles (Blattner, 1964). Cohen (1963) encountered in one heart interstitial infiltrates of histiocytes and lymphocytes, with and without related foci of necrosis of myocardial fibres. He found characteristic multi-nucleated Warthin–Finkeldey giant cells in the lungs, thymus and lymph nodes, but not in the heart.

References

Blattner, R. J. (1964). 'Myocarditis in prodromal measles.' (Editorial) *J. Pediat.* **65**, 144

Christensen, P. E., Schmidt, H., Bang, H. O., Anersen, V., Jordan, L. B. and Jensen, O. (1953). 'An epidemic of measles in southern Greenland, 1951. Measles in virgin soil, II. The epidemic proper.' *Acta med. scand.* **144**, 430

Cohen, H. A. (1963).'Myocarditis in prodromal measles.' *Am. J. clin. Path.* **40**, 50

Degan, J. A. (1937). 'Visceral pathology in measles: A clinico-pathologic study of 100 cases.' *Am. J. Med. Sci.* **194**, 104

Giustra, F. X. and Nilson, D. C. (1950). 'Final report on a case of myo-carditis following measles.' *Am. J. Dis. Child.* **79**, 487

Goldfield, M., Bayer, N. H. and Weinstein. L. (1955). 'Electrocardio-graphic changes during the course of measles.' *J. Pediat.* **46**, 30

Ross, L. S. (1952). 'Electrocardiographic finding in measles.' *Am. J. Dis. Child.* **83**, 282

SMALLPOX

Reports of cardiac involvement following smallpox are extremely uncommon. Anderson *et al.* (1951) reported that five young nurses, none of whom had been vaccinated, but all previously in excellent health, died of smallpox contracted during an epidemic. All of them manifested clinical evidence of myocarditis, and the cause of death in each case was acute cardiac failure. Complement-fixation tests were positive and the virus was cultured from skin lesions.

Reference

Anderson, T., Foulis, M. A., Grist, N. R. and Landsman, J. B. (1951). 'Clinical and laboratory observations in a smallpox outbreak.' *Lancet* **2**, 1248

VACCINIA

Dolgopol, Greenberg and Aronott (1955) described mononuclear cell infiltration in one fatal case of vaccinia. Myocarditis as a specific complication of anti-smallpox vaccination has been reported by Dalgaard (1957), Finlay-Jones (1964) and Caldera *et al.* (1961). The latter workers isolated vaccinia virus from the myocardium of an $11\frac{1}{2}$ month old girl who died 12 days after vaccination. Because the myocardium had been in contact with other organs (including the skin, prior to cultivation) they felt they could not definitely state that the myocarditis was vaccinial, even though they thought such an origin likely.

Characteristically, the myocarditis is diffuse with a mixed infiltrate of mononuclear cells and lesser numbers of lymphocytes, eosinophils and neutrophils. The infiltrations are present mainly in oedematous intramuscular septa, but also between degenerating muscle fibres. An occasional focus of necrotic muscle, surrounded by inflammatory cells, chiefly eosinophils, was observed by Finlay-Jones (1964).

References

Caldera, R., Sarrut, S., Mallet, R. and Rossier, A. (1961). 'Are there any cardiac complications in vaccine?' *Sen. Hôp. Paris* **37**, 1281

Dalgaard, J. B. (1957). 'Fatal myocarditis following smallpox vaccination.' *Am. Heart J.* **54**, 56

Dolgopol, V. B., Greenberg, M. and Aronott, R. (1955). 'Encephalitis following smallpox vaccination.' *Archs Neurol. Psychiat., Chicago* **73**, 216

Finlay-Jones, L. R. (1964). 'Fatal myocarditis after vaccinations for smallpox.' *New Engl. J. Med.* **270**, 41

INFECTIOUS MONONUCLEOSIS (GLANDULAR FEVER)

Cardiac complications have often been reported to attend infectious mononucleosis; the incidence of such complications has not been established, owing to the frequency of uncertainty in the diagnosis of mononucleosis. Custer and Smith (1948) have reported nine necropsies of patients with mononucleosis, in which the findings consisted chiefly of atypical lymphocytes in the peripheral blood. Aggregates of these cells may be found sparsely distributed within the myocardium, in the vicinity of small intramyocardial blood vessels or beneath the endocardium.

Fish and Barton (1958) described a case where myocardial necrosis was also present, associated with mononuclear cell infiltrates.

Hoagland (1956, 1964) has, however, reviewed these articles reporting a relatively high incidence of cardiac complications in infectious mononucleosis and has confirmed the opinion of many clinicians that there is little to fear from the cardiac complications of this disease and that minor electrocardiogram disturbances should not cause concern to clinician or patients. In a series of 419 patients, he found only 3 with cardiac symptoms, 2 with palpitations and 1 with dyspnoea on exertion, although there were 338 patients with abnormal electrocardiogram tracings (Hoagland, 1964).

References

Custer, R. P. and Smith, E. B. (1948). 'The pathology of infectious mono-nucleosis.' *Blood* 3, 830

Fish, M. and Barton, H. R. (1958). 'Heart involvement in infectious mononucleosis.' *Archs intern. Med.* **101**, 636

Hoagland, R. J. (1956). 'Cardiac involvement in infectious mononucleosis.' *Am. J. med. Sci.* **232**, 252

— (1964). 'Mononucleosis and heart disease.' *Am. J. Med. Sci.* **248**, 1

RABIES

In the last two cases of rabies occurring in the United Kingdom (cases 7 and 8, Macrae, 1969), an associated myocarditis was found at necropsy (Cheetham *et al.*, 1970).

The first patient was a 39 year old Pakistani woman bitten by a rabid dog in Pakistan, who was being given a 20-day prophylactic course of anti-rabies vaccine, but collapsed suddenly on day 18 of the course, following a generalized convulsion. Macroscopically the heart appeared normal, but microscopically it was seen to be infiltrated by lymphocytes, histiocytes and occasional neutrophils. This infiltrate was mainly in the interstitial tissue of the myocardium and around necrotic muscle fibres, but also involved the pericardium and the endocardium. There were inflammatory cells within and adherent to the walls of many vessels in the heart.

The second patient was a 46 year old Indian who had been bitten by a supposedly rabid dog in India some six months before. He had started on a course of 14 intramuscular injections of anti-rabies vaccine the following day. When in England he fell while drunk and collapsed and died some days later, after being admitted to

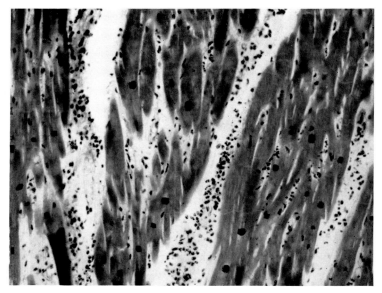

Figure 8.4. Active myocarditis caused by rabies. The myocardium is diffusely infiltrated with lymphocytes, histiocytes and a few neutrophils. This infiltrate is found mainly within the interstitial tissue (haematoxylin and eosin × 200, reduced to 2/3). (Reproduced from Cheetham et al. (1970) by courtesy of the authors and Editor of the Lancet)

hospital without recovering consciousness. On x-ray some cardiac enlargement was seen. At autopsy the heart was macroscopically normal (350 g), but microscopically the myocardium was diffusely infiltrated with lymphocytes, histiocytes and occasional neutrophils. The infiltration was mainly in the interstitial tissue of the myocardium and around the necrotic muscle fibres, but also involved the pericardium and the endocardium. There were also some areas of interstitial fibrosis (*Figure 8.4*). The diagnosis of rabies in these cases was confirmed by an examination of cerebral tissue, where in both cases Negri bodies were demonstrated, and the virus subsequently isolated by animal inoculation (Macrae, 1969).

In the only other case previously reported, where histological changes were found in the heart (Ross and Armentrout, 1962), a similar picture of an active myocarditis was seen.

It is not certain if the myocarditis in any of these cases was due to direct involvement of the heart by the rabies virus, as no attempts to isolate the virus from myocardial tissue were carried out. Although immunofluorescent tests on paraffin sections of case 1 of Cheetham *et al.* (1970) were negative, this does not exclude the presence of rabies virus (WHO, 1966).

In all the cases of rabies myocarditis, there was clinical evidence of this condition: in the two described by Cheetham *et al.* (1970) there was marked pulmonary oedema, tachycardia and hypotension, while in that of Ross and Armentrout (1962) there was tachycardia, gallop-rhythm and also hypotension.

It thus seems probable that myocarditis may well play an important part in the terminal stages of rabies but that cardiac lesions have very probably been overlooked by investigators in the past, as these people have concentrated largely on the central nervous system, especially as the heart appears macroscopically to be uninvolved.

References

Cheetham, H. D., Hart, J., Coghill, N. F. and Fox, B. (1970). 'Rabies with myocarditis. Two cases in England.' *Lancet* **1**, 921

Macrae, A. D. (1969). 'Rabies in England.' *Lancet* **2**, 1415

Ross, E. and Armentrout, S. A. (1962). 'Myocarditis associated with rabies.' *New Engl. J. Med.* **266**, 1087

World Health Organization. (1966). 'Laboratory Techniques in Rabies.' Monograph Series No. 22

YELLOW FEVER

In most fatal cases of yellow fever the heart is flabby and rarely displays petechial haemorrhage in the epicardial and endocardial surfaces. Fatty alteration of the myocardial fibre is most severe in the subendocardium and occasional foci of myocardial necrosis may be seen.

In 2 of 29 cases examined by Connell (1928) there was also a cellular response in association with the damaged muscle fibre.

Bugher (1951), however, reported minimal cellular infiltration or fibro-elastic proliferations in the cases which he described. Lloyd (1931) observed in experimental yellow fever in monkeys, degenerative changes throughout the heart, including fatty and granular degeneration of the myofibres, occasional areas of hyalinization, and isolated areas of necrosis of muscle fibres surrounded by foci of lymphocytes and occasionally polymorphs.

References

Bugher, J. C. (1951). 'The pathology of yellow fever.' In *Yellow Fever*. Ed. by G. K. Strode, pp. 137–163. New York: McGraw Hill
Connell, D. E. (1928). 'Myocardial degeneration in yellow fever.' *Am. J. Path.* **4**, 431
Lloyd, W. (1931). 'The myocardium in yellow fever. II. Myocardial lesions in experimental yellow-fever.' *Am. Heart J.* **6**, 504

VARICELLA (CHICKENPOX)

The rare involvement of the heart in varicella was thought to be non-specific until Hackel (1953) reported myocarditis in seven patients who had died during the course of acute varicella. There were no clinical signs of myocarditis, and death in all cases had been attributed to pneumonia. The hearts microscopically exhibited focal lesions consisting of interstitial oedema, collections of mono-nuclear cells and lymphocytes, and occasional plasma cells, poly-morphs and eosinophils. Focal necrosis of muscle fibres was also present, together with inclusion bodies. Hackel felt that in the absence of a history of rheumatic fever or endocarditis, focal myocarditis might be explained on the basis of a viral aetiology. Sampson (1959) described similar findings of viral myocarditis in a child. Tatter *et al.* (1964) encountered varicella myocarditis in a three year old girl with chickenpox, who died suddenly six days after the appearance of the rash. Her heart displayed hypertrophy, haemorrhagic streaking and stipplings, diffuse interstitial and peri-vascular infiltration of large histiocytes, plasma cells and occasional lymphocytes. Intranuclear inclusions were also present in myocardial fibres, and cellular infiltration extended to both endocardium and epicardium. Unfortunately, viral studies were not carried out on the cardiac tissue, but the formation of intranuclear inclusion bodies in several human viscera is a well-recognized property of this virus.

References

Hackel, D. B. (1953). 'Myocarditis in association with varicella.' *Am. J. Path.* **29**, 369
Sampson, C. C. (1959). 'Varicella myocarditis—report of a case.' *J. natn. med. Ass.* **53**, 138

Tatter, D., Gerard, P. W., Silverman, A. H., Wane, C. and Pearson, H. E. (1964). 'Fatal varicella pericarditis in a child.' *Am. J. Dis. Child.* **68**, 88

HERPES SIMPLEX

Ross and Stevenson (1961) reported the cardiac changes found in a mixed series of paediatric and adult cases of herpes simplex meningo-encephalitis and stated that such cases made up 19·3 per cent (6/31) of all cases of meningo-encephalitis studied during the period by serological methods.

Macroscopically the heart is unremarkable, but microscopically the myocardium shows an interstitial myocarditis of chronic inflammatory cells which is masked by numerous cardiac histiocytes. There are also areas of increased fibrosis.

References

Ross, C. A. and Stevenson, J. (1961). 'Herpes simplex meningo-encephalitis.' *Lancet* **2**, 682

POLIOMYELITIS

Saphir and Wile (1942) reported myocarditis in 6 of 7 patients with acute poliomyelitis and, subsequently (Saphir, 1945), in 10 of 17 additional cases. Myocarditis was reported also by Ludden and Edwards (1949) in 14 of 28 cases. Jungeblut and Edwards (1951) isolated the causative virus from the hearts of three patients with poliomyelitis. Histologically only neutrophils are seen in the early stages but later focal areas of myocardial necrosis and infiltrates of lymphocytes and macrophages are visible. Laake (1951) found electrocardiogram abnormalities in 31 per cent of 265 patients with acute poliomyelitis and Kipkie and McAuley (1954) estimated, on the basis of reports in the literature, that myocarditis occurs in approximately 42 per cent of patients with poliomyelitis.

References

Jungeblut, C. W. and Edwards, J. E. (1951). 'Isolation of poliomyelitis virus from the heart in fatal cases.' *Am. J. clin. Path.* **21**, 601

Kipkie, G. F. and McAuley, S. M. (1954), 'Acute myocarditis occurring in bulbar polio.' *Can. med. Ass. J.* **70**, 315

Laake, H. (1951). 'Myocarditis in poliomyelitis.' *Acta med. scand.* **140**, 159

Ludden, T. E. and Edwards, J. E. (1949). 'Carditis in poliomyelitis.' *Am. J. Path.* **25**, 357

Saphir, O. (1945). 'Visceral lesions in poliomyelitis.' *Am. J. Path.* **21**, 99

Saphir, O. and Wile, S. A. (1942). 'Myocarditis in poliomyelitis.' *Am. J. med. Sci.* **203**, 781

GONOCOCCAL MYOCARDITIS

Myocarditis may occur as an extension of the rare ailment, gonococcal endocarditis. Williams (1938) reported focal suppurative myocardial necrosis in 6 of 10 patients who had died from acute or subacute gonococcal endocarditis. In the absence of cultural studies a history of gonococcal arthritis or urethritis and demonstration of intracellular Gram-negative, bean-shaped diplococci in the lesions, permits a diagnosis of gonococcal myocarditis (Saphir, 1958).

References

Saphir, O. (Ed.) (1958). 'A text on systemic pathology.' In *Heart: Classification of Myocarditis*, Vol. 1, pp. 64–70. New York: Grune and Stratton
Williams, R. H. (1938). 'Gonococcic endocarditis.' *Archs intern. Med.* **61**, 26

TULARAEMIA

Although tularaemia may be associated with cardiac disability, accompanying myocardial lesions have been observed only infrequently (Saphir, 1960). Goodpasture and Wandhouse (1928) described focal perivascular mononuclear infiltrates in the heart attending tularaemia.

Among 14 cases of tularaemia, Lillie and Francis (1936) described focal myocardial degeneration in 3 instances and diffuse interstitial myocarditis in 1. They had difficulties, however, in producing cardiac lesions in rabbits, only one out of 28 rabbits with acute tularaemia revealed focal necrosis. Experimentally, in late acute or subacute infection focal granulomatous lesions were found. Only 13 of 64 rabbits with more prolonged illness produced tuberculoid foci.

References

Goodpasture, E. and Wandhouse, S. J. (1928). 'Pathologic anatomy of tularaemia in man.' *Am. J. Path.* **4**, 213
Lillie, R. D. and Francis, E. (1936). 'The pathology of tularaemia.' *National Institute of Health Bulletin 167*, pp. 217. US Treasury Department Public Health Services
Saphir, O. (1960). 'Non-rheumatic inflammatory disease of the heart.' In *Pathology of the Heart*, Ed. by S. E. Gould, pp. 778–823. Springfield, Ill: Thomas

HEPATITIS

INFECTIOUS HEPATITIS

Infectious hepatitis is found most frequently in children and young adults and is spread by faecal contamination. The disease shows a seasonal incidence especially in the winter and autumn and the incubation period is 15–45 days. Suspected cases of the disease not showing jaundice can be detected by the transaminase test. The

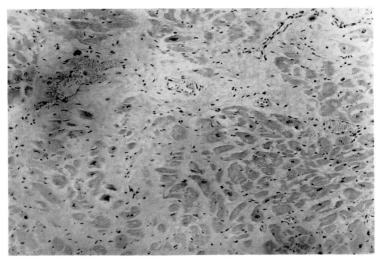

Figure 8.5. The myocardium from a patient who died from infective hepatitis. Some of the myocardial fibres are necrotic and are surrounded by much oedematous interstitial tissue, which contains few inflammatory cells—largely lymphocytes (haematoxylin and eosin × 42, reduced to 2/3)

mortality in reported series appears to be about 1 per cent, but in certain outbreaks has been considerably higher.

Saphir, Ambomin and Yokoo (1965) reported the finding of myocarditis in 4 of 6 patients who had died of infectious hepatitis, the most characteristic features of which were minute foci of necrosis of isolated muscle bundles, together with diffuse serous inflammation. The necrotic foci were often surrounded by lymphocytes, myocardial reticulocytes and a few polymorphonuclear leucocytes. Minute isolated necrotic muscle fibres not surrounded by inflammatory cells were also seen. There was also an increase in fibrous tissue present (*Figure 8.5*). Most interesting was the isolated muscle

fibre necrosis involving the left bundle of His with the presence of a
few lymphocytes and polymorphs in three of the four patients. In
Lucke's review (1944) of 125 fatal cases of epidemic hepatitis from
the US army in World War II however, no myocardial changes
were found, except for the frequent finding of small haemorrhages
between the endocardium and pericardium.

SERUM HEPATITIS

Serum hepatitis affects adults and is acquired by the parenteral
route. It has an incubation period of about 2–5 months, and shows

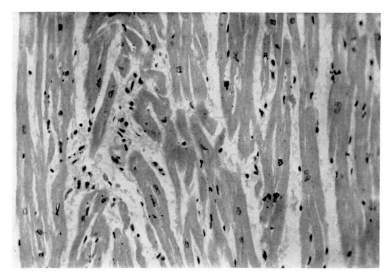

*Figure 8.6.   Section of the myocardium from a patient who died from serum
hepatitis showing diffuse infiltrations with lymphocytes together with marked
oedema of the interstitial tissue (haematoxylin and eosin × 260, reduced to 2/3)*

no seasonal variation. Infection is caused by the entry of the virus
through the intact skin, usually by way of the administration of
infected blood or pooled plasma. The mortality rate is about 10 per
cent but as no electrocardiogram studies have been carried out on
patients with this disease the exact incidence of cardiac involvement
is not known. There are no reported cases of any myocardial
changes being found in autopsies in patients with the disease, but I
have personally seen several cases in which the myocardium was
diffusely infiltrated with chronic inflammatory cells. In these cases
the myocardial interstitial tissue is markedly odematous (*Figure 8.6*).

The above two forms of hepatitis are very similar clinically but caused by different virus strains, which do not give cross-immunity. Although fully characterized neither virus has yet been propagated in culture.

References

Lucke, B. (1944). 'The pathology of fatal epidemic hepatitis.' *Am. J. Path.* **20**, 471

Saphir, O., Ambomin, G. D. and Yokoo, H. (1956). 'Myocarditis in viral (epidemic) hepatitis.' *Am. J. med. Sci.* **231**, 168

Nine

Rickettsial, bacterial and spirochaetal infections

RICKETTSIAL INFECTIONS

TYPHUS

Wolbach, Todd and Palfrey (1922) described inflammatory changes in the myocardium caused by typhus as nodular, predominantly mononuclear, interstitial infiltrates, most prominent in the deepest parts of the ventricular wall (*Figure 9.1*), and frequently with thrombosis of small arterioles and venules (*Figure 9.2*). Similar lesions were described by Herzog and Rodriguez (1936) in 97 per cent of 103 patients with typhus.

Collections of small red intracytoplasmic bodies seen in some cardiac muscle fibres are rickettsia and may be shown by using Macchiavello's stain (*Figure 9.3*).

SCRUB TYPHUS

Macroscopic changes in the heart caused by scrub typhus (tsutsugamushi disease) are minimal (Settle, Pinkerton and Corbett, 1945). Microscopically focal or diffuse mononuclear infiltrates associated with endothelial swelling in small vascular channels have been observed. Similar changes were reported by Levine (1946) in all of 31 cases, in approximately one half of which such findings were associated with focal necrosis.

Allen and Spitz (1945) recorded abnormal myocardial findings in 99 of 110 patients (90 per cent) with rickettsial infections. These were present in 93 per cent of 74 patients with scrub typhus; in 83 per cent of 84 patients with epidemic typhus; and in 73 per cent of 12 with Rocky Mountain spotted fever. Microscopically interstitial infiltrates were usually apparent and, less often, periarterial infiltrates; both were composed of plasma cells, neutrophils and Anitschkow cells. Polymorphonuclear cells were most often present in spotted fever and in this condition isolated necrotic muscle fibres were only rarely noted.

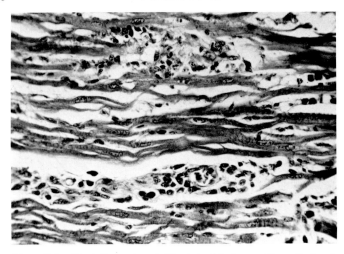

Figure 9.1. The inflammatory infiltrate in this disease (from the heart of a young Indian) usually takes the form of nodular, predominantly mononuclear interstitial infiltrates (× 240, reduced to 6/10). (Reproduced by courtesy of Major-General Sacks)

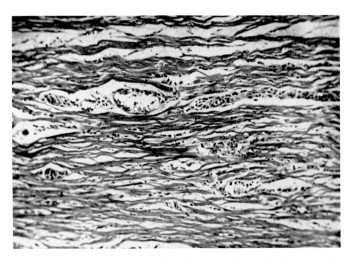

Figure 9.2. There is frequently focal necrosis of muscle fibres together with thrombosis of some small blood vessels (× 240, reduced to 6/10). (Reproduced by courtesy of Major-General Sacks)

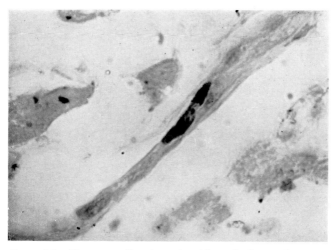

Figure 9.3. The myocardium in typhus (from the heart of a young Indian). A collection of small red intracytoplasmic bodies in a muscle fibre which are Rickettsia (Macchiavello's stain × 800, reduced to 6/10). (Reproduced by courtesy of Major-General Sacks)

Q FEVER

Wendt (1953) described myocarditis in Q fever; its frequency in the infection is, however, unknown.

In the case of a 60 year old man described by Evans, Powell and Barrell (1959), who died from endocarditis associated with Q fever, the cardiac changes were as follows; apart from the presence of friable vegetation in the aortic valve.

Macroscopically the pericardium was seen to contain a few petechial haemorrhages while the wall of the left ventricle was thickened. The endocardium of the posterior wall of the left ventricle showed an area of pallor 3 cm in diameter. Numerous greyish-white spots, 0·5–1 cm in diameter, were distributed throughout the muscle of the left ventricle.

Microscopically the left ventricle showed subendocardial collagen formation. The white foci seen macroscopically were areas where the muscle fibres had become necrotic and swollen. Groups of muscle fibres were disrupted and oedematous. There were irregular areas of fibrosis. A small branch of the left coronary artery was entirely occluded by thrombus.

A few red coccobacillary forms were seen amongst the necrotic fibres near the endocardial surface of the left ventricle.

To demonstrate rickettsia histologically the best stain to use is Macchiavello's. The stain shows obvious brownish-red intracytoplasmic organisms. These organisms vary from coccobacillary forms, about 0·5 μm in diameter, to large irregular ovoids about 3 μm in diameter.

To isolate rickettsia, suspensions of the myocardium and spleen are diluted 1/5, 1/10, 1/50 and 1/250 and then inoculated into guinea-pigs. Two guinea-pigs are used for each dilution. At 4 and 6 weeks serum from these animals is tested for rickettsia antibodies. When these animals die or are killed after 6 weeks, impression smears are taken from the spleen and then stained into Macchiavello's stain. If the test is positive, large numbers of rickettsial-like bodies are seen intracellularly.

References

Allen, A. C. and Spitz, S. (1945). 'A comparative study of the pathology of scrub typhus (Tsutsugamushi disease) and other rickettsial diseases.' *Am. J. Path.* **21**, 603

Evans, A. D., Powell, D. E. D. and Barrell, C. D. (1959). 'Fatal endocarditis associated with Q. Fever.' *Lancet* **1**, 864

Herzog, E. and Rodriguez, H. (1936). 'Die Beteiligung des Myocardi beim Fleckfieber.' *Beitr. path. Anat.* **96**, 431

Levine, H. D. (1946). 'Pathologic study of 31 cases of scrub typhus fever with special references to the cardiovascular system.' *Am. Heart J.* **31**, 314

Settle, E. B., Pinkerton, H. and Corbett, J. A. (1945). 'A pathologic study of the tsutsugamushi disease (Scrub typhus) with notes on clinical pathological correlations.' *J. Lab. clin. Med.* **30**, 639

Wendt, M. L. (1953). 'Myokarditis bei Q. Fieber.' *Z. ges. inn. Med.* **1**, 93

Wolbach, S. B., Todd, J. L. and Palfrey, F. W. (1922). *The Etiology and Pathology of Typhus*, pp. 222. Cambridge: Harvard University Press

BACTERIAL INFECTIONS

INFECTIONS OF THE UPPER RESPIRATORY TRACT

Myocarditis may develop during an upper respiratory tract infection, especially tonsillitis, and its incidence is much higher than is appreciated at the autopsy table.

Scherf (1940) stated that clinically detectable myocarditis developed among 10–15 per cent of patients with tonsillitis. Candel and Wheelock (1945) reported the post-mortem findings in one case of acute myocarditis secondary to tonsillitis which they believed to be the first reported case of myocarditis in this disease. The inflammatory reaction in the myocardium consisted of a diffuse infiltration with polymorphs but no bacteriological studies were carried out. Lustock, Chase and Lubitz (1955) encountered 13 instances of myocarditis among 45 patients with upper respiratory tract infection. Gore and Saphir (1947) while studying 1402 cases of myocarditis at the Armed Forces Institute of Pathology found it to be associated with upper respiratory tract infection in 35 cases (2·5 per cent); acute tonsillitis in 12, and acute nasopharyngitis in 23 instances. All were males between 20 and 30 years of age and the duration of the illness was 4–38 days. In all cases the cause of death was cardiac failure: fifteen of the patients had died unexpectedly—all of them within two weeks after the onset of the infection. Grossly the hearts showed grey streaks with red or yellow mottling and a softened flabby or friable myocardium. The characteristic findings were necrosis of myocardial fibres together with interstitial infiltrates, consisting chiefly of lymphocytes but also of macrophages, neutrophils and Anitschkow myocytes. In some cases these workers noted a diffuse type where the interstitial cellular exudate was associated with extensive muscle-cell necrosis, an interstitial type where muscle necrosis was not prominent and a mixed type. The authors did not believe that these myocardial changes were the result of septicaemia and were unable to demonstrate organisms in stained sections.

In persons who had died more than two weeks after the onset of the respiratory infection, the loss of muscle fibres was associated with early fibroblastic proliferation,

Bacteriological examinations were not adequately carried out, and it is possible that some of these cases were of viral origin. Four of these cases showed fibrinoid necrosis and could have been rheumatic cases in the prodromal stage of the disease. Thirteen of these cases also had pneumonia.

References

Candel, S. and Wheelock, M. C. (1945). 'Acute non-specific myocarditis.' *Ann. intern. Med.* **23**, 309

Gore, I. and Saphir, O. (1947). 'Myocarditis. A classification of 1402 cases.' *Am. Heart J.* **34**, 831

Lustock, M. J., Chase, J. and Lubitz, J. M. (1955). 'Myocarditis. Clinical and pathogenic study of 45 cases.' *Dis. Chest* **28**, 243

Scherf, D. (1940). 'Myocarditis following acute tonsillitis.' *Bull. N. Y. med. Coll.* **3**, 252

DIPHTHERITIC MYOCARDITIS

Myocardial damage is a well known and sometimes fatal complication of diphtheria, which manifests itself clinically in disorders of rhythm including heart block, cardiac failure and sudden death.

Indeed, Gore and Saphir (1947) found, in examining 221 cases of diphtheria, that 144 had myocarditis; while in another study Gore (1948) found myocarditis in 143 of 205 fatal cases. There are numerous studies on the pathology of diphtheritic cardiac damage.

Very often cardiac signs do not develop immediately at the onset of the illness but, after four or five days, electrocardiogram signs are commonly found. Some days later arrythmias and cardiomegaly are often found; the patient develops rapidly progressive congestive heart failure which often proves resistant to the accepted methods of treatment. Apart from the isolation of corynebacteria from throat or nasal swabs, most other laboratory tests are negative, except for the serum glutamic oxalacetic transaminase, which may be raised to a level of about 100–150 units.

Mallony (1908) believed that there were two kinds of damage to the heart, one resulting from direct injury to the myocardial fibres, and a second type where an interstitial myocarditis was present, which was not dependent on initial damage to the myocardial fibres. This view is not now generally accepted and it is now believed, on the basis of experimental and post-mortem studies, that the primary lesion consists of toxic myocardial damage and that the cellular changes are secondary (Warthin, 1924; Gukelberger, 1936).

At autopsy the heart is enlarged and dilated, pale and flabby, and the myocardium has a typical 'streaky' appearance. The most common microscopic change is a fatty infiltration of some myocardial cells and this is found in more than half of the cases.

Other forms of damage include hydropic change and the most severe form of damage results in myocytolysis and hyaline necrosis of muscle fibres. This severe type of damage is associated with an interstitial cellular exudate, consisting mainly of histiocytes, plasma cells and lymphocytes. Polymorphs and eosinophils are rare. Numerous large mononuclear cells with eosinophilic cytoplasm are present within the areas showing hyaline necrosis of muscle fibres. Periodic acid Schiff stains show a decrease in positive staining when compared with normal myocardium. By the end of the third week fibrosis occurs and adjacent to the fibrotic areas are hypertrophied muscle cells with large distorted nuclei. Eosinophilic infiltrate has also been described (Tanaka, 1912; Nuzum, 1919). The gaps left by the damaged muscle cells are replaced by fibrous tissue.

Stains for succinic and beta-hydroxybutyric dehydrogenase usually reveal extensive areas of early myocardial damage, especially in those areas of marked necrosis where there is considerably reduced activity of both enzymes.

The conducting system of the heart has been extensively studied in an attempt to show a connection between disorders of rhythm, especially heart block, and anatomical lesions. Various changes similar to but not parallel in degree to the changes in the myocardium have been reported. These include fatty change, necrosis of fibres and cellular infiltration.

The Purkinje fibres frequently have a large pale cellular appearance in cross section, with less oxidative enzyme activity than in normal myocardium. There is usually a complete loss of enzyme activity in the conducting fibres, which often show a 'ghost cell' appearance in enzyme preparations.

The relationship of the degree of damage to the type of organism has been investigated by McLeod, Orr and Woodcock (1938). Fatty change occurred in cases surviving more than five days and was not any more severe in the gravis as compared with the mitis type, but in general, the toxic effects were more frequent in the gravis and intermedius types.

Using immunofluorescent antibody technqiues diphtheria toxin can be visualized in the myocardium (Burch et al., 1968). The toxin is seen to be mainly localized within the large mononuclear cells in the necrotic areas which have previously been mentioned to have intensely eosinophilic cytoplasm in haematoxylin and eosin-stained sections. Within the myocardial fibres the toxin shows a patchy distribution and no toxin can be seen in areas of advanced necrosis.

Electronmicroscopy shows fragmentation of some myocardial fibres and degeneration of some of the mitochondria, while in other areas lipid droplets can be seen in some myocardial fibres.

Peripheral circulatory failure or congestive cardiac failure sometimes occurs in the course of diphtheria if the prognosis is grave. Sudden death may also occur, possibly from involvement of the conduction system. When recovery takes place the disorders of chronic rhythm usually disappear but sometimes heart block persists (Perry, 1939).

References

Burch, G. E., Shih Chien Sun, Sowal, R. S., Kang chv/cmv and Cozcozovgh, W. L. (1968). 'Diphtheritic myocarditis. A histochemical and electron microscopic study.' Am. J. Cardiol. 21, 261

Gore, I. (1948). 'Myocardial changes in fatal diphtheria. A summary of observations in 221 cases.' Am. J. Med. Sci. 215, 257

— and Saphir, O. (1947). 'Myocarditis. A classification of 1402 cases.' Am. Heart J. 34, 827

Gukelberger, M. (1936). 'Neue experimentelle Arbeiten über Beginn und Ausbreitung der diptheritischen Schadigung des Herzmuskels.' Z. ges. exp. Med. 97, 749

Mallony, F. B. (1908). *Bacteriology of Diphtheria*. Cambridge: Nuttall and Graham-Smith

McLeod, J. W., Orr, J. W. and Woodcock, E. de C. (1938). 'The morbid anatomy of gravis intermediate and mitis diphtheria.' *J. Path. Bact.* **48**, 99

Nuzum, F. (1919). 'Eosinophillous myocarditis in diphtheria.' *J. Am. med. Ass*, **73**, 1925

Perry, C. B. (1939). 'Persistent conduction defects following diphtheria.' *Br. Heart J.* **1**, 117

Tanaka, T. (1912). 'Ueber die Vercauderringen der Herzmusculatar vor allem der Atrio ventrikular bundels bei Diphtherie.' *Virchows Arch. path. Anat. Physiol.* **207**, 115

Warthin, A. S. (1924). 'The myocardial lesions of diphtheria.' *J. infect. Dis.* **35**, 32

STREPTOCOCCAL INFECTIONS

β-Haemolytic

Myocarditis is a frequent finding in fatal scarlet fever. Brody and Smith (1936) reported cardiac involvement in over 90 per cent of 44 patients with scarlet fever and 15 with other streptococcal infections. The lesions reported consist of focal or diffuse infiltrates in the interstitial tissue with mononuclear cells and occasional polymorphs, or infiltration with mononuclear cells beneath the endothelium of the ventricles or Thesbean veins. It is characterized by small foci of myocardial necrosis and interstitial as well as subendocardial infiltrates of lymphocytes (Gore, 1948).

Rantz, Boisvert and Spink (1945) observed non-specific myocarditis in 20 out of 185 patients (11 per cent) with haemolytic streptococcal infections. Gore and Saphir (1947) also found myocarditis in 24 of 44 cases of fatal scarlet fever. Unfortunately, bacteriological studies were not carried out, but organisms were sometimes detected in stained sections.

Benetsson, Birke and Wingstrand (1951) reported that among 3·9 per cent of 3069 patients with scarlet fever, non-fatal myocarditis developed during their first week of illness and lasted one to several weeks. Schenken and Coleman (1951) reported acute myocarditis attended by progressive heart failure in a five year old boy as a result of infection with a haemolytic micro-aerophilic streptococcus.

Viridans

Saphir, Katz and Gore (1950) who studied 76 fatal cases in which histological and electrocardiographical data could be correlated, showed that the major changes in *Streptococcus viridans* bacterial endocarditis are: (1) direct extension of the suppurative process from the valve into the adjacent myocardium; (2) ischaemic sequelae arising from the embolization of the coronary arteries or localized end arteritis; (3) toxic changes exhibited by granular or hyaline degeneration of muscle fibres, or interstitial myocarditis; (4) micro-abscesses arising from bacterial seeding; and (5) the presence of Aschoff bodies from a pre-existing rheumatic myocarditis. Saphir (1946) observed, among a series of 55 cases of subacute bacterial endocarditis, Aschoff nodules in 19 and granulomatous reactions to calcific emboli arising from healing vegetations in 4; the latter lesions had not been seen in persons during the era ante-dating sulphonamide or penicillin therapy. Acute bacterial endocarditis may sometimes complicate valvuloplasty and, in such instances, may extend into the myocardium.

References

Benetsson, E., Birke, G., and Wingstrand, H. (1951). 'Acute non-specific myocarditis in scarlet fever and acute haemolytes tonsillitis,' *Cardiologia* **18**, 360

Brody, A. and Smith, L. W. (1936), 'Visceral pathology in scarlet fever and related streptococcal infections.' *Am. J. Path.* **12**, 373

Gore, I. (1948). 'Myocarditis in infectious diseases.' *Am. Practnr. Philad.* **1**, 292

— and Saphir, O. (1947). 'Myocarditis associated with acute naso-pharyorgitis and acute tonsillitis.' *Am. Heart J.* **34**, 831

Rantz, L, A., Boisvert, P. J. and Spink, W. W. (1945). 'Etiology and pathogenesis of rheumatic fever.' *Archs intern. Med.* **76**, 131

Saphir, O. (1946). 'Myocardial granuloma in sub-acute bacterial endocarditis.' *Archs Path.* **42**, 574

— Katz, L. N. and Gore, I. (1950). 'The myocardium in sub-acute bacterial endocarditis.' *Circulation* **1**, 1155

Schenken, J. R. and Coleman, F. C. (1951). 'Microaerophilic streptococcus as a cause of acute isolated myocarditis.' *Am. J. clin. Path.* **21**, 451

INFECTION OF THE LOWER RESPIRATORY TRACT

Myocarditis is an infrequent complication of acute laryngo-tracheo-bronchitis. Saphir (1945) reported the unexpected death of five children with severe largyngeal oedema involving the epiglottis and glottis. Three of the five children also had an early broncho-pheumonia. The myocarditis was interstitial and primarily serous, with infiltrating lymphocytes and only occasional neutrophils.

Stone (1922) found myocarditis associated with both lobar pneumonia (3 per cent of 34 patients) and bronchopneumonia (3 per cent of 37 patients). Among 67 patients who had had broncho-pneumonia involving at least one entire lobe, Saphir and Amromin (1948) found myocarditis in 26 (39 per cent): the myocarditis was acute in 15, acute serous in 3 and subacute in 8. All the patients developed classic clinical symptoms and 6 had electrocardiogram abnormalities. Saphir (1943) found myocarditis in 8 of 152 patients with bronchiectasis; 3 of the 8 had died unexpectedly. Of clinical significance was the discrepancy between the accelerated pulse rate and the slight degree of the accompanying fever. He also described myocarditis in one of three patients with bronchial asthma who died unexpectedly.

References

Saphir, O. (1943). 'Myocarditis in bronchiectasis.' *Archs intern. Med.* **72**, 775

— (1945), 'Laryngeal oedema, myocarditis and unexpected death (early acute laryngo-tracheobronchitis).' *Am. J. med. Sci.* **210**, 296

— and Amromin, G. D. (1948). 'Myocarditis in instances of pneumonia.' *Ann. intern. Med.* **28**, 963

Stone, W. J. (1922). 'Heart muscle changes in pneumonia with remarks on digitalis therapy.' *Am. J. med. Sci.* **163**, 659

MENINGOCOCCAL MYOCARDITIS

In 1936 Saphir encountered myocarditis in 2 of 10 cases of meningococcal septicaemia. The cardiac lesions were characterized by focal areas of muscle necrosis with a cellular reaction of polymorphs and mononuclears. Sometimes the lesions were haemorrhagic and organisms were identified within the inflammatory areas.

In rapidly fatal meningococcal infections Moritz and Zamcheck (1946) reported myocarditis in 37 of 81 patients dying within 24 hours of becoming ill. In 14 of these cases myocarditis was the only finding. Among 256 cases of acute meningococcal septicaemia, 97 (43 per cent) were complicated by myocarditis. Although patients who survive the acute illness usually present no cardiac disability, Holman and Angevine (1946) encountered an instance in which cardiac failure followed bacteriological cure. Death occurred after 33 days and there was extensive necrosis in the outer zone of the myocardium with focal areas of necrosis elsewhere.

Lukash (1963) noted evidence of myocarditis, a gallop rhythm and electrocardiogram changes on the fifth day of treatment, of a case of meningococcal pericarditis with effusion.

Friderichsen-Waterhouse Syndrome

This syndrome is frequently caused by fulminating meningococcal septicaemia. The usual findings in the heart are cloudy swelling, severe fatty change, occasionally focal muscle necrosis (d'Agate and Murangoni, 1945) and in a few instances an acute myocarditis has been reported (Saphir, 1949). It is probable that many cases die before a cellular inflammatory reaction develops.

References

d'Agate, V. and Murangoni, B. A. (1945). 'The Waterhouse-Friderichsen syndrome.' *New Engl. J. Med.* **232**, 1

Holman, D. V. and Angevine, D. M. (1946). 'Meningococcal myocarditis; report of two cases with anatomied and clinical characteristics.' *Am. J. med. Sci.* **211**, 120

Lukash, W. M. (1963). 'Massive pericarditis effusion due to meningococcis pericarditis (myocarditis also present).' *J. Am. med. Ass.* **185**, 598

Moritz, A. R. and Zamcheck, N. (1946). 'Sudden and unexpected deaths of young soldiers.' *Archs Path.* **42**, 459

Saphir, O. (1936). 'Meningococcus myocarditis.' *Am. J. Path.* **12**, 677

— (1949). 'Myocarditis associated with the Waterhouse-Friderichsen syndrome.' *Studies in Pediatrics and Medical History*, Abraham Levinson Anniversary Volume. Ed. by S. R. Kagen, pp. 57–64. New York: Froben Press

PERTUSSIS AND HAEMOPHILUS INFECTION

Myocarditis occurs only rarely in infections caused by *Bordetella pertussis*, *Haemophilus influenzae* and *H. para-influenzae*. Obendorfer (1914) reported myocarditis as the cause of the unexpected death of a seven year old girl, a few weeks after the onset of whooping cough. Vischer (1924) described interstitial myocarditis in a patient with active whooping cough and histologically the myocardium was found to be infiltrated with lymphocytes, a few neutrophils and plasma cells.

Few reports have been published of myocarditis caused by *H. influenzae*, and it is probable that most instances of myocarditis recorded during the 1918 influenza epidemic were due to the virus of influenza, rather than to this bacillus. Wolbach and Frothingham (1923) found myocarditis in 1 out of 27 patients who died of influenza, and Craven, Poston and Orgian (1940) encountered myocarditis in two instances of myocarditis caused by *H. para-influenzae*.

References

Craven, E. B., Jnr, Poston, M. A. and Orgian, E. S. (1940). 'Haemophilus para-influenzae endocarditis.' *Am. Heart J.* **19**, 434

Obendorfer, I. (1914). 'Pathologisch-anatomische Demonstrationen.' *Mschr. Kinderheilk.* **13**, 356

Vischer, M. (1924). 'Beitrag zur Myokarditis in Klurdesatten.' In *Czerny: Abhandlungen aus der Kinderheilkunde und ihren Grenzgebieten.* p. 86. Berlin: Karger

Wolbach, S. B. and Frothingham, L. (1923). 'Influenzae epidemic at Camp Devins in 1918.' *Archs intern. Med.* **32**, 571

SALMONELLA

The heart appears to withstand occasional bacteraemic states more effectively than do most other tissues of the body, and salmonella infection of the heart is rare.

There may be a slight pericardial effusion and sometimes a fibrinous deposit on the surface of the pericardium. The heart is usually flabby and slightly dilated, but of normal weight. Mural thrombi may be found attached to the endocardium, and to have shed emboli into the lungs and systemic circulation. In most cases the inflammatory response is composed predominantly of small lymphocytes and macrophages, and involves the entire thickness of the ventricular wall.

Acute myocarditis as the dominant feature of a salmonella infection is exceedingly rare (Hennigar *et al.*, 1953). However, a careful examination of autopsy reports from cases of salmonella endocarditis reveals an underlying myocarditis (Saphir, 1947; Deswiet, 1949; Stumpe and Barody, 1951; Levin and Hosier, 1961).

Typhoid and paratyphoid infections usually show only moderate degenerative changes such as fatty change and hydropic change. Occasional changes have been reported with muscle necrosis or a true myocarditis but Gore and Saphir (1947) did not find any histological evidence of myocarditis in 80 cases of typhoid and 30 cases of bacillary dysentery.

Salmonella choleraesius is the type of salmonella infection most commonly found to involve the heart. Sapha and Winter (1957) found this organism in half of twenty cases of salmonella endocarditis which they investigated. Over half of these cases had focal cardiac lesions (abscesses), and in this type of bacterial infection myocardial rupture may occasionally be seen. If the infection is associated with another disease involving the myocardium, such as the metasatic deposits of lymphosarcoma present in Sanders and Misanic's case (1964), this is more likely to occur.

References

Deswiet, J. (1949). 'Sub-acute bacterial endocarditis due to salmonella typhimurium.' *Br. med. J.* **2**, 1155
Gore, I. and Saphir, O. (1947). 'Myocarditis. A classification of 1402 cases.' *Am. Heart J.* **34**, 831
Hennigar, G. R., Thabet, R., Bundy, W. E. and Sutton, L. E. (1953). 'Salmonellosis complicated by pancarditis.' *J. Pediat.* **43**, 524

Levin, H. S. and Hosier, D. M. (1961). 'Salmonella pericarditis. Report of a case and review of the literature.' *Ann. intern. Med.* **55**, 817

Sanders, V. and Misanic, L. F. (1964). 'Salmonella myocarditis, report of a case with ventricular rupture.' *Am. Heart J.* **68**, 682

Sapha, I. and Winter, J. W. (1957). 'Clinical manifestations of Salmonellosis in man.' *New. Engl. J. Med.* **256**, 1128

Saphir, O. (1947). 'Myocarditis, a general review with an analysis of 240 cases.' *Archs Path.* **32**, 1000

Stumpe, A. R. and Barody, N. R. (1951). 'Salmonella endocarditis.' *Archs intern. Med.* **88**, 679

TUBERCULOSIS

The myocardium is rarely involved in tuberculosis. Horn and Saphir (1935) in a review of the literature found 19 cases in 7683 autopsies (1·24 per cent) of patients with generalized tuberculosis. In a similar review, Auerbach and Guggenheim (1937) found 29 examples amongst 10 165 fatal cases of tuberculosis.

Among 96 children with myocarditis, 4 were infected with pulmonary tuberculosis and in 2 of them tubercules were present in the myocardium accompanied by diffuse non-specific inflammation (Saphir, Wile and Reingold, 1944). Occasionally, both tubercular and rheumatic lesions may occur simultaneously (Masugi, Murasawa and Ya-Shu, 1937; Roberts and Lisa, 1937). It must not be forgotten that patients with tubercle may develop myocarditis from other causes (Saphir, 1958). Sudden death occurred in a case reported by Neuman (1952). Exceptional complications of tuberculous myocarditis include ventricular aneurysm (Jones and Tilden, 1942) and endocardial thrombosis with systemic embolization (Beebe and Coleman, 1945). Myocardial involvement in tuberculosis may be nodular (tuberculoma), miliary or diffusely infiltrative (Rosenbaum and Linn, 1948).

Miliary Type

The heart is involved in miliary tuberculosis to a variable degree, the post-mortem incidence depending to some extent on the amount of material examined. The appearances are similar to miliary tuberculosis elsewhere.

Nodular Type

The most frequent form of myocardial involvement is the nodular type; tuberculomata occur as yellow-grey rounded circumscribed firm nodules 5–70 mm in diameter (Rauchwebber and Rogers,1947). These may involve any portion of the heart—most frequently the right atrium (Rosenbaum and Linn, 1948). Histologically the lesions show caseation with giant cells, while tubercle bacillus usually can be visualized in sections.

Diffuse Type

The diffuse type is uncommon but shows an extensive infiltration of the myocardium with epithelioid cells and lymphocytes. Histological diagnosis in this type is not reliable and bacteriological examination is required to demonstrate the tubercle bacillus. It must be differentiated from diffuse sarcoidosis or giant-cell myocarditis.

In addition to these types a non-specific myocarditis consisting of focal collections of lymphocytes and monocytes has been described (Saphir, Wile and Reingold, 1944). When this occurs in the absence of demonstrable tuberculous lesions in the myocardium, it is doubtful if it is a manifestation of tuberculosis.

References

Auerbach, O. and Guggenheim, A. (1937). 'Tuberculosis of the myocardium. Review of literature and report of six new cases.' *Q. Bull. Sea View Hosp.* **2**, 264

Beebe, R. A. and Coleman, G. H. (1945). 'Embolic thrombosis of the abdominal aorti with tuberculous (histologic) lesions of the heart containing giant cells with radial inclusions.' *Am. Heart J.* **29**, 539

Horn, H. and Saphir, O. (1935). 'The involvement of the myocardium in tuberculosis, a review of the literature and report of three cases.' *Am. Rev. Tuberc. pulm. Dis.* **32**, 492

Jones, K. P. and Tilden, I. L. (1942). 'Tuberculous myocardial aneurysm with rupture and sudden death from tampoinade.' *Hawaii med. J. inter-Isl. Nurs. Bull.* **1**, 295

Masugi, M., Murasawa, S. and Ya-Shu (1937). 'Ueber das Vorkommen von aschoffschen Knotchen in Phthisikerherzen; pathologische anatomische Bertrage zur Frage des Zusammen raugerzurischen Tuberculose und Rheumatisum.' *Virchows Arch. path. Anat. Physiol.* **299**, 426

Neuman, H. A. (1952). 'Tuberculous lesions of the conducting system.' *Am. J. Path.* **28**, 919

Rauchwebber, S. N. and Rogers, R. J. (1947). 'Tuberculoma of the myocardium.' *Am. Heart J.* **34**, 280

Roberts, J. E. and Lisa, J. R. (1937). 'The heart in pulmonary tuberculosis.' *Am. Rev. Tuberc. pulm. Dis.* **47**, 253

Rosenbaum, H. and Linn, H. J. (1948). 'Tuberculoma of the myocardium in a patient with tuberculous meningitis treated with streptomycin.' *Am J. clin. Path.* **18**, 162

Saphir, O. (1958). *A Text on Systemic Pathology*. Vol. 1, pp. 64–70. New York: Grune and Stratton

— Wile, S. A. and Reingold, I. M. (1944). 'Myocarditis in children.' *Am. J. Dis. Child.* **67**, 294

Ten

Fungal infections

AETIOLOGICAL FACTORS

Fungal infections are 'opportunistic', that is to say they attack subjects with lowered resistance; thus diabetes mellitus may be associated with phycomycosis and deep-seated coccidioidomycosis; leukaemia and lymphomas with histoplasmosis, cryptococcosis, coccidioidomycosis, blastomycosis, nocardiasis, and aspergillosis. Antecedent treatment with antibiotics, steroids and cytostatic drugs are also common aetiological factors.

Most patients suffer only a minor illness but resistance varies greatly.

DIAGNOSTIC TESTS

Complement-fixation and precipitin tests are of value in that they both demonstrate the presence of antibodies to a particular fungus. The coccidioidin skin test, which comprises an antigen to demonstrate delayed hypersensitivity is of no use in assessing the patient's prognosis. It does indicate that the patient has been exposed to infection, at some time previously, with coccidioidomycosis. It does not indicate the state of activity of the disease and thus is analogous to the Mantoux test. Skin tests are also useful for indicating exposure to infection in histoplasmosis and North American blastomycosis, but are not of value in detecting chromoblastomycosis, sporotrichosis or maduramycosis. Aspergillosis may produce precipitin antibodies.

Cryptococcus neoformans has a thick polysaccharide capsule (demonstrable histologically in nigrosin preparations) and a capsular antigen which can be detected by the latex test at an early stage of the disease. Later, when the capsular antigen titre level falls, the antibody titre, as demonstrated by the complement-fixation test, rises. There is, therefore, an inverse relationship between these two serum factors.

ASPERGILLOSIS

Generalized aspergillosis is rare, but is increasing in frequency. A case involving the endocardium and myocardium was described by Grekin, Cawley and Zheutiln (1950).

Sporulating hyphae of *Aspergillus fumigatus* have been found within granuloma in the myocardium and subendocardium (Courvoisier, Löffler and Schuppli, 1958) in a 22 year old male with disseminated aspergillosis. Aspergillus endocarditis and myocarditis have been reported as complications of lung abscess in an 18 year old male with a history of repeated upper respiratory tract infections who had been treated wih steroids (Welsh and Buchners, 1955) and myocardial involvement has been encountered in 1 out of 25 patients who suffered from leukaemia or lymphoma and secondary mycosis (Gruhn and Sanson, 1963).

DIAGNOSIS

Diagnosis depends on the identification of the fungus by culture. Pepys and Longbottom (1964) at the Institute of Diseases of the Chest in London developed a serodiagnostic gel diffusion test for serum antibodies to Aspergillus; the serum was placed in a central well and the two diagnostic antigens and saline in the outer wells; the plate was incubated at 28°C for 2–7 days, and examined daily for precipitin lines. These could be brought out if unclear by removing the gels, soaking it in daily changes of sodium-azide-saline for a week, drying at 40°C and staining with a protein stain, e.g., azocarmine and differentiating with acetic acid to clear the background. Finally, the gel is soaked in 10 per cent glycerol in ethanol and blotted dry. (The antigen is now available commercially.)

References

Courvoisier, E., Löffler, A. and Schuppli, R. (1958), 'Über einen Fall von eosinophiler Myokarditis bei Asthma bronchiale.' *Allergie Asthma* 4, 325

Grekin, R. H., Cawley, E. P. and Zheutiln, B. (1950). 'Generalised Aspergillosis.' *Archs Path.* 49, 387

Gruhn, J. C. and Sanson, J. (1963). 'Mycotic infection in leukaemic patients at autopsy.' *Cancer* 16, 61

Pepys, J. and Longbottom. Joan L. (1964). 'Preliminary aspergillosis; diagnostic and immunologic significance of antigen and c-substance in Aspergillus fumigatus.' *J. Path. Bact.* 8, 141

Welsh, R. A. and Buchners, J. M. (1955). 'Aspergillus endocarditis, myocarditis and lung abscess.' *Am. J. clin. Path.* 25, 782

HISTOPLASMOSIS

Histoplasmosis, like tetanus, anthrax and some salmonella infections is a telluric (earth) disease. Its cause (*Histoplasma capsulatum*) lives in the soil especially when this is moist and warm and richly organic, as in the river valleys of the American middle west; it also contaminates bird droppings. It is endemic in certain areas of the USA, but a few cases have been reported in Britain and elsewhere.

Histoplasmosis is non-sporing in culture at 22°C but it has characteristic tuberculate chlamydospores.

Procknow (1967) described a family of 8 people, living on a farm in Indiana; in 1950, 6 developed histoplasmosis from a semiderelict silo, the wife and daughter-in-law escaped infection because they never went in it. All 6 recovered but showed x-ray calcification.

Histoplasmosis may occasionally cause myocarditis (Kuzma, 1947). Cardiac involvement is uncommon but Merchant *et al.* (1958) described 2 cases of endocarditis and found 9 others in the literature. In a few myocardial lesions were also present. Organisms could be demonstrated in the vegetations. Crawford *et al.* (1961) reported acute myocarditis and pericarditis in two siblings who had developed respiratory symptoms and fever, and yielded positive complement-fixation tests for histoplasmosis. In one child serial electrocardio-grams revealed flattened or inverted T waves which persisted for about one year and examination disclosed persistent tachycardia, a friction rub, and roentgenographic evidence of cardiac enlargement. Granulo-matous lesions in the myocardium have been described by Humphrey (1940) and Binford (1955) in which organisms were demonstrated.

Several cases of pericarditis have also been described and Wooley and Hosier (1961) described a case of constrictive pericarditis which they believed resulted from histoplasmosis.

Histoplasma capsulatum usually occur in yeast form, which may be up to 16 μm in diameter but are usually much smaller—2–4 μ. These smaller mycotic forms may be found in histiocytes and stain pink with PAS. They may also be demonstrated by Gridley's stain.

DIAGNOSIS

A positive histoplasmin skin test is useful in indicating a previous exposure to the organisms, but is not of use in demonstrating if the infection is at present active and the organisms may be grown from blood culture.

The complement-fixation test is of value and can demonstrate rising titre if infection is active.

References

Binford, C. H. (1955). 'Histoplasmosis. Tissue reactions and morphological variations of the fungus.' *Am. J. clin. Path.* **25**, 25

Crawford, S. E., Crook, W. G., Harrison, W. W. and Somerville, B. (1961). 'Histoplasmosis as a cause of acute myocarditis and pericarditis.' *Pediatrics, Springfield* **28**, 92

Humphrey, A. A. (1940). 'Reticuloendotheliol cytomycosis (histoplasmosis of Darling).' *Archs intern Med.* **29**, 139

Kuzma, J. F. (1947). 'Histoplasmosis: The pathologic and clinical findings.' *Dis. Chest* **13**, 338

Merchant, R. K., Louria, D. B., Geisler, P. H., Edgcomb, J. H. and Utz, S. P. (1958). 'Fungal endocarditis. Review of the literature and report of three cases.' *Ann. intern. Med.* **48**, 242

Procknow, J. J. (1967). 'Pulmonary histoplasmosis in a farm family, 15 years later.' *Am. Rev. resp. Dis.* **95**, 171

Wooley, C. F. and Hosier, D. M. (1961). 'Constrictive pericarditis due to histoplasma capsulatum.' *New Engl. J. Med.* **264**, 1230

ACTINOMYCOSIS

Infection may be spread by the blood or by extension from adjacent structures (Kirch, 1927). Because actinomycotic infection is rarely disseminated throughout the body, the heart is seldom affected; myocardial involvement having been reported in only 5 of 475 cases of actinomycosis, which Kasper and Pinner (1930) reported. Edwards (1931) described myocardial actinomycotic abscesses in a 10 year old boy with primary bronchiolar actinomycosis.

Cornell and Shookoff (1944) described 3 cases and analysed other reported cases. The pericardium was involved in all 3 cases and the myocardium in 2. The lesions are suppurative and diagnosis depends on identification of the organisms.

Endocarditis due to actinomycosis has been reported by Uhr (1939) and Wedding (1947).

The organism may reach the pericardium by direct spread from the lungs or they may be carried by the blood stream. Usually there is an obvious focus of infection elsewhere.

References

Cornell, A. and Shookoff, H. B. (1944). 'Actinomycosis of the heart simulating rheumatic fever. Report of three cases of cardiac actinomycosis with a review of the literature.' *Archs intern. Med.* **74**, 11

Edwards, A. B. (1931). 'Actinomycosis in children.' *Am. J. Dis. Child.* **41**, 1419

Kasper, J. A. and Pinner, M. (1930). 'Actinomycosis of the heart: report of a case with actinomycotic emboli.' *Archs Path.* **10**, 687

Kirch, E. (1927). 'Pathologie des Herzens.' *Ergeben. allg. Path. path. Anat.* **22**, 65

Uhr, N. (1939). 'Bacterial endocarditis. Report of a case in which the cause was Actinomyces bovis.' *Archs intern. Med.* **64**, 84

Wedding, E. S. (1947). 'Actinomycotic endocarditis. Report of two cases with a review of the literature.' *Archs intern. Med.* **79**, 203

BLASTOMYCOSIS

According to Kirch (1927) the heart is seldom involved in generalized blastomycosis. Organisms have been identified within a caseous, tuberculoid, myocardial lesion (Medlar, 1927) and lesions in the pericardium, myocardium and endocardium have been reported in a series of 9 patients with blastomycosis; suggesting that the lymphatics served as the route of infection (Martin and Smith, 1939). Baker and Brian (1937) described two cases in which pericarditis was present and penetration to the myocardium had occurred in both. The lesions showed caseation and tubercle formation and organisms were demonstrated. Merchant *et al.* (1958) collected four cases of endocarditis from the literature.

References

Baker, R. D. and Brian, E. W. (1937). 'Blastomycosis of the heart. Report of two cases.' *Am. J. Path.* **13**, 139

Kirch, E. (1927). 'Pathologie des Herzens.' *Ergeben allg. Path. path. Anat.* **22**, 65

Martin, D. S. and Smith, D. T. (1939). 'Blastomycosis.' *Am. Rev. Tuberc. pulm. Dis.* **39**, 275

Medlar, E. M. (1927). 'Pulmonary blastomycosis; its similarity to tuberculosis.' *Am. J. Path.* **3**, 305

Merchant, R. K., Louria, D. B., Geisler, P. H., Edgcomb, J. H. and Utz, S. P. (1958). 'Fungal endocarditis. Review of the literature and report of three cases.' *Ann. intern. Med.* **48**, 242

CRYPTOCOCCUS (TORULOSIS)

Cryptococcus neoformans is a pathogenic fungus found in soil and in pidgeon excreta. Human infection may cause disseminated crypto-coccosis which may be associated with the reticuloses; meningeal and cerebral infection may be fatal, but pulmonary infection is often self-limiting. The disease was reviewed by Littman (1959).

A case of endocarditis due to *C. neoformans* was reported by Lombardo, Rabsen and Dodge (1957). It occurred in a patient suffering from rheumatic heart disease and was superimposed on a damaged valve. Lesions were also present in the myocardium.

Cryptococcal infection of the myocardium was reported in a man with reticulum cell sarcoma (Littman and Zimmerman, 1956), and in 2 of 16 patients with disseminated cryptococcosis complicating cancer (Hutter and Collins, 1962). Severe tachycardia and heart failure were reported by Jones, Nassau and Smith (1965) in a 31 year old male who had palpitations for four months, severe shortness of breath for two days and paroxysmal ventricular tachycardia; quinidine restored normal rhythm. He recovered partially but suffered relapses in the ensuing six months, eventually being found dead in bed at home. Necropsy revealed miliary lesions in the lungs; the hilar and tracheal lymph nodes were caseous and calcified and the heart was flabby; and showed greyish streaks. Microscopy showed epitheliod granulomata with giant cells in the myocardium, lungs and hilar nodes; *C. neoformans* was demonstrated in the lesions by Grindley's stain and by PAS staining.

References

Hutter, R. V. P. and Collins, H. S. (1962). 'The appearance of opportunistic fungus infections in a cancer hospital.' *Lab. Invest.* **11**, 1035

Jones, I., Nassau, E. and Smith, P. (1965). 'Cryptococcosis of the heart.' *Br. Heart J.* **27**, 462

Littman, M. I. (1959). 'Cryptococcosis (Torulosis). Current concepts and therapy.' *Am. J. Med.* **27**, 976

— and Zimmerman, L. E. (1956). *Cryptococcosis, torulosis or European blastomycosis.* p. 205. New York: Grune and Stratton

Lombardo, T. A., Rabsen, A. S. and Dodge, H. T. (1957). 'Mycotic endocarditis: Report of a case due to Cryptococcus neoformans.' *Am. J. Med.* **22**, 664

CANDIDIASIS (MONILIASIS)

Candida albicans and other candida species are of low pathogenicity. With the increased use of antibiotics and steroids for various diseases and the combined use of antibiotics, steroids and antimetabolites in the treatment of leukaemia, an increase in the number of cases of generalized candidiasis and other fungal infections has been reported (Zimmerman, 1955; Lannigan and Meynell, 1959; Craig and Farber, 1963). Infections may occur in infancy, pregnancy, skin diseases, endocrine disorders, malnutrition, malabsorption, therapy with steroids and antibiotics, post-operation states, agranulocytosis, aplastic anaemia and in malignant disease. Thrush due to *Candida* may indicate a deep-seated disease such as endocrine or malignant disease. Susceptibility varies from person to person and it is not known why some persons get infected while others, with similar predisposing factors, do not. In many of the reported cases the portal of entry of the organism is known but in others no primary source can be identified. Sometimes the fungus grows on the skin to produce a granuloma with much hyperkeratosis, on the hands or scalp of children with diabetes or other predisposing causes, or sometimes, even in the healthy.

The heart is involved in a proportion of cases, the most common type of involvement being endocarditis.

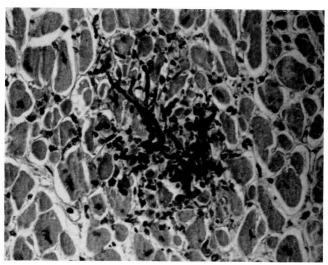

Figure 10.1. Small myocardial abscess with a Candida albicans *(PAS × 400, reduced to 2/3). (Reproduced from Chatty and Deodhar (1969) by courtesy of the authors and Editor of the* Archives of Pathology)

A patient with systemic candidiasis, endocarditis and acute interstitial myocarditis was found to have a massive vegetation containing candida organisms, leucocytes and fibrin on the non-coronary cusp of the aortic valve. The vegetation bulged into the right atrium and perforated the atrial septum just above the septal leaflet of the tricuspid valve (Joachim and Polayes, 1941). Merchant *et al.* (1958) reviewed 11 cases: in 5 there was a history of drug addiction, the organisms being probably introduced by dirty syringes; and in 3 antibiotics were being administered and may have contributed to the development of the disease. Myocardial lesions are sometimes found (*Figure 10.1*) and these consist of rounded abscesses (Zimmerman, 1955). Myocardial involvement was reported in 5 patients among 74 with disseminated candidiasis (Hutter and Collins,

1962) and in 2 patients among 25 with leukaemia or lymphoma (Gruhn and Sanson, 1963). *Candida endocarditis* infections have also been described following cardiac surgery (Hyun and Collier, 1960) and Kay *et al.* (1961) reported a case following surgical excision of the lesion. Clayton and Noble (1966) made a large scale epidemiological survey of oral and fungal infections, using Sabouraud's dextrose agar with 0·05 per cent actidione and streptomycin for culture at 37°C (or 26°C for skin infections). The study included 376 adults and 73 children in hospital, 375 boarding school children and 277 healthy young adults. Mouth fungi were present in 16·4–32·9 per cent of patients and in 5·4–8·6 per cent of healthy people, whereas finger fungi were found in only 6·8–7·7 per cent of patients compared to 1·7 per cent in young adults and 0·5 per cent of boarding school boys. Carrier rates were thus higher inside hospital than outside, and spread was similar to that of Staphylococci.

DIAGNOSIS

Several workers have reported up to nine antigens in *C. albicans*, some specific and others shared with other species. Serum agglutinins are usually greater than 1 : 320 in systemic candidiasis but sometimes high titres may also be found in normal subjects. In general, therefore, these tests are not of much diagnostic value. Serum precipitins may also indicate systemic candidiasis (Winner, 1966); Stallybrass (1964) described a serum precipitin test using a formanide extract of the fungus but high-precipitin titres may also be found in normal people, and, like agglutinin levels, are of little practical value.

References

Clayton, Yvonne and Noble, W. C. (1966). 'Observations on the epidemiology of Candida albicans.' *J. clin. Path.* **19**, 76

Craig, J. M. and Farber, S. (1953). 'The development of disseminated visceral mycosis during therapy for acute leukaemia.' *Am. J. Path.* **29**, 601

Gruhn, J. C. and Sanson, J. (1963). 'Myocardial infections in leukaemic patients at autopsy.' *Cancer* **16**, 61

Hutter, R. V. P. and Collins, H. S. (1962). 'The occurrence of opportunistic fungus infection in a cancer hospital.' *Lab. Invest. N.Y.* **11**, 1035

Hyun, B. H. and Collier, F. C. (1960). 'Mycotic endocarditis following intra-cardiac operations. Report of four cases.' *New Engl. J. Med.* **263**, 1339

Joachim, H. and Polayes, S. H. (1942). 'Subacute endocarditis and systemic mycosis (Monilia).' *J. Am. med. Ass.* **115**, 205

Kay, J. H., Bernstein, S., Feinstein, D. and Biddle, M. (1961). 'Surgical cure of Candida albicans infection with open heart surgery.' *New Engl. J. Med.* **264**, 903

Lannigan, R. and Meynell, M. J. (1959). 'Moniliasis in acute leukaemia.' *J. clin. Path.* **12**, 157

Merchant, R. K., Louria, D. B., Gersler, P. H., Edgcombe, J. H. and Utz. S. P. (1958). 'Fungal endocarditis. Review of the literature and report of three cases.' *Ann. intern. Med.* **48**, 242

Stallybrass, F. C. (1964). 'Candida precipitins.' *J. Path. Bact.* **87**, 89

Winner, H. I. (1966). 'Candida infections.' *Medical News* September **9**, 8

Zimmerman, L. E. (1955). 'Fatal fungus infections complicating other diseases.' *Am. J. Clin. Path.* **25**, 46

COCCIDIOIDOMYCOSIS

Gore and Saphir (1947) listed cardiac lesions in 11 of 48 cases of generalized coccidioidomycosis. Reingold (1950) found granuloma in the myocardium in 4 patients with disseminated coccidioidomycosis; 3 hearts contained non-specific, mononuclear, interstitial and perivascular infiltrates and degenerating myocardial fibres having indistinct cross striations and 1 heart with discrete granuloma of the fungi.

Merchant *et al.* (1958) described a case of generalized coccidioidomycosis in which there was an adhesive pericarditis and an abscess at the base of the mitral valve involving the myocardium. The lesion was granulomatous and showed caseation; organisms were also demonstrated.

References

Gore, I. and Saphir, O. (1947). 'Myocarditis. A classification of 1402 cases.' *Am. Heart. J.* **34**, 827

Merchant, R. K., Louria, D. B., Geisler, P. H., Edgecombe, J. H. and Utz, S. P. (1958). 'Fungal endocarditis. Review of the literature and report of three cases.' *Ann. intern. Med.* **48**, 242

Reingold, I. M. (1950). 'Myocardial lesions in disseminated coccidioidomycosis.' *Am. J. Path.* **20**, 1044

Eleven

Parasitic infections

PROTOZOAL

CHAGAS' DISEASE

Chagas' disease is caused by *Trypanosoma cruzi*, a tiny protozoon which may inhabit the blood and tissues of both man and animals. The disease may lead to an extensive myocarditis and the destruction of ganglion cells in the peripheral autonomic nervous system, which may produce, as a result, marked enlargement of the heart, oesophagus, colon and other hollow viscera. The natural history of Chagas' disease is only partially known but is characterized by an acute phase, a period of latency and a chronic phase. Its most important clinical manifestation is a late-developing, chronic myocarditis and, much less frequently, an early acute myocarditis, which together result in a greater morbidity and mortality than does the involvement of all other organs together. During the latent phase, there is serological indication of trypanosomal infection but there is usually no evidence of visceral involvement.

Trypanosoma cruzi was first described in Brazil in 1909 by Carlos Chagas. The organism is transmitted to human beings by the bite of haematophagus insects of the reduviidae family (Triatomidae bugs) who have become infected after feeding on infected animals. The various changes which occur in this trypanosome during its life cycle in animal and Triatomidae in man, are shown in *Figure 11.1*. The armadillo is the most common animal-host but racoons, skunks and the opossum are frequently found to be infected. Approximately 100 species have been described; nearly all of them in the American continent. The insect of most importance is *Triatoma infestans* because of its exclusive domestic habitat. This insect is known popularly, in the Argentine, as 'vinchuca', meaning 'to let oneself drop'. These insects live in holes and crevices in the walls and roofs of mud huts, from which they emerge at night—being night feeders—

and drop from the ceiling on to the beds where people are sleeping underneath, commonly biting the individual about the eyes or mouth, especially young children.

The importance of Chagas' disease in the American continent is primarily due to the severe myocardial involvement it produces.

In 1960 a World Health Organization study group estimated that 7 million people in southern and central America were infected with

Trypanosome cycle

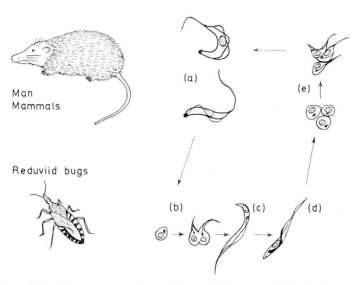

Man
Mammals

Reduviid bugs

Figure 11.1.   The trypanosome form of T. cruzi (a) is seen in the blood of man and animals. When ingested by a reduviid the trypanosomes undergo metamorphosis in the insect's gut wall to the leishmanial form (b). This transforms to a crithidial (c) and an infective metacyclic form (d). These infect the animal via the insect faeces and establish leishmanial forms (e) in the tissue cells. These transform to the free swimming blood trypanosomes. (Reproduced from Woody and Woody (1961) by courtesy of the authors and Editor of the Journal of Paediatrics)

Chagas' disease and that 35 million people are exposed to the infection (WHO Technical Report, 1960).

Infection occurs as a result of contamination of the feeding site by the animals' faeces which are loaded with trypanosomes which then subsequently penetrate in to the body of the host. In about half the cases the portal of entry is the conjunctive of the eye (Prata, 1968), producing 'Romama's sign' (*Figure 11.2*). In other cases the route of entry is through the skin, often producing a 'chagoma'

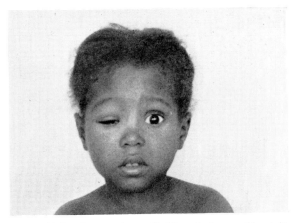

Figure 11.2. A young boy with Chagas' disease. The right eyelid being swollen and oedematous and showing the early signs of a bite by a reduviid bug (Romama's sign). (Reproduced by courtesy of Dr A. Prata)

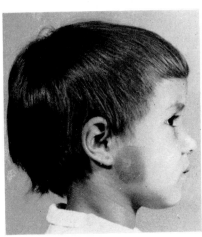

Figure 11.3. Photograph of the face of a young girl to show an 'inoculation chagoema'. (Reproduced by courtesy of Dr A. Prata)

(*Figure 11.3*), but in many cases it is not known. (Most of the parasites which have haematophagus insects as vectors are transmitted by inoculation when the insect bites the host, because the infectious forms are located in the salivary glands of the insect (Mazza, 1951).)

A chagoma usually forms at the site of the inoculation and here the organisms multiply in the leishmania form before eventually developing in to the flagellar form. These protozoa travel within the blood stream in the flagellar form, but on invading somatic cells they undergo transformation to Leishmania, which divide by binary fission to form intracellular colonies or cell 'nests' (*Figure 11.4*) (Johnson, 1943; Woody and Woody, 1961). These parasites then soon change into trypanosomal forms (*Figure 11.5a* and b) and then

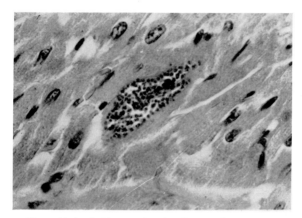

Figure 11.4.   Leishmania 'nest' in hamster heart muscle.

emerge for future migration. They may wander locally or travel by the blood or lymph stream to invade more distant cells and repeat the process.

The disease has been found only in the western hemisphere, particularly in South America, and in some countries it constitutes one of the most important public health problems; indeed in some places 50 per cent of the population are infected. It is most common in rural areas but is prevalent from Mexico to the Argentine; and two cases of acute Chagas' disease have even been reported from the southern USA—Texas (Woody and Woody, 1955; Greer, 1955).

Infected triatomids have been found in many parts of the southern and western USA (Lorenzana, 1967) so there is always a possibility that the disease may extend further. However, in some areas, despite the existence of poor living conditions, of many infected bugs, and of vertebrates infected with *T. cruzi*, the insects do not adapt themselves to human housing and consequently cases of Chagas' disease are uncommon. Three phases should be considered in Chagas' disease: acute, chronic and latent.

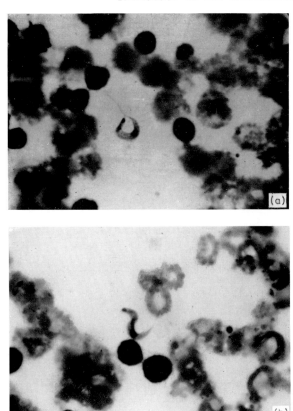

Figure 11.5. Leishmania in the 'chagoma' soon change into trypanosomal forms and emerge for future migration. Characteristic C (a) and S (b) shapes of T. cruzi, *showing anterior flagellum, central nucleus and posterior kinetoplast*

ACUTE CHAGAS' DISEASE

The acute phase of Chagas' disease can occur at any age but is most common in the first years of life. Indeed, 70 per cent of cases of acute Chagas' disease are seen in the first decade of life but it can appear occasionally at a later age. It usually develops in the hot summer months (Laranja *et al.*, 1956; Rosenbaum, 1964).

Rosenbaum estimates that in the initial stages of infection, i.e., in the first few months, only one per cent of those infected will develop clinical signs (Rosenbaum, 1964). These signs include fever, malaise, muscle pains, sweating, vomiting and diarrhoea; generalized oedema and hepatosplenomegaly; unilateral oedema of the eyelid; 'Romama's sign' (Laranja *et al.*, 1956). The sign of entry develops when the portal of entry is the eye, consisting of unilateral palpable oedema, of purplish colour, with conjunctival hyperaemia and lymphadenopathy on the side of the lesion. There may be some induration, erythema and slight tenderness with occasional ulceration or necrosis in the area of the skin, or mucosa where the parasite entered the body. This is called a 'chagoma'. The classic-clinical picture is the syndrome of ocular entry, which consists of unilateral oedema of the eyelid, lasting 30–60 days with swelling of the regional lymph nodes rarely marked. Nondescript findings in the acute cases are those which are usually seen. In some cases symptoms and signs of cardiac and central nervous system involvement (acute meningo-encephalitis) may be apparent. In such cases the laboratory findings may arouse suspicion of trypanosomiasis. The lymphocytes, many of them young forms, may comprise 70–90 per cent of the white cells, giving a 'pseudo-leukaemic' picture. After the first week most infants have a white cell count which usually exceeds 18 000 and may reach 30 000 with a marked lymphocytosis, elevated erythrocyte sedimentation rate and the demonstration of trypanosomes in peripheral blood smears. In very young infants eosinophilia may occur.

Some degree of cardiac involvement probably occurs in virtually all cases of acute Chagas' disease but is usually not detected clinically. The mortality from acute myocarditis or meningo-encephalitis varies from 2 to 10 per cent of those with clinical disease at this stage, that is 2–10 out of every 10 000 infected persons.

In Laranja's series of 235 acute cases, the mortality rate was 9·4 per cent, with death due to congestive heart failure, convulsive seizures or associated infections (Laranja *et al.*, 1956). However, when the subclinical cases are considered the mortality rate falls below one per cent.

The clinical manifestations of acute Chagasic myocarditis are similar to myocarditis of other aetiological causes. In most cases transient cardiac insufficiency occurs with slight reversible cardiac enlargement. More severe right or left-sided failure may occur with pulmonary and systemic congestion, rapid heart rate, gallop rhythm, arrhythmias and decreased blood pressures. In the majority of patients with acute Chagas' disease, symptoms disappear after a few months, although some patients (probably about 15 per cent) continue to have abnormal electrocardiograms.

In the acute stage, invasion of the heart by *T. cruzi* is associated with invasion of myocardial fibres by the parasites. Within the individual muscle cell rapid binary multiplication of the parasites produces an expanding cyst-like structure, which ultimately leads to destruction of the cell and release of the contained organisms (Crowell, 1923). Many cardiac cells parasitized with *T. cruzi* appear to be well preserved (Lundeberg, 1938; Kean, 1946) and are free of surrounding inflammatory cells; upon rupture of the parasitic cyst an intense myocarditis ensues. Infiltration with lymphocytes, plasma cells and other mononuclear cells then follows. Monocytes containing leishmania may be seen in some cases, but usually are extremely difficult to find. This myocarditis is histologically characterized by a diffuse subacute exudative reaction, in which many myocardial fibres are compressed and separated by the infiltrate and exhibit fragmentation, loss of striations, hyalinization and vacuolization and oedema (Crowell, 1923). The inflammation, although less severe, usually extends into the endocardium which may harbour inflammatory foci and extend into the subendocardial muscle and nerve bundles; sometimes leading to mural thrombus formation and in the epicardium giving rise to pericardial effusion (Winslow and Chaffee, 1965). Indeed, Mazza (1951) stressed that the epicardium is always affected in some cases exhibiting fibrinous exudates and increased volume of fluid in the pericardial sac. Typically also, the perineum of small sensory nerves in the epicardium is also infiltrated by mononuclear cells (Enos and Elton, 1950).

Transient and shifting disturbances of the conducting system may also be present. Laranja *et al.* (1956) noted that, in the grossest cases, the myocarditis may produce profound heart failure, unattended by conspicuous irregularities of rhythm and often followed by death. Such cases are accompanied by pronounced dilatation of all four chambers, a flaccid myocardium, and sometimes by massive pericardial effusion. Indeed, there are a considerable number of reports of fatal cases of acute Chagasic myocarditis in the literature and, although many of them are incomplete, they may be summarized as follows. In nearly all the cases there is a severe myocarditis with serious disturbances in the myocardial fibres and considerable interstitial cellular infiltration. There is also a panmyocarditis in most of the cases reported. In half the cases described many of the cardiac muscle fibres contain parasites, while in most of the other cases they were not numerous; but in a few cases fibres containing parasites could not be found.

In still other instances, however, the patients apparently recover entirely from their acute cardiac involvement—only to develop signs of chronic heart disease as late as 10–20 years afterwards.

CHRONIC CHAGAS' MYOCARDIOPATHY

It is generally agreed that Chagas' disease goes unrecognized in the majority of individuals at the time of infection: 99 per cent of people acquire the disease without knowing it (Rosenbaum, 1964), a fact of great importance in the understanding of the development, many years later, of the chronic form of this disease.

Although necrotizing panmyocarditis is unusual in the initial phase, it may slowly develop after a long relatively asymptomatic interval, which is usually 10–20 years after the initial infection.

De Freitas reported that about 10 per cent of individuals in endemic areas have chronic Chagas' myocarditis with 15–30 per cent of those from 30–60 years of age so affected (De Freitas, 1960). Others have also testified to the great prevalence of chronic Chagas' disease in Brazil, Argentina and Venezuela (Laranja *et al.*, 1956; Rosenbaum, 1964; Puigbo *et al.*, 1966).

In Chile, myocardial involvement is much less severe than in countries of the Atlantic coast and is usually confined to a few scattered valleys in the northern Andes (Arribade, 1970, personal communication). These clinical findings depend chiefly on the severity and number of myocardial lesions and the presence of heart failure and arrhythmias. The most frequent types of arrhythmias are ventricular extrasystoles, atrioventricular block and bundle branch block. Right bundle branch block is not commonly found but left bundle branch block is not infrequent. These irregularities of enductum may also be responsible for sudden death, which is commonly seen in patients suffering from the disease. Sudden death is extremely common in Chagas' disease and occurs in about seven per cent of patients so affected. On physical examination there may be signs of cardiac enlargement, irregularities of rhythm and systolic murmurs, due to functional mitral or tricuspid regurgitation. There may be marked increase in systemic venous pressure and hepatomegaly, and the systolic blood pressure is normal in most cases as is the pulse pressure.

In some parts of South America Chagas' disease accounts for nearly 30 per cent of deaths (Koberle, 1958). *Figure 11.6* shows the distribution of this cardiomyopathy according to sex and age in 1000 autopsy cases of chronic Chagas' disease. The highest incidence is found between 20 and 50 years, of age, especially in males.

In some endemic areas there is a high incidence of mega-oesophagus and megacolon (Brazil, 1955; Koberle, 1958; Jung, 1959; Ferreira-Santos, 1961; Ferreira-Santos and Carril, 1964; Raeder and Simao, 1969) and occasionally dilatation and/or aperistalsis of other

hollow viscera, such as the stomach, duodenum, ureter and bronchi
may occur.

Pathological Findings

The great majority hearts with Chagas' cardiomyopathy show
marked alterations in size and frequently in form as well. In exceptional cases the heart may appear to be normal in size and shape. All

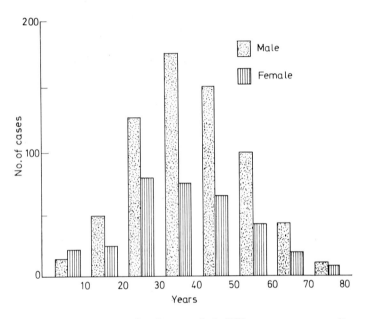

*Figure 11.6.   Frequency of cardiomyopathy in 1000 autopsy cases according
to sex and age (Koberle, 1968)*

degrees of enlargement of the heart may be found, mainly affecting
the right heart, and in particular the right atrium (*Figure 11.7*).
However, the gross anatomical changes include dilatation and muscular flaccidity of all chambers and hypertrophy of the myocardium
(Anselmi *et al.*, 1966) (*Figure 11.8*). Ventricular aneurysmal dilatation
occurs as a compensatory mechanism for the function and efficiency
of the damaged myocardial fibres (*Figure 11.9*). Dilatation is most
pronounced in the area of greatest fibrosis and destruction of myocardium. The heart typically weighs between 400 and 600 g, and

occasionally up to 800 g (Rosenbaum, 1964). At times there is increased thickness of the wall, especially of the left ventricle. The increase in weight is due chiefly to hypertrophy of the myocardial fibres, which lengthen to permit maximum function. However, once the fibres stretch beyond certain limits, their working capacity diminishes accounting for the decreased cardiac contractions observed fluoroscopically in advanced cases with marked cardiac

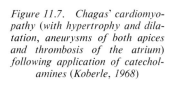

Figure 11.7. Chagas' cardiomyo-pathy (with hypertrophy and dila-tation, aneurysms of both apices and thrombosis of the atrium) following application of catechol-amines (Koberle, 1968)

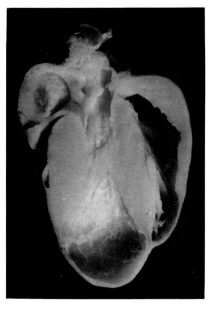

dilatation. The heart can take an almost globular shape but a separation of the left and right apex is found in more than 68 per cent of cases, giving the heart the characteristic appearance of 'cor bifidum'. This appearance is almost pathogenic of Chagas' disease. The epicardium may show small white plaques or tiny white granules along the coronary vessels (fibrous pericarditis 'in-rosary').

Endocardial fibrosis and thinning of the wall may occur principally at the apex of the left ventricle where aneurysm formation is often seen (Carvalhal *et al.*, 1954) (*Figure 11.10*). More than fifty per cent of cases show a very unusual appearance at the apex since it has not been observed in other heart diseases. The lesion consists of thinning and bulging of the apical region mainly of the left ventricle (*Figure 11.11*), and is known variously as infarct of the apex, ventricular

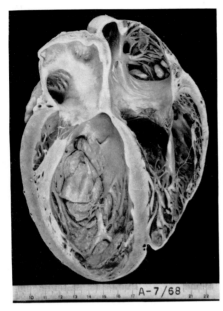

*Figure 11.8. Chronic Chagas'
cardiomyopathy with hypertrophy
and dilatation of the heart, separation of the apex (cor bifidum),
aneurysm of both apices with
thrombosis of the right atrium
(Koberle, 1968)*

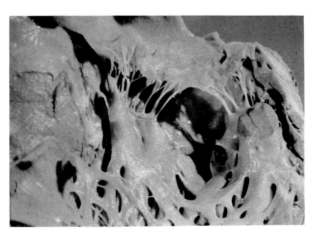

*Figure 11.9. Aneurysmal dilatation, 4 × 3 cm located at the
posterosuperior zone of the left ventricle wall immediately below
the AV sulcus as seen from the interior of the chamber of the left
ventricle; the wall is translucent at the subvalvular mitral area.
Wall thickness was 1 mm and consisted of a fibrous plaque. Heart
weight was 320 g and dilatation was most marked in the right
chambers (Anselmi et al. 1966)*

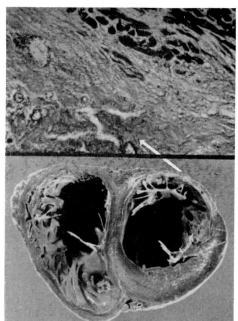

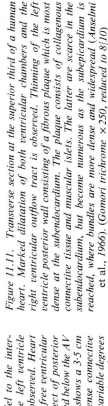

Figure 11.11. Transverse section at the superior third of a human heart. Marked dilatation of both ventricular chambers and the right ventricular outflow tract is observed. Thinning of the left ventricle posterior wall consisting of a fibrous plaque which is most dense at the subendocardium. The plaque consists of collagenous connective tissue and muscular islets. The latter are scarce in the subendocardium, but become numerous as the subepicardium is reached, where bundles are more dense and widespread (Anselmi et al., 1966). (Gomori trichrome ×250, reduced to 8/10)

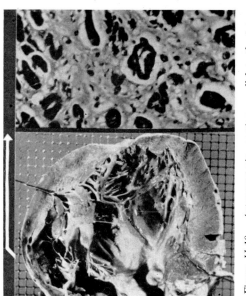

Figure 11.10. Anteroposterior section parallel to the interventricular septum. Marked dilatation of the left ventricle chamber and an increase in trabeculation is observed. Heart weight was 785 g. Significant dilatation of the free ventricular wall seen at the apex and in the superior aspect of posterior wall of the left ventricle. The latter one, localized below the AV sulcus and behind the posterior mitral leaflet, shows a 3·5 cm aneurysm. Histologically, this consisted of dense connective tissue with islets of muscular fibres undergoing variable degrees of degeneration (Anselmi et al. 1966). (Gomori trichrome ×320, reduced to 8/10)

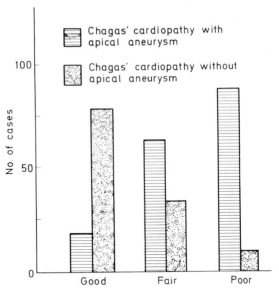

Figure 11.12. Frequency of the aneurysms in chronic Chagas' cardiomyopathy according to the coronary circulation (grades as good, fair or poor). (Koberle, 1968)

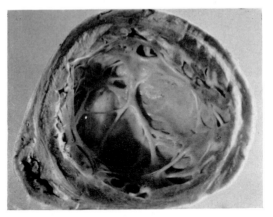

Figure 11.13. Transverse section at the level of the inferior heart of a heart with chronic myocarditis of T. cruzi origin. Marked dilatation of the left ventricle is observed with an increase in trabeculation and significant thinning of the wall. Heart weight was 498 g. There is an extensive and dense fibrotic plaque at the lateral aspect of the wall, and smaller fibrous plaques dispersed through the muscular tissue. The apex of the left ventricle is translucent as a result of thinning of the foliaceous type consisting of collagenous connective tissue. (Anselmi et al., 1966)

aneurysm, or thinning of the apex, its frequency being shown by *Figure 11.12*. The diameter of these aneurysms does not usually exceed 5 cm and the wall may consist only of endocardium and epicardium, and appears translucent (*Figure 11.13*). Thrombosis within these aneurysms is very common but, even without aneurysm formation, extensive mural thrombosis in the lower part of the left ventricle may be seen. Necrosis of the apex is thought by Byington (1969) to appear at an advanced stage when the cardiac area is already greatly enlarged. Mural thrombus formation in the apex of the left ventricle or in the right atrium is frequent (Mott and Hagstrom, 1965). Adequate demonstration of the characteristic lesions requires a special technique for opening the heart. In cases with marked cardiomegaly a massive thrombus of the right auricle is amost invariably present. The heart is injected with a formalin solution at 100 cm of mercury and after fixation for 24 hours is opened, cutting from the apex to the base and thus dividing the heart into anterior and posterior halves.

Microscopical Findings

Diffuse inflammation of the myocardium involving all walls, including the septum, was present in all the 21 hearts studied by Laranja *et al.* (1956). The cellular reaction is both diffuse and focal, consisting of lymphocytes, plasma cells and macrophages. Fibrotic foci composed of collagen fibres are usually most severe in the left ventricle (*Figure 11.11*) but the valves and coronary arteries are uninvolved.

Leishmania are usually difficult to find in chronic cases, but a diligent search will often reveal a parasite in one or more fibres (Winslow and Chaffee, 1965).

Pathogenesis

The pathogenesis of chronic Chagas' disease is controversial. It is generally accepted that the disease represents a chronic myocarditis caused by *T. cruzi*. However, for each myocardial fibre involved and destroyed by parasites, there are thousands damaged or destroyed without leishmania and the observation therefore raised hypotheses, other than those of direct invasion and destruction of myofibres by the organism. The parasites may cause myocardial destruction indirectly by elaborating a toxic substance or by causing an immunological reaction.

Koberle believes that the cardiomegaly is caused by the same basic toxic effect or that involving intrinsic neurological innervation, as he showed in his classic experiments to produce megacolon and mega-oesophagus (Koberle, 1958, 1963) and there is evidence to support this concept (Annotation—Lancet, 1965; Mott and Hagstrom, 1965). He postulates that, during the acute phase of the disease, destruction of leishmania causes the release of a neurotoxin which selectively attacks and destroys the parasympathetic cells of the heart and other hollow viscera.

Rosenbaum (1964) and others believe that this neurotoxin hypothesis is unlikely for several reasons; principally because there is no

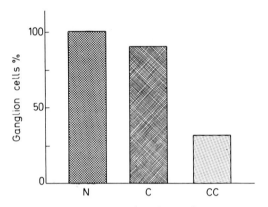

Figure 11.14. Result of ganglion cell counting in normal hearts (N), Chagas' hearts without cardiomyopathy (C) and Chagas' hearts with cardiomyopathy (CC). (Koberle, 1968)

inflammatory reaction around the intact fibres containing parasites and because, to date, investigations have been unable to identify a specific neutrotoxin produced by *T. cruzi*. They favour an immunoallergic mechanism somehow connected with the presence of leishmania in some of the fibres. As yet neither the toxic nor the immunoallergic theory has been proved, but the facts prevail: (1) that a diffuse inflammation of the myocardium is associated with loss of myofibrils; and (2) that there is a destruction of the intrinsic musculature of the heart. The subject is still very unsettled.

In conclusion it can be stated that it is *not* known, as yet, whether the late manifestations of this disease are caused by damage to the nervous system or are secondary to the myocarditis.

Prognosis

The prognosis in patients with clinically apparent myocarditis is grave. Many have syncope and some die suddenly from the effects of the disease in the conductive system of the heart, while others develop progressive cardiac failure. The disease appears to have a prevalance for selectively attacking the cardiac ganglia (*Figure 11.14*).

As is evident from the above description of the clinical picture of this disease suspicion should be aroused when an infant or child, resident in an endemic area, develops a persistent or irregular fever in association with one or more of the following.

(1) Oedema, facial or pedal, without urinary abnormalities.
(2) Unilateral conjuctivitis with pre-auricular lymphadenitis.
(3) Cellulitis and induration at the site of an insect bite.
(4) Otherwise unexplained hepatosplenomegaly.
(5) Tenderness and swelling of the buccal fat pad in nurslings.
(6) Tender, indurated, subcutaneous nodules.
(7) 'Non-specific' myocarditis.
(8) Meningoencephalitis.
(9) Leucocytosis.

Although *T. cruzi* trypanosomes are present in the blood during the acute stages, they are not always easily demonstrated, especially after the fever has subsided. In the most severe cases during the febrile period, the blood is almost literally swimming with trypanosomes and they are easily demonstrated by the procedures listed below.

(1) *Wet coverglass preparation*—This is made by placing a drop of blood (plain, citrated or heparinized) on a slide and covering it with a coverglass. Under low-power magnification the frantically mobile trypanosomes may be seen jostling their way around the red cells. Brought under high power the organism is seen to have a 'snapping' kind of twisting and turning motion.

(2) *Thick-file preparation from the buffy layer*—These films are made from citrated or heparinized blood which has been spun down in a Wintrobe haematocrit. A portion of the buffy layer is set up as a wet preparation and examined for mobile forms. If none are seen thick-film smears are stained with Wright's or Giemsa's stains. At least three such films should be searched with an immersion lens. The stained organism is characteristically C- or S-shaped (*Figure 11.5a* and b). The cytoplasm is stained blue and the nucleus and Kinetoplast are stained red or pink.

(3) *Phytohaemagglutination* (*concentration test*)—The test is technically more involved but quite practical. It consists of the application of a substance to agglutinate and remove red blood cells. Since larger samples of blood can be studied, it has value when the

number of parasites present is low (Yaeger, 1960). A thorough and competent search by the other three methods on successive days and during times when the temperature is elevated will usually reveal parasites. Failure to find *T. cruzi* by direct methods does not exclude infection and more complicated methods for their diagnosis may then have to be undertaken.

(4) *Blood culture*—One millilitre of fresh or heparinized blood should be inoculated on slopes of WNN medium (Novy and MacNeil, 1904; Nicolle, 1908) in screw-cap culture bottles. At least four bottles should be inoculated. They are then incubated in a cool, dark place. They may be checked after two weeks but should not be discarded as negative until after 90 days.

(5) *Xenodiagnosis*—This requires a colony of laboratory reared triatomes. Both a direct method (where the insects feed on the patient) and an indirect technique (where they are fed heparinized blood) can be used (Brumpt, 1914; Nussenzveig and Sonntag, 1952). In either case, within 60 days, if trypanosomes have been consumed with the blood the organism will have multiplied in the gut and can be demonstrated in faeces of the insect.

(6) *Demonstration of fluorescent antibodies*—As Essenfeld and Fennell (1964) have shown, the fluorescent-antibody technique (introduced by Coons *et al.* (1942)) may be employed as either a direct or an indirect method. The direct technique involves the application of a conjugate containing the antibody to a smear or section.

The indirect technique involves the application of a specific antibody when, bound to the antigens, it is identified by staining with a conjugate containing an antigen against the specific antibody. Girelda, Martini and Milic (1965) found a 96 per cent correlative between the fluorescent-antibody test, performed on slides with antigens from culture forms and the complement-fixation test.

Alvarez, Cerisola and Rohwedder (1967) evaluated the immuno-fluorescent method in comparison with the complement-fixation and the indirect haemagglutination techniques with 1083 sera. They concluded that, in the chronic stage, the fluorescent test was as sensitive as the haemagglutination method and slightly superior to the complement-fixation method. In the acute stage, the fluorescent method was far more sensitive than either of the other two methods.

(7) *Indirect haemagglutination*—The first to be introduced was the method of Muniz (1949) in which immodified red cells are used with a polysaccharide fraction of *T. cruzi* as antigen.

Later, in 1950, he introduced a modification in which complement was added to the antigen/antibody complex (red cells were sensitized with trypanosome polysaccharides and placed in contact with the patient's serum), effecting a specific haemolysis. Bouisset, Ducos and Ruffie (1960) were the first to use red cells, modified at their surface with tannic acid, to absorb a soluble antigen of *T. cruzi*. These studies were conducted in laboratory animals, but Cerisola and Lazzari (1962) introduced this reaction for use in routine examination of human sera. He compared the results with those stained by complement-fixation. The test is regarded by Cerisola, Lazzari and Dioorleto (1964) to be an excellent diagnostic method of notable simplicity and speed. Neal and Miles (1968) employed a technique adapted from that of Gill (1964). They found no cross-reactions with sera from patients with malaria, tuberculosis, syphilis, or amoebiasis. Titres of sera from patients with Chagas' disease varied from 1:1000 to 1:512 000.

References

Alvarez, M., Cerisola, J. A. and Rohwedder, R. W. (1967). 'Test de immunofluorescencia para el diagnostico de la enfermedad de Chagas.' *Primer Congreso Latinoarmericano de Parasitologia*, p. 32. Santiago de Chile, Resumenes

Annotation (1965). 'Cardiac nerve lesions in Chagas' disease.' *Lancet* **2**, 375

Anselmi, A., Pifano, F., Suarez, J. A. and Curdirol, O. (1966). 'Myocardiopathy in Chagas' disease. I. Comparative study of pathologic findings in chronic human and experimental Chagas' myocarditis.' *Am. Heart J.* **72**, 469

Atias, A., Neghime, A., Mackay, L. A. and Jarpa, S. (1963). 'Megaesophagus, megacolon and Chagas' disease in Chile.' *Gastroenterology* **44**, 433

Bouisset, L., Ducos, J. and Ruffie, J. (1960). 'Passive haemagglutination technique in research on trypanosomian immunization.' *Path. Biol.*, *Paris* **8**, 91

Brazil, A. (1955). 'Aperistolsis of the oesophagus.' *Revta bras. Gastroent.* 7, 21

Brumpt, E. (1914). 'Le Xénodiagnostic. Application au diagnostic de quelques infections parasitaires et en particulier à la Trypanosomose de Chagas.' *Bull. Soc. Path. exot.* **7**, 706

Byington, C. A. B. (1969). *Veetocardiographia em Doenca de Chagas Anaes. de Congresso International sobre a Doenca de Chagas.* Vol. 1, pp. 357–374. Rio de Janeiro: Oficina Grafica da Universiolade de Brazil

Carvalhal, S. *et al.* (1954). 'Alterações do complexo QRS nas derivações precordiais e seu substrato anatômico em pacientes portadores de miocardite chagásica crônica.' *Rev. Paulista Med.* **45**, 161

Cerisola, J. A. and Lazzari, O. (1962). 'Resultados obtenidos con el test de hemaglutinacion para diagnostico de la enfermedad de Chagas.' *Proceedings of the Seventh International Congress of Tropical Medicine and Malaria.* Vol. 2, pp. 242–243. Rio de Janeiro

Cerisola, J. A. and Lazzari, J. and Dioorleto, C. A. (1964). 'Nuestra experiencia con el test de hemaglutinacion para el diagnostico de la enfermedad de Chagas.' Primeras Journadas Enf. Trans. Carlos Paz (Cordoba).

Coons, A. H., Creech, H. J., Jones, R. N. and Berliner, E. (1942). 'The demonstration of Pneumococcal antigen in tissues by the use of fluorescent antibody.' J. Immun. 45, 159

Crowell, B. C. (1923). 'The acute form of American trypanosomiasis: notes in its pathology with autopsy reports and observations on trypanosomiasis cruzi in animals.' Am. J. trop. Med. Hyg. 3, 425

De Freitas, J. L. (1960). 'Importance of Chagas' disease for public health.' Bol. Offic. Sanit. Panamer. 49, 552

Enos, W. F. and Elton, N. W. (1950). 'Fatal acute Chagas' disease in a North American in the Canal Zone.' Am. J. trop. Med. Hyg. 30, 829

Essenfeld, E. and Fennell, R. H., Jnr (1964). 'Immunofluorescent study of experimental Trypanosoma cruzi infection.' Proc. Soc. exp. Biol. Med. 116, 728

Ferreira-Santos, R. (1961). 'Aperistalsis of the esophagus and colon (megaesophagus and megacolon) etiologically related to Chagas' disease,' Am. J. dig., Dis. 6, 700

— and Carril, C. F. (1964). 'Acquired megacolon in Chagas' disease.' Dis. Colon Rectum 7, 353

Gill, B. S. (1964). 'A procedure for the indirect haemagglutination test for the study of experimental Trypanosoma evansi infections.' Ann. trop. Med. Parasit., 58, 473

Girelda, R., Martini, G. J. W. and Milic, A. (1965). 'La reaccion de inmuno-fluorescencia en el diagnostico de la enfermedad de Chagas.' Segundas Jornadas Entomoepidem. Salta, Argentina

Greer, D. A., Snr (1955). Texas Public Health Report, Texas, USA

Johnson, C. M. (1943). 'American trypanosomiasis.' Med. Clins N. Am. 27, 822

Jung, R. C. (1959). 'Chagas' disease—a possible cause of megaesophagus and megacolon.' Am. J. Gastroent., N.Y. 72, 311

Kean, B. H. (1946). 'Fatal Chagas' disease,' Am. J. clin. Path. 16, 81

Koberle, F. (1958). 'Megaoesophagus.' Gastroenterology 34, 460

— 'Enteromegaly and cardiomegaly in Chagas' disease.' Gut 4, 399

— (1968). 'Chagas' heart disease—pathology.' Cardiologia 52, 82

Laranja, F. S., Dias, E., Nobrega, G. and Miranda, A. (1956). 'Chagas' disease: A clinical, epidemiologic and pathologic study.' Circulation 14, 1035

Lorenzana, R. (1967). 'Chronic Chagas' myocarditis—Report of a case.' Am. J. clin. Path. 48, 39

Lundeberg, K. R. (1938). 'A fatal case of Chagas' disease occurring in a man of 77 years of age.' Am. J. trop. Med. Hyg. 18, 185

Mazza, S. (1951). 'Chagas' disease' In Clinical Tropical Medicine. Ed. by R. B. H. Gredwohl, L. B. Soto and O. Felsenfeld, pp. 127–155. St. Louis: Mosby

Mott, K. E. and Hagstrom, J. W. (1965). 'The pathologic lesions of the cardiac autonomic nervous system in chronic Chagas' myocarditis.' *Circulation* **31**, 273

Muniz, J. (1950). 'A hemolise condicionada como um fenomeno de ordem mais geral.' Quinto Congresso Internacional Microbiologia, Abstracts, pp. 144–145

Neal, R. A. and Miles, R. A. (1968). 'An indirect haemagglutination test for *Trypanosoma cruzi* (Chagas' disease).' *Trans. R. Soc. trop. Med. Hyg.* **62**, 7

Nussenzveig, V. and Sonntag, R. (1952). 'Xenodiagnostica artificial, Novo processo. Primeires resoltidos positives.' *Revta paul. Med.* **40**, 41

Prata, A. (1968). 'Introduction to Chagas' heart disease.' *Cardiologia* **52**, 79

Puigbo, J. J., Rhode, J. R., Barrios, H. G., Suárez, J. A. and Yepez, C. G. (1966). 'Clinical and epidemiological study of chronic heart involvement in Chagas' disease.' *Bull. Wld. Hlth. Org.* **34**, 655

Raeder, M. M. and Simao, Clovis (1969). 'Chagas' myocardiomyopathy.' *Semin. Roentgenol.* **4**, 374

Rosenbaum, M. B. (1964). 'Chagasic myocardiopathy.' *Prog. cardiovasc. Dis.* **7**, 199

WHO Technical Report (1960). 'Chagas' disease—Report of a study group (1960).' *Tech. Rep. Ser. Wld. Hlth. Org.* **202**, 1

Winslow, D. J. and Chaffee, E. F. (1965). 'Preliminary investigations on Chagas' disease.' *Milit. Med.* **130**, 826

Woody, N. C. and Woody, H. B. (1955). 'American trypanosomiasis (Chagas' disease). First indigenous case in the U.S.A.' *J. Am. med. Ass.* **159**, 676

—— (1961). 'American trypanosomiasis. I. Clinical and epidemiologic background of Chagas' disease in the United States.' *J. Pediat.* **58**, 568

Yaeger, R. G. (1960). 'A method of isolating trypanosomes from the blood.' *J. Parasit.* **96**, 288

AFRICAN TRYPANOSOMIASIS

Much continues to be written about the cardiac lesions in Chagas' disease, but little attention has been devoted to those occurring in African trypanosomiasis. Cardiac signs, such as cardiomegaly or abnormal electrocardiograms, are frequent but the symptoms complained of in African trypanosomiasis are usually minor.

It has been suspected for over half a century that both species of African trypanosomiasis (*Trypanosoma gambiense* and *Trypanosoma rhodesiense*) may involve the heart. A review of some early accounts of post-mortem examinations discloses the presence of lymphocytic infiltration of the myocardium together with associated pleural effusions (Lau and Castellani, 1903; Thomas and Breinl, 1905).

West African trypanosomiasis is caused by *Trypanosoma gambiense* and East African infections by the much more virulent *Trypanosoma rhodesiense*.

Clinical cardiac insufficiency is exceptional in Gambian trypanosomiasis, but is more frequent in the Rhodesian trypanosomiasis.

Most often the only abnormality is found in the electrocardiogram, typically the T waves. Extrasystoles and blocks are much less frequent than in Chagas' disease.

Macroscopically the size of the heart may be normal or enlarged; enlargement is caused more by dilatation than hypertrophy. No lesion comparable to the apical lesion of Chagas' disease has been seen. Two types of lesion have been described in African trypanosomiasis. Hawking and Greenfield (1941) studied two cases of Rhodesian trypanosomiasis, one apparently of an acute variety, and the other subacute, and uninfluenced by treatment. In each instance the pericardial sac contained 500 ml of slightly turbid yellowish, serous fluid in which trypanosomes were easily found. The heart was small in both cases (170 and 200 g), and soft and flabby in one. The epicardium was considerably thickened by a subacute inflammatory reaction. The striking feature, however, was the state of the myocardium, which microscopically exhibited groups of shrunken and degenerated muscle fibres, and an intense infiltrate of macrophages, plasma cells, lymphocytes and polymorphs.

The histopathological lesions that have been described are mainly inflammatory changes, consisting of: (1) infiltrates of lymphocytes, histiocytes and plasma cells; and (2) oedema (WHO Report, 1969). These changes can progress to fibrosis. These lesions always involve the myocardium and may involve the endocardium and pericardium.

The infiltrates are most often involved in perivascular locations, but may also be seen around nerve fibres. The muscle fibres are rarely involved by the interstitial inflammatory exudates.

Lavier and Leroux (1939) have described two cases of long-standing T. gambiense infection in which the lesions were characterized by hyaline-like fibrosis of the epicardium, considerable perivascular fibrosis in the myocardium with extensive inflammatory exudates, and some endocardial sclerosis. There was also arteritis of branches of the coronary arteries in the hearts. Parasites, however, were not seen. The patients came from the Congo (Kinshasa).

As far as is known, parasites have been demonstrated in only one case—a patient with T. rhodesiense infection (Hawking and Greenfield, 1941). The lesions were comparable but more advanced than those recorded by Perruzzi (1927) in monkeys, where severe, frequently fatal myocarditis occurred in experimentally inoculated animals. The lesions were due to massive deposits of trypanosomes, which multiplied in myocardial fibres external to small intramyocardial blood vessels.

These workers suggested that the increased severity of the disease in the human heart could be explained by the fact that the disease evolved much more slowly in man.

Clinical myocarditis with decompensation may respond to both specific and general treatment, as in the cases reported by Manson-Bahr and Charters (1963): two patients with myocarditis thought to be due to Rhodesian trypanosomiasis.

In view of the cardiac disturbances, sudden deaths and premature fatal issue noted frequently in human infections due to *T. rhodesiense*, it is extremely probable that, in acute cases, the cardiac lesions are very severe and may be much more important to the patient's survival than involvement of the nervous system.

Ash and Spitz (1945) acknowledge this in their statement: 'The most notable features grossly evident in *T. rhodesiense* infections are the pronounced polyserositis and myocarditis as shown by flabbiness, areas of haemorrhage, and necrosis and, in later stages, fibrosis of the myocardium.'

Armengaud and Diop (1960) reported seven cases of cardiomyopathy with heart failure from Dakar. Trypanosomes were identified in the blood of those patients who responded to antitrypanosomal treatment. Trypanosomes were seldom found in the cerebrospinal fluid of these patients, but immuno-electrophoresis showed a marked increase in macroglobulins.

Bertrand *et al.* (1967) described cardiac involvement in 100 patients with African trypanosomiasis seen in Abidjan, Ivory Coast. Symptoms in most were of doubtful significance and the major electrocardiographic changes were of T wave abnormalities. Autopsy findings in three patients showed considerable inflammatory reaction with an infiltrate of histiocytes, lymphocytes and plasma cells that, in some areas, formed true granulomas, affecting the myocardium, pericardium and endocardium. The absence of parasites, classical inflammatory histological appearances of the heart and raised macroglobulins (Mattern, 1964), in cases of trypanosomal myocarditis due to *T. gambiense*, would suggest an immunological basis for the cardiomyopathy.

Francis (1972), in a case report on visceral complications in Gambian trypanosomiasis, describes a patient who presented in a stuporose condition and with signs of tachycardia, congestive heart failure and marked cardiomegaly. Numerous active trypanosomes were found on examining a wet film of pericardial fluid. On admission the electrocardiogram showed T wave inversion suggestive of myocardial damage. These changes persisted until day 40 of hospitalization when they reverted to normal—from shortly after admission the patient had been treated. In this patient the IgM and IgA were raised.

To summarize the lesions are usually interstitial and inflammatory and represent only a diffuse cardiac localization of an inflammatory disease; they cannot be considered as being specific for trypanosomiasis.

TABLE 11.1

Cardiac Manifestations of Trypanosomiasis

Manifestation	American trypanosomiasis T. cruzi	African trypanosomiasis T. gambiense and T. rhodesiense
Cardiac enlargement	Very common	Common
Cardiac failure	Very common	Very rare
Arrhythmias	Very common	Rare
Conduction defect	Very common	Rare
Thrombo-embolism	Common	Exceptional
Electrocardiogram ST–T changes	Common	Common

Table 11.1 compares the cardiac manifestations of the two forms of Trypanosomiasis (Technical Report, 1969).

References

Armengaud, M. and Diop, B. (1960). *Bull. Mem. Fac. Nat. Med. Rharm. Dakar* **8**, 263

Ash, J. E. and Spitz, S. (1945). *Pathology of tropical diseases. An Atlas.* p. 186. Philadelphia: Saunders

Bertrand, E., Baudin, L., Vacher, P., Sentiches, L., Ducasse, B. and Veyret, V. (1967). WHO/FAO publication. Tryp/Ent. **62**, 24, 2

Francis, T. I. (1972). 'Visceral complications of Gambian trypanosomiasis in a Nigerian.' *Trans. R. Soc. trop. Med. Hyg.* **66**, 140

Hawking, F. G. and Greenfield, J. G. (1941). 'Two autopsies on Rhodesiense sleeping sickness, visceral lesions and significance of changes in cerebrospinal fluid.' *Trans. R. Soc. trop. Med. Hyg.* **35**, 155

Lau, C. L. and Castellani, A. (1903). 'Report on sleeping sickness from its clinical aspects.' *Rep. sleep. Sickn. Commn. R. Soc.* **5**, 14

Lavier, G, and Leroux, R, (1939). 'Lésions cardiaques dans la maladie du sommeil.' *Bull. Soc. Path. exot.* **32**, 927

Manson-Bahr, P. E. C. and Charters, A. D. (1963). 'Myocarditis in African trypanosomiasis.' *Trans. R. Soc. trop. Med. Hyg.* **57**, 119

Mattern, P. (1964). 'Techniques et intérét épidêmiologique du diagnostic de la trypanosomiase humaine africaine par la recherche de la beta-macroglobuline dans le sang et dans le L.C-R.' *Annls Inst. Pasteur, Paris* **107**, 415

Perruzzi, M. (1927). *Final Report of the League of Nations. International Committee on Human Trypanosomiasis.* Publications of the League of National (III) health. 1927. 111, 13, CH, 629, pp. 245–324

Technical Report Series of the World Health Organization (1969). 'Comparative studies of American and African Trypanosomiasis.' No. 411

Thomas, H. W. and Breinl, A. (1905). 'Report on trypanosomes, trypanosomiasis and sleeping sickness.' *Mem. Lpool Sch. trop. Med.* **16**, 66

TOXOPLASMOSIS

Toxoplasmosis is due to infection by a minute coccoidal protozoon *Toxoplasma gondii*, which was first described by Nicolle and Manceaux in 1908. Wolfe and his colleagues established the syndrome of intra-uterine infection of the unborn foetus by *T. gondii* via the placenta (Wolf and Cowen, 1937; Wolf, Cowen and Paige, 1939), while Beckett and Flynn (1953) demonstrated *T. gondii* in the placenta. Adult infection is now recognized as a cause of myocarditis and of a syndrome resembling glandular fever or lymphoma. Many adult infections must go unnoticed as they are often asymptomatic. Beverley and Beattie (1952) estimated that by 20 years of age one quarter or more of the population had had an infection. Hutchison *et al.* (1969) and Frenkel, Dubey and Miller (1970) have demonstrated the cat to be the definitive host in whose intestines the toxoplasma undergoes a sexual stage division to form oöcysts, which are excreted in the faeces and are infective.

The organism is an obligate intracellular parasite which occurs in masses to form cysts in host tissue cells. These cysts are visible in haematoxylin and eosin stained sections with the low power of the microscope. The parasite has a low viability outside the body except in its cystic form as the oöcyst which, in the presence of moisture, is resistant to temperatures varying from 0 to 45°C. It can be cultivated in mice, guinea-pigs or fertile hens' eggs. Garnham, Baker and Bird (1962) studied the cysts in the brains of mice and rats by means of electron microscopy and found that they were true cysts of at least 100 μm in diameter. Toxoplasma has a complex structure including a two-layered pellicle, a well-defined micropyle, convoluted tubes, nucleus with nucleoli, a large mitochondrian and a strong tip for penetrating the host cell. Henry and Beverley (1969) inoculated 34 mice with the virulent 'Rh' strain and 24 (71 per cent) developed cardiac lesions, comprising interstitial oedema, myocardial necrosis, cell infiltration and pericarditis; toxoplasma cysts were found in the myocardial cells of two mice on day 10. Of 52 mice given the low virulence (Beverley) strain, 41 (71 per cent) developed cardiac lesions and 23 (44 per cent) skeletal muscle lesions; the cardiac lesions were less florid than in the first experiment but showed more necrotic muscle cells; pericarditis occurred in 4 and mural endocarditis in 1. The lesions were maximal at 17 days and then regressed leaving scars; only one toxoplasmic cyst was seen. Skeletal muscle also showed necrosis of isolated muscle cells and toxoplasmic cysts were found in two mice. Toxoplasma infection is widespread and this parasite is found in a wide variety of other domestic and wild animals. Dogs appear to be less susceptible as they grow older but they may have extensive gastro-intestinal ulceration and yet appear healthy. Human infection can arise from insect or animal scratches and bites, but most human infections probably arise from eating contaminated food. Laboratory workers run a special risk of infection when handling this organism.

Foetal infection arises from a mother who develops the disease in the last six months of pregnancy. The mother is often symptom-free but may have lassitude, a maculopapular rash, alimentary upsets with cramp-like abdominal pains, vaginal haemorrhage, laryngitis or bronchitis. If the maternal infection occurs in the first trimester, foetal infection can occur only if the mother has active disease during pregnancy and therefore no children in subsequent births will be affected.

CONGENITAL TOXOPLASMOSIS

Toxoplasma gondii reaches the foetus via the placenta and invades the foetal lungs, myocardium, liver, kidneys, muscles, testes, ovaries, adrenals, thyroid and particularly the eyes and central nervous system.

Sabin (1941) described toxoplasmosis in two cases presenting as meningo-encephalitis and in 1942 he published the well-known tetrad of the disease: hydrocephalus, choroidoretinitis, convulsions and intracerebral calcification. Any one of this tetrad may occur alone, especially choroidoretinitis. Considerable literature has now accumulated: the clinical and pathological features have been well documented by Sabin and Feldman (1949), Cathie and Dudgeon (1949), Hutchinson (1949), Wyllie and Cathie (1950) and others.

The manifestations may be four-fold.

(1)   Central nervous system: whence the disease often presents as convulsions.

(2) In the eye as bilateral macular choroidoretinitis.

(3) Intracranial calcification.

(4) Internal hydrocephalis.

It can be seen that toxoplasma infections are comparatively common from the fact that Montgomery, Donnison and Jolly (1958) were able to find over 50 reports in the British literature, to which they added a further two cases.

Laboratory Diagnosis

(1) Intracerebral or intraperitoneal inoculation into mice of suspect material, e.g., cerebrospinal fluid, blood, saliva, lymph node or other tissue.

(2) The dye test of Sabin and Feldman (1949) depends on the observation that toxoplasma organisms lose their affinity for methylene blue in the presence of specific antibody and a heat labile 'accessory factor' (not complement) present in certain human sera.

(3) Complement-fixation test (CFT) using an antigen already made from cultures of the organism in fertile eggs.

(4) Intradermal toxoplasmin skin test correlates with the dye test. Jirovec and Jira (1961) used material prepared from peritoneal exudates of infected mice, and ground up until innocuous to mice; it was injected intracutaneously over the deltoid area. Positive re-action was indicated by erythema and induration in 24–28 hours.

(5) Biopsy of a lymph node is usually done in cases of erroneous diagnosis of a lymphoma.

(6) The haemagglutination test has been used by Mitchell and Green (1960) for toxoplasma antibodies and they found positive results in over 60 per cent of 446 sera from blood donors over the age of 70; but there are no quantitative agreements with the dye tests.

(7) The immunofluorescent antibody tests are elegant and reliable but have not replaced the CFT in many laboratories. The technique is simple; smears of *T. gondii* (obtained from passages in white mice at intervals of 3–4 days) are made on glass slides, dried and stored at $-70°C$. They are then incubated in serial dilution of the test serum, washed and then covered by fluorescein-conjugated, anti-luminous gamma-globulin and examined by dark ground ultraviolet microscopy for green fluorescence, the intensity of which is proportional to the strength of the antibody.

Early reports came from Kelen, Ayllon-Leindl and Labzoffsky (1962), Mandras, Vanini and Ciarlin (1962), and Fulton and Voller (1964) who found the test correlated well with the dye, direct agglutinatious and complement-fixation tests. It was more specific and showed no cross reactions with trypanosomiasis, malaria, kala azar, sarcosporidiosis, leptospirosis, syphilis, schistosomiasis or filariasis.

Fletcher (1965) also recommended it; the point was sharp; no accessory factor serum was needed; protozoa undetected by the dye test were strongly positive at screening dilutions.

Remington (1967) introduced an immunofluorescent test to detect the foetal antibody which forms in foetal infection. Test serum was mixed with *T. gondii* and fluorescent animal serum antibody, known to react with foetal antibody; agglutination occurred and was detected by fluorescent microscopy.

The organism is readily transferrable so that the tests for toxoplasma infections require great caution and experience. Goldman (1956) said that exact results in the dye test required standard toxoplasma suspension and a standard accessory factor.

In Britain tests are performed in references laboratories. The public health laboratories at Cardiff give the following interpretation of tests.

(1) The dye tests for normal adults (20–40 per cent) have a titre of 1/8–1/128. One per cent have a titre of 1/258. Any titre, however low, indicated toxoplasma infection sometime in the past.

(2) CFT for normal adults (5 per cent) have a titre of $\frac{1}{4}$ or more. This is specific and usually indicates a relatively recent or active infection.

(3) For ocular toxoplasmosis some cases have a dye test of 1/256 or higher, in the majority the titres are 1/8–1/128. Negative results are uncommon.

(4) Acquired toxoplasmosis is usually an acute illness rarely proved except in laboratory workers, or when the disease is remembered as a cause of lymphadenopathy, resembling lymphoma or glandular fever.

Fatal cases may present with myocarditis, interstitial pneumonia, or a blood dyscrasia resembling acute leukaemia. Myocardial involvement may be found incidentally on clinical examination of those cases as cardiomegaly or after the patient has presented with congestive heart failure and the patients are then found to have a significantly high level of toxoplasma antibodies in their blood.

(5) For laboratory infection several well-documented cases have been published; the first by Bengtsson (1950) and Ström (1951); but only one has proved fatal, although others have shown signs of cardiac abnormality such as T wave inversion on the electrocardiogram.

(6) The cases of non-laboratory infection in adults reported have presented with lymphadenopathy, raising the suspicion of a

lymphoma or glandular fever especially as the blood picture may show abnormal monocytes or lymphocytes.

(7) Cysts of *T. gondii* and focal necrosis have been reported several times in the myocardium of fatal cases of acute generalized toxoplasmosis, as part of multiple infection involving other organs such as the brain, spleen and lungs.

Great interest was aroused by the report of Paulley *et al.* (1954) of three cases of myocardial toxoplasmosis. The heart of the first patient, a man of 24 who died in heart failure, weighed 960 g and showed extensive areas of yellow mottling or fibrosis. At the apex, where there was a large mural thrombus, microscopy showed interstitial fibrosis and hypertrophy of the remaining muscle fibres. There was no inflammation and no pseudocysts. The case of a man aged 47, with an enlarged heart, presented with a sudden occlusion of the aortic bifurcation; autopsy showed coarse myocardial fibrosis but no coronary artery disease. The arterial bifurcation obstruction was due to an embolism.

It has been suggested that attacks of Stokes–Adams syndrome may be due to toxoplasmosis (Shee, 1964).

Pathological Changes Found in the Heart

In severe disseminated infection, the heart has been described as dilated (not hypertrophied) and displaying petechial haemorrhage and grey areas of necrosis. The microscopic changes consist of focal interstitial infiltrates containing lymphocytes, plasma cells, histiocytes and occasionally eosinophils (Pinkerton and Weinman, 1940). In some places the myocardial fibres exhibit swelling, loss of striations, varying degrees of necrosis, and clumps of parasites varying from 8 to 100 in number. Because necrosis and inflammation are not encountered in the vicinity of parasitized fibres (*Figure 11.15*), the inflammatory response is attributed to rupture of the parasitized fibres, rather than to the presence of parasites within the fibre. The cysts of those parasites that are found, incidentally, at autopsy (*Figure 11.16*) are usually not associated with inflammatory lesions (Kean and Grocott, 1947). Zuelzer (1944) has given us one of the clearest descriptions of the detailed histology in toxoplasma myocarditis. In the heart of an 11 day old baby dying of infantile toxoplasmosis, he found widespread infiltration of the myocardial fibres and interstitium with chronic inflammatory cells. The infiltrates were mainly focal but poorly circumscribed. In most of the foci, the myocardial fibres had undergone hyaline necrosis and fragmentation. The process was slightly more marked in the inner layers of the

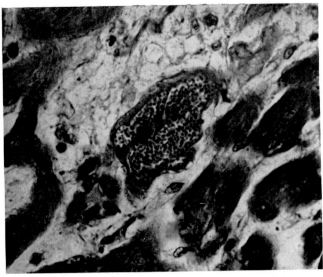

Figure 11.15. Toxoplasma gondii *involving myocardial fibres.* (*Haematoxylin and eosin and counterstained with methylene blue* × 600, *reduced to 2/3.*) (*Reproduced from Chatty and Deodhar (1969) by courtesy of the authors and Editor of the* Archives of Pathology)

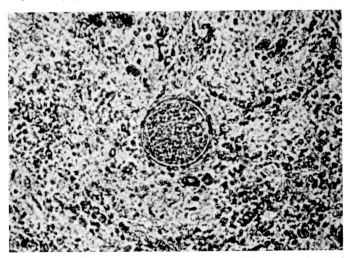

Figure 11.6. Histological section of myocardium showing a pseudocyst of Toxoplasma gondii. *Microphotograph taken with immersion lens.* (*Reproduced from Arribada and Escobar (1968) by courtesy of the authors and Editor of the* American Heart Journal)

myocardium than elsewhere. Many fairly well-preserved fibres contained collections of characteristic toxoplasma. The parasitized fibres, around the largest collections of parasites, were usually smaller and had lost their transverse striations close to the parasitic aggregations. Necrosis or inflammatory changes were almost never encountered in the vicinity of parasitized cardiac muscle fibres.

Single parasites were often found in areas of incipient necrosis and cellular infiltration. Some of the fibres, in otherwise intact areas, contained fine droplets of fat. The small blood vessels were often surrounded by inflammatory cells and the endothelium was swollen. A few cellular foci were present in the connective tissue underlying the endocardium. Durgé, Baqai and Ward (1967) describe the results of post-mortems on two patients whom they previously considered to have myocardial toxoplasmosis (Ward et al., 1964).

The first was a 30 year old man who lived and worked for 4 years after the diagnosis was made, even though the heart gradually increased in size. The toxoplasma dye test was finally positive at 1/256. His heart weighed 847 g. No evidence of coronary artery disease was found and microscopic examination of the myocardium showed a diffuse fibrosis. No cysts were found and investigation for toxoplasmosis was negative.

The second case was that of a 29 year old man in which a diagnosis of cardiac toxoplasmosis was made in 1965 when the dye test was 1/1024. Pronounced cardiomegaly then appeared fairly rapidly and he died from pulmonary embolic infection in 1966 (his heart weighing 840 g). Microscopy showed much diffuse interstitial fibrosis, with scattered chronic inflammatory cells throughout the myocardium. No toxoplasma 'cysts' were found despite examination of several sections. Incubation, however, with pepsin digested heart muscle was positive in one of the four cases.

It may be difficult for tissue sections to distinguish the parasite from other less common organisms such as Sarcocystis. To establish the diagnosis, therefore, one should supplement the histological examinations with serological tests and attempt to isolate the parasites.

Pericarditis has been reported to have been associated with toxoplasmosis in several instances, only one of which has been documented at post-mortem. It seems that pericarditis may, in some instances, be the predominant clinical manifestation of cardiac toxoplasmosis; however the pathological characteristics of this type of lesion have not been conclusively demonstrated as yet (Jones, Kimball and Kean, 1965; Arribada, 1971, personal communication).

Toxoplasmosis, for the present, should be considered as a cause of idiopathic cardiomyopathy.

References

Arribada, A. and Escobar, E. (1968). 'Cardiomyopathies produced by *Toxoplasma gondii.*' *Am. Heart J.* **76**, 329

Beckett, R. S. and Flynn, F. J., Jnr (1953). 'Toxoplasmosis: Report of two new cases with classification and with a demonstration of the organisms in the human placenta.' *New Engl. J. Med.* **249**, 345

Bengtsson, E. (1950). 'Affection of the heart in toxoplasmosis.' *Cardiologia* **17**, 289

Beverley, J. K. A. and Beattie, C. P. (1952). 'Standardisation of the dye test for toxoplasmosis.' *J. clin. Path.* **5**, 350

Cathie, I. A. and Dudgeon, J. A. (1949). 'The laboratory diagnosis of Toxoplasmosis.' *J. clin. Path.* **2**, 259

Chatty, A. Eyad and Deodhar, S. D. (1969). 'Myocardial changes and kidney transplantation.' *Archs Path.* **88**, 602

Durgé, N. G., Baqai, M. U. and Ward, R. (1967). 'Myocardial Toxoplasmosis.' (Letter) *Lancet* **2**, 155

Fletcher, S. (1965). 'Indirect fluorescent antibody technique in the serology of *Toxoplasma gondii.*' *J. clin. Path.* **18**, 193

Frenkel, J. K., Dubey, J. P. and Miller, N. L. (1970). '*Toxoplasma gondii* in cats: fecal stages identified as coccidian oöcysts.' *Science, N.Y.* **167**, 893

Fulton, J. D. and Voller, A. (1964). 'Evaluation of immunofluorescent and direct agglutination methods for detection of specific toxoplasma antibodies.' *Br. med. J.* **2**, 1173

Garnham, P. C. C., Baker, J. R. and Bird, R. G. (1962). 'Fine structure of cystic form of *Toxoplasma gondii.*' *Br. med. J.* **1**, 83

Goldman, M. (1956). 'Observations on some problems encountered in the routine performance of the dye test for toxoplasmosis.' *J. clin. Path.* **9**, 55

Henry, L. and Beverley, J. K. A. (1969). 'Experimental toxoplasma myocarditis.' Communication to the 118th meeting of the Pathological Society of Great Britain and Ireland. January 2–4 London: Pathological Society

Hutchinson, J. H. (1949). 'Congenital toxoplasmosis: Report of two cases.' *Arch. Dis. Child.* **24**, 303

Hutchison, W. M., Dunachie, J. F., Siim, J. and Work, K. (1969). 'Life cycle of *Toxoplasma gondii.*' *Br. med. J.* **4**, 806

Jirovec, O. and Jira, I. (1961). 'A contribution to the technique of intracutaneous testing with toxoplasmin.' *J. clin. Path.* **14**, 522

Jones, T. C., Kimball, A. C. and Kean, B. H. (1965). 'Pericarditis associated with Toxoplasmosis: Report of the case and review of the literature.' *Ann. intern. Med.* **62**, 786

Kean, B. H. and Grocott, R. G. (1947). 'Asymptomatic Toxoplasmosis.' *Am. J. trop. Med. Hyg.* **27**, 745

Kelen, A. E., Ayllon-Leindl, L. and Labzoffsky, N. A. (1962). 'Indirect fluorescent antibody method in sero-diagnosis of toxoplasmosis.' *Can. J. Microbiol.* **8**, 545

Mandras, A., Vanini, G. C. and Ciarlin, E. (1962). 'La reazione di unmanoflorescensa pal la demarstrazione degli anticarpi carta "Toxoplasma gondi.' ' *Ig. mod.* **55**, 636

Mitchell, R. G. and Green, C. A. (1960). 'The haemagglutination test for toxoplasma antibodies.' *J. clin. Path.* **13**, 331

Montgomery, R. D., Donnison, B. and Jolly, N. (1958). 'Congenital toxoplasmosis.' *J. clin. path.* **11**, 114

Nicolle, C. and Manceaux, L. (1908). 'Sur une infection à corps de Leishman (ou organismes voisons) du gondi.' *C. r. hebd. Séanc. Acad. Sci., Paris* **147**, 763

Paulley, J. W., Jones, R., Green, W. P. D. and Kane, E. P. (1954). 'Myocardial toxoplasmosis.' *Lancet* **2**, 624

Pinkerton, H. and Weinman, D. (1940). 'Toxoplasma infection in man.' *Archs Path.* **30**, 374

Remington, J. S. (1967). 'A rapid test for toxoplasmosis may lead to speedier treatment.' *Medi. miscellanea* **1**, 5, 1

Sabin, A. B. (1941). 'Toxoplasmic encephalitis in children.' *J. Am. med. Ass.* **116**, 801

— and Feldman, H. A. (1949). 'Chorioretinopathy associated with other evidence of cerebral damage in childhood.' *J. Pediat.* **35**, 296

Shee, J. C. (1964). 'Stokes-Adams attacks due to toxoplasma myocarditis.' *Br. Heart J.* **26**, 151

Ström, J. (1951). 'Toxoplasmosis due to laboratory infection in two adults.' *Acta med. scand.* **139**, 244

Ward, R., Durgé, N. G., Arya, J. and Baqai, M. U. (1964). 'Myocardial toxoplasmosis.' *Lancet* **2**, 723

Wolf, A. and Cowen, D. (1937). 'Granulomatous encephalomyelitis due to encephalitozoon (Encephalitozonic encephalomyelitis); new protozoan disease of man.' *Bull. neurol. Inst. N.Y.* **6**, 306

— — and Paige, Beryl (1939). 'Human toxoplasmosis; occurrence in infants as an encephalomyelitis verification by transmission to animals.' *Science N.Y.* **89**, 226

Wyllie, W. G. and Cathie, I. A. B. (1950). 'Congenital toxoplasmosis.' *Q. Jl. Med.* **19**, 57

Zuelzer, W. W. (1944). 'Infantile toxoplasmosis, with report of 3 new cases, including 2 in which patients were identical twins.' *Archs Path.* **38**, 1

MALARIA

Cardiac involvement caused by malaria depends primarily on the type of infecting parasite and is divided into two types.

(1) The 'benign' tertian form of malaria caused by *Plasmodium vivax*, the quartan form due to *Plasmodium malariae*, and that caused by *Plasmodium ovale* show very little effect on the heart, apart from changes which may result from any severe anaemia—fatty 'tabby-cat' markings of the interior of the musculature. The pigment liberated when the parasitized red blood cells rupture is taken up by

the reticulo-endothelial cells and resembles 'formalin-fixation' pigment, but the granules are of uniform size and shape, and are not refractile. However, tissue for histology is best fixed in formalin-free fluid, such as Zenker's fixative or alcohol.

Simonson and Keys (1950) infected 12 young men with *Plasmodium vivax* and detected slight changes in T waves, ST depression and other minor changes when compared with pre-infection tracings, but these were still within normal limits.

(2) The 'malignant' tertian form of malaria, due to *Plasmodium falciparum*, is a serious disease which is frequently fatal if untreated, because—besides anaemia—the parasitized cells accumulate and plug the capillaries in the brain (cerebral malaria) and other organs. In the heart there may be fatty changes, small haemorrhages and infiltration with lymphocytes, plasma cells and macrophages around foci of degenerative muscle associated with the plugged capillaries.

MACROSCOPICAL CHANGES

As early as 1900 Marchiafava and Bignami reported flaccid, dilated hearts with subepicardial haemorrhages in fatal cases. Ewing (1901) was impressed with the pallor and flaccidity of the myocardium which may be more or less discoloured by malaria pigment. Mohr (1940) in a detailed study of 260 fatal cases of malaria, described only minimal cardiac damage, such as flabbiness of the myocardium and slight dilatation of the chambers. In the hearts which I have seen, I have never been able to recognize grossly any specific changes.

HISTOLOGICAL CHANGES

Mohr (1940) observed microscopic lesions so numerous as sometimes to cause significant myocardial injury. The finer capillaries were partially and sometimes completely blocked by an accumulation of parasites, resulting in injury to the endothelium and malnutrition of the muscle tissue supplied by these choked vessels.

In fatal, untreated malaria, the myocardial capillaries are often distended with parasitized erythrocytes (Spitz, 1946).

Amoeboid forms of the parasites may also adhere to the walls of the vessels, and at their bifurcations clumps of amoeboid cells may plug the lumen. Parasites as well may be found along the walls of larger vessels, particularly of the venules. The parasitized erythrocytes are often arranged as mounds along the same side of the walls of different vessels, suggesting that some of the clumps observed may be a post-mortem phenomenon. Within the myocardial capillaries, thrombi may also sometimes be found.

Alterations of the myocardial fibres are inconstant and varied, and include loss of striations with translucency of the cytoplasm and severe fatty degeneration. This may be diffuse or irregular; the fat chiefly in the form of fine droplets (together with interstitial oedema) and small areas of haemorrhage either diffuse or subendocardial. In some instances myocardial damage may be focal, and may resemble micro-infarcts with scarring. A high parasite count is sometimes attended by an irregularly distributed interstitial myocardial infiltrate, containing lymphocytes, plasma cells and macrophages.

The plugging of myocardial capillaries with resulting anoxic changes in the myocardial fibres, constituting a form of coronary occlusive disease, has been observed by Merkel (1946) and Spitz (1946). The latter has also described thrombosis in coronary capillaries resulting from the tendency of the infected red cells and of the free amoeboid forms of the parasite to adhere to the endothelium, forming heaped up mounds, particularly at the bifurcation of small vessels.

Rojas and Deza (1947) have also observed cardiac capillary thrombosis in a fatal case of malaria and, like Spitz (1946), have described foci of interstitial collagenous hyperplasia, as well as interfibrillar oedema and interstitial infiltration with large, pigment-free macrophages, plasma cells and Anitschkow myocytes.

Micheletti (1930), however, while describing myolysis in malignant tertian malaria, found no endotholial changes or evidence of parasitic phagocytosis in the heart.

The cause of the concentration of the parasites within these capillaries is not known. Knisley, Stratman-Thomas and Elliot (1941) experimentally demonstrated the 'sludging phenomenon', during which parasitized erythrocytes tended to adhere to the walls of the vessels, accompanied by considerable slowing of the capillary flow. This observation, added to the interference by parasitized erythrocytes with normal exchange of oxygen, suggests that anoxia may be responsible for many of the clinical manifestations of the disease.

In addition, Merkel (1946) also showed that the endothelial cells of the affected capillaries were swollen and many contained phagocytosed myocardial pigment. He believed that when these occlusions were present, the heart muscle must experience anoxia proportional to the extent of the area involved. He also believed that, in fatal cases of malaria, anoxic ischaemia of the myocardium (resulting in acute micro-infarcts, dilatation and collapse) may be as important as the better known finding of occlusion of cerebral blood vessels.

Maegraith (1948) described two types of degenerative change in heart muscle: (1) perinuclear 'fat' globules—so called brown-atrophy; and (2) toxic fatty degeneration of the muscle cells. Both changes are presumably caused by relative anoxia.

In summary, from certain evidence presented in the literature, it seems fairly certain that malaria, particularly massive infections of the malignant tertian variety, may cause injury to the heart by the specific mechanism of coronary capillary occlusion, resulting in myocardial ischaemia. In a few well-documented cases, this mechanism appears to have been the direct cause of death. However, in the remainder of cases which have been published, in which cardiac muscular injury has been reported, it does not seem possible to distinguish between the effects which stem from the actual presence of the parasite within the vasculature of the heart, and those due to the less well-understood factors such as 'toxaemia', profound anaemia and haemolysis. It must also be remembered that it has never been conclusively demonstrated that malaria is the cause of chronic heart disease, aside from those myocardial changes which are known to accompany severe and prolonged anaemia.

References

Ewing, J. (1901). 'Contribution to the pathological anatomy of malarial fever.' *J. exp. Med.* **6**, 119

Knisely, M. H., Stratman-Thomas, W. K. and Elliot, T. S. (1941). 'Observations on circulating blood in the small vessels of internal organs in living Macaeus rhesus infected with malarial parasites.' *Anat. Rec.* **79**, 90

Maegraith, B. G. (1948). *Pathological Processes in Malaria and Blackwater Fever.* p. 430. Springfield; Ill: Thomas

Marchiafava, E. and Bignami, A. (1900). *Malaria in 20th Century Practice of Medicine.* Ed. by W. Wood, Vol. 18. New York: Stedman

Merkel, W. C. (1946). 'Plasmodium falciparum malaria; the coronary and myocardial lesions observed at autopsy in two cases of acute fulminating plasmodium, falciparum infection.' *Archs Path.* **41**, 290

Micheletti, E. (1930). 'Il contenuto parassitario degli organi nelle forme malariche perniciose.' *Annali Med. nav. colon.* **2**, 365

Mohr, W. (1940). 'Herz-gefässstörungen bei Malaria.' *Arch. Schiffs- u. Tropenhyg.* **44**, 521

Rojas, R. A. and Deza, D. (1947). 'Cardiac changes in malarial patients.' *Am. Heart J.* **33**, 702

Simonson, E. and Keys, A. (1950). 'Experimental malaria in man. III. The changes in the electrocardiogram.' *J. clin. Invest.* **29**, 68

Spitz, S. (1946). 'The pathology of acute falciparum malaria.' *Milit. Surg.* **99**, 555

SARCOSPORIDIOSIS

Sarcosporidiosis is a very common protozoal, parasitic disease of animals invading muscle fibres both skeletal and myocardial. The organism was described by Miescher (1843). Man is rarely infected—eight human cases were collected from the literature by Feng (1932), who added a personal case. Most reports of cardiac sarcosporidiosis in human beings have probably been cases of toxoplasmosis (Kean and Grocott, 1945).

McGill and Goodbody (1957) reported the case of a 60 year old man who had the infection in India—proved by muscle biopsy. At necropsy there were large vegetations on the tricuspid valve spreading to the atria and ventricles. These heart lesions proved to be mainly-fibrinous and free of parasites, but some pulmonary lesions were like peri-arteritis nodosa. The authors concluded that the pulmonary lesions were manifestations of peri-arteritis nodosa resulting from a reaction to sarcosporidia cyst material. They also traced seventeen acceptable cases of sarcosporidiosis from the literature.

Infection is probably by mouth from food contaminated by animal faeces. In man the infection is attributed to *Sarcocystis lindemanni*, despite the lack of conclusive evidence that the parasite differs from *Sarcocystis tenella* or any of the many other types which have been discussed. Ingested parasites reach the striated muscle and form cysts up to 5 mm long in individual muscle fibres. The cyst is subdivided into chambers by septae, and contains many sickle-shaped spores.

DIAGNOSIS

A diagnosis may be established by muscle biopsy, and by the serum complement-fixation test of Awad and Lainson (1954)

PATHOLOGY

Gross findings have been conspicuously absent from reports on involved hearts.

Lambert (1927), however, did describe numerous subendocardial haemorrhages 'of considerable size' in the septal portion of the left ventricle. Gilmore, Kean and Posey (1942), likewise, mentioned small subendocardial haemorrhages in the papillary muscles but felt that these were more likely to be terminal in origin.

The parasite usually occupies a muscle fibre in the form of an elongated cyclindrical cyst that varies in length from 25 μm to several millimetres, and may enlarge the width of the fibre to 50 μm. The wall of the cyst, which is approximately 1 μm thick, is laminated and may be radially striated. Individual cysts may contain hundreds of crescent shaped organisms which, when stained by Romanowsky's method, reveal a light blue cytoplasm, and a basophilic eccentrically placed nucleus. In addition, trabeculae may be seen crossing the cyst.

Pathological Features

The most striking pathological feature is the absence of any inflammatory reaction; there is no cellular infiltration surrounding parasitized muscle fibres, nor are there any degenerative changes in adjacent fibres (Gilmore, Kean and Posey, 1942; Reich, 1954).

Though no myocardial necrosis or fibrosis was noted in tissues adjoining these organisms, the individual host fibres, in general, may appear swollen to about twice the size of their normal neighbours (Manifold, 1924).

In man, the cysts may either be few in number and confined chiefly to the left ventricular wall, or so numerous that they are visible in almost every high-power field; occasionally they may be found in Purkinje's tissue.

In Hewitt's case (1933) cysts were seen in every section of the ventricular wall examined, with an average of 10–12 'tubes' per low-power field. Despite the absence of an inflammatory reaction, the fibres which were invaded were 2–3 times their normal size.

CONCLUSION

There is no evidence whatsoever that sarcosporidiosis has ever been responsible for any clinical manifestations or morbidity in man.

Darling (1919) believed that this infection is an example of a parasitic 'blind alley', wherein the parasite has accidentally reached a strange host from which it is unable to escape for continuation of its life cycle. Therefore, at present, sarcosporidiosis must be considered to be an example of aberrant parasitism which is, apparently, well tolerated by the human body.

References

Awad, F. I. and Lainson, R. (1954). 'A note on the serology of sarcosporidiosis and toxoplasmosis.' *J. clin. Path.* **7**, 152

Darling, S. T. (1919). 'Sarcosporidiosis in an East Indian.' *J. Parasit.* **6**, 98

Feng, L. C. (1932). 'Sarcosporidiosis in man; report of a case in a Chinese.' *Chin. med. J.* **46**, 976

Gilmore, H. R., Kean, B. H. and Posey, F. M. (1942). 'Sarcosporidiosis with parasites found in the human heart.' *Am. J. trop. Med. Hyg.* **22**, 121

Hewitt, J. A. (1933). 'Sarcosporidiosis in human cardiac muscle.' *J. Path. Bact.* **36**, 133

Kean, B. H. and Grocott, R. G. (1945). 'Sarcosporidiosis or toxoplasmosis in man and guinea pig.' *Am. J. Path.* **21**, 467

Lambert, S. W., Jnr (1927). 'Sarcosporidial infection of the myocardium in man.' *Am. J. Path.* **3**, 663

McGill, R. J. and Goodbody, R. A. (1957). 'Sarcosporidiosis in man with periarteritis nodosa.' *Br. med. J.* **2**, 333

Manifold, J. A. (1924). 'Report of a case of sarcosporidiosis in a human heart.' *Jl. R. Army med. Cps.* **42**, 275

Miescher, F. (1843). 'Ueber eigenthümliche Schläuche in der Muskel einer Hausmaus.' *Ber. Verh. naturforsch. ges. Basel* **5**, 198

Reich, N. E. (1954). *Uncommon Heart Diseases.* p. 227. Springfield, Ill: Thomas

METAZOAL DISEASES

SCHISTOSOMIASIS

Although approximately 200 million people are infected with one of the three main species of schistosomes to which man may be host, cardiac involvement in schistosomiasis is rare; an astonishing fact in as much as the infection is disseminated in its earliest phase in the blood stream, and the eggs may reach any organ. Schistosomiasis may involve the human heart in any of four ways: (1) by presence of the adult fluke; (2) by presence of the ova; (3) by back pressure on the right heart, secondary to obstruction of the lesser circuit in pulmonary schistosomiasis; and (4) possibly by the production of a toxic or allergic myocarditis. Following the invasion of the skin or mucous membranes by cercariae released from infected snails, immature schistosomes circulate throughout the entire body, causing fever, pneumonitis and eosinophilia.

Although electrocardiogram changes may be induced by this process, parasites have not been found in the heart, nor are cardiac lesions apparent at this stage of the disease. About six weeks after infection when parasites reach adulthood, *Schistosoma mansoni* and *S. japonicum* take residence in the portal circulation; and *S. haematobium* in the systemic veins around the urinary bladder. In a few instances these parasites may reach ectopic vessels, including those of the heart.

DIAGNOSIS

Precise laboratory diagnosis can usually be made by microscopy of urine or faeces, according to the infecting species and supplemented by serological tests, of which the CFT (using an antigen from cercariae) and the fluorescent antibody test are the most helpful.

In summary, although schistosomiasis is one of the most widespread parasitic diseases in the world, cardiac involvement is relatively rare, except in the South American variety caused by *S. cruzi*. Involvement by the adult fluke is so rare as to be a pathological curiosity only. The production of miliary myocardial granulomata surrounding ova, which reach the heart by the systolic route is more common as a complication of this disease and may be a potential cause of heart failure. On the other hand, considerable doubt has been cast on the supposed schistosomal aetiology of toxic or allergic myocarditis, which lacks specific histopathological changes.

PRESENCE OF ADULT FLUKE

El Gazayerli (1939) reported the finding of an adult *S. haematobium* in the circumflex branch of the left coronary artery, and mature flukes have been seen in the cardiac chambers in man and other primates—occupying these sites without having caused any myocardial lesions.

PRESENCE OF OVA

Although the eggs from any species from time to time may reach the myocardium, they rarely seem to produce any cardiac manifestations.

Lesions produced by schistosome eggs, wherever localized, are essentially the same: a zone of acute focal necrosis develops, accompanied by infiltrates of neutrophils which degenerate, and are then replaced by plasma cells, lymphocytes, monocytes and eosinophils. Either as a result of secretions produced by developing miracidia within the ova, or following release of toxic material by dead parasites, a zone of diffuse acellular eosinophilic necrosis may be seen soon after the egg has been deposited in the tissue.

There then follows the formation of pseudotubercles (*Figure 11.17*) with fibroblasts arranged in concentric fashion about the ova, which, although persisting for many months, are eventually absorbed. These findings are illustrated in the schistosomal granuloma discovered as an incidental finding in a Rhodesian African, who, although suffering from bilharziasis, died from chronic heart failure caused by cardiomegaly of unknown origin (McKinney and Ashworth, 1973). Giant cells may be present and often fragments of egg-wall may be seen within their cytoplasm. Eventually a simple scar, sometimes containing deposits of calcium, constitutes the only evidence of the former presence of an egg.

Africa and Santa Cruz (1939) described pseudotubercles caused by the eggs of *S. japonicum* in the interventricular septum, and Thomas,

Bracken and Bang (1946) reported that, in a fatal acute case in an American soldier, eggs of *S. japonicum* in the heart had caused thrombosis and hyaline necrosis of coronary arteries and venules, finally leading to a massive infarction of the interventricular septum, mural thrombosis and death from pulmonary embolism.

Clark and Graef (1935) first found direct invasion of the myocardium of both ventricles by small numbers of eggs, which were

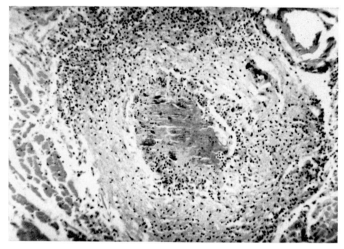

Figure 11.17. Schistosomiasis granuloma in myocardium. The ova are in the centre of the granuloma and are associated with an infiltrate of lymphocytes, plasma cells and eosinophils. A zone of fibrosis separates the granuloma from the adjacent myocardium (haematoxylin and eosin × 12, reduced to 6/10). (Reproduced by courtesy of Dr T. G. Ashworth, Rhodesia)

surrounded by inflammatory cells and miliary foci of interstitial fibrosis. Armbrust (1949) reported the histopathological finding of many bilharzial tubercles in the myocardium, each containing a single centrally placed egg of *S. mansoni*. The heart was macroscopically normal except for slight right ventricular hypertrophy. Microscopically, however, the eggs were encircled by multiple small necrotic areas which were surrounded in turn by epithelioid cells, lymphocytes, and eosinophils. Eggs were also seen in the lumina of small blood vessels. Other reported instances of *S. mansoni* eggs located in the myocardium include two instances reported by Jaffé (1943) from a series of more than 400 autopsies of Manson's schistomiasis. A most dramatic example of the possible consequences of myocardial involvement by schistosomal eggs is illustrated in the case reported from Egypt by Al Zahawi and Shukri (1956), who described schistosomal myocarditis in a 13 year old boy who had entered hospital with the clinical picture of far advanced congestive heart failure, and who died within sixteen hours of admission. At autopsy the heart weighed 460 g and the right side was dilated. The myocardium of the left ventricle contained small isolated dark red foci of necrosis, the largest being 3 mm in diameter. Microscopically, these foci contained eggs of *S. haematobium*. There were also perivascular collections of mononuclear cells and eosinophils, but the absence of fibrosis or myocardial degeneration in any part of the heart indicated the acute onset of these changes. Because there were no other findings to explain the clinical condition, the authors thought that the heart failure was due to the focal bilharzial myocarditis. They felt certain that the eggs had reached the myocardium from the primary site of infection in the bladder by way of anastomotic connections with veins in the pelvic venous plexus.

PULMONARY SCHISTOSOMIASIS

In contrast to the rarity of direct involvement of the heart by adult flukes or their eggs, schistosomiasis in man is much more likely to cause pulmonary hypertension, due to the formation of bilharzial granulomata in the lungs with secondary pulmonary fibrosis and cardiac changes, than to any direct myocardial involvement. Thus, Bedford, Aidaros and Girgis (1946) found cor pulmonale in six (2·1 per cent) of 282 consecutive autopsied cases with *S. haematobia* infection, and Le Faria (1954) 5·5 per cent positive in 180 necropsies of verified cases of schistosomiasis. In heavily infected areas the condition is often of great practical importance. The pulmonary lesions in these cases are interesting. In addition to the formation of numerous granulomata with extensive scarring and diminution of the pulmonary vascular bed, the eggs may be responsible for the formation of very many small arteriovenous aneurysms following the development of pulmonary arteritis and arteriolitis.

TOXIC OR ALLERGIC MYOCARDITIS

In those parts of the world where schistosomiasis is an important disease (as in Egypt and Brazil) a syndrome known as bilharzial myocarditis has been described. These patients exhibit clinical evidence of heart disease with electrocardiogram abnormalities including bundle branch block, notching of the QRS complex and T wave changes. These changes are almost certainly caused by the toxic effects of some of the anti-schistosomal drugs on the myocardium—

probably due to their high antimony content, and not to any cardiac changes due to the direct action of schistosomes or their eggs.

I have performed autopsies on two patients who died suddenly while undergoing treatment with antimony-containing drugs for schistosomiasis. At autopsy the septal regions of the hearts of these patients contained about five times as much antimony as other parts of the heart—that is in the region of the conduction tissues in the heart.

References

Africa, C. M. and Santa Cruz (1939). 'Ova of Schistosoma japonicum in the human heart.' In Vol. Jubilare pro Professor Sadao Yoshida, Osaka, Japan 2, 113

Al Zahawi, S. and Shukri, N. (1956). 'Histopathology of fatal myocarditis due to ectopic schistosomiasis.' Trans. R. Soc. trop. Med. Hyg. 50, 166

Armbrust, A. de F. (1949). 'Miocardite esquitossomótica (forma granulomatosa);' nota prévia. Hosp. Rio de Janeiro 36, 213

Bedford, D. E., Aidaros, S. M. and Girgis, B. (1946). 'Bilharzial heart disease in Egypt; cor pulmonale due to bilharzial pulmonary endarteritis.' Br. Heart J. 8, 87

Clark, E. and Graef, I. (1935). 'Chronic pulmonary arteritis in Schistosomiasis mansoni associated with right ventricular hypertrophy.' Am. J. Path. 11, 693

El Cazayerli (1939). 'Unusual site of a schistosome worm in the circumflex branch of the left coronary artery.' J. Egypt. med. Ass. 22, 34

Jaffé, R. (1943). 'Cardiac schistosomiasis consideraciones sobre la patogenia de la miocarditis.' Revta Sanid. Assist. soc., Caracas 8, 85

Le Faria, J. L. (1954). 'Cor pulmonale in Manson's Schistosomiasis I. Frequency in Necroscopy material; pulmonary vascular changes caused by schistosoma ova.' Am. J. Path. 30, 167

McKinney, B. and Ashworth, T. G. (1973). 'Spontaneous cardiomyopathy found in African in Rhodesia.' (In press)

Thomas, H. M., Jnr, Bracken, M. M. and Bang, F. B. (1946). 'The clinical and pathological picture of early acute schistomiasis japonica.' Trans. Ass. Am. Physns 59, 75

ECHINOCOCCOSIS (HYDATID DISEASE)

In Australia (Cole, 1947), New Zealand and in parts of South America and the Mediterranean area, echinococcal disease is frequently found. Infections with this parasite are also often seen in parts of North America (Magath, 1941) and in Wales, particularly the more northern parts (Jonathan, 1960). Publications relative to cardiac localization have been few, one of the first being that of Grulee (1905). It seems, however, that the condition is more frequent than supposed because cysts located in the territory of distribution of the systemic circulation (spleen, kidneys, brain and muscle) are not uncommon.

AETIOLOGY, PATHOGENESIS AND INCIDENCE

Echinococcus disease in man is caused by the development of the larval stage of *Echinococcus granulosus*, a cystode tapeworm, whose definitive host is the dog in most instances. The dog is infected, when fed, with cyst-bearing organs (such as lungs or liver) of intermediate hosts which are usually sheep. These cysts contain scolices (tapeworm heads), usually numbered in hundreds, which develop in the intestine of the dog into the adult form of the worm. The worm, usually of rather small size (4–5 mm), has a head, a neck and three proglottides. The last proglottis, containing the sexual organs, when distended by the ova, is shed in the faeces of the dog, thus contaminating grass and water that may be ingested by another intermediate host, such as a sheep. Owing to close contact with infected dogs in rural areas, man may become readily infected.

The chitinous shell of the ova of *Echinococcus granulosus* is dissolved in the gastro-intestinal tract of the intermediate host (i.e., sheep or man), thus liberating a hexacanth embryo which then passes through the intestinal wall to reach the portal circulation and the liver, the organ most frequently involved by echinococcal disease. Occasionally the liver may be spared, because of the rather small size of the hexacanth embryo and the distensibility of the hepatic capillaries. If so, the embryo goes on its way down the pulmonary capillary circulation, where it may be blocked. Pulmonary cysts are second to hepatic cysts in incidence. This second capillary barrier may also be passed, however, by the parasite.

It was originally believed that echinococcal disease of the heart was predominantly, or exclusively secondary to rupture of a primary hydatid cyst elsewhere in the body; and encystation of the hexacanth embryo on the endocardial surface of the right-heart chambers, which is more commonly involved than the left (Peters, Dexter, and Weiss, 1945). From its original endocardial graft the embryo would be able to reach any other region of the heart by active movements.

However, according to Dew (1928) and to most other modern writers (Devé, 1946), the hexacanth embryo, after passing through the capillary networks of the liver and lungs, arrives in the left heart chambers, enters the coronary circulation and become lodged in the tissue of the myocardium of any of the four cardiac chambers or the cardiac septa.

Devé also pointed out that the primary cardiac cyst is most frequently located in the wall of the left, rather than the right, side of the heart because of the richer coronary circulation on this side. This distribution has been confined by the reports of other workers (Diehiero *et al.*, 1958). Although Devé's views on the pathogenesis of echinococcal disease of the heart have usually been generally accepted, some workers (such as Jorge and Modre, 1946) have proposed the theory that the hexacanth embryo can reach the heart via the lymphatic system. This is based on the observation that many cases of cardiac echinococcal infection do not have concomitant hepatic cysts. They also accept the possibility of transendocardial migration of the embryo after it has arrived in the right heart chamber.

INCIDENCE OF INVOLVEMENT OF THE MYOCARDIUM

Various authors state that cardiac cysts are seen in 0·5–2 per cent of all cases of echinococcus infection in humans. It has also been shown (Diehiero *et al.*, 1958) that the incidence is higher in men than in women (2:1). It is also found that most cases occur in the second to fifth decade in patients living in cattle-raising areas (Dumont, 1918; Dew, 1928). In a case reported by D'Abreau (1950) it is illustrated that an intra-cardiac hydatid cyst may be successfully removed. This patient lived for several years after the operation and, although she had a splenectory for another hydatid cyst in the spleen, had no further symptoms or signs of cardiac disease. The patient eventually died of renal disease.

PATHOLOGY

A few weeks after its arrival in the interstitial tissue of the myocardium from any part of the body, the hexacanth embryo becomes vesicular and grows slowly but steadily into a unilocular hydatid vesicle, with an outer elastic membrane duplicated by an inner germinal layer containing clear fluid (*Figure 11.18*). The hydatid vesicle thins out the myocardial wall during its process of growth (*Figure 11.19*) and exerts pressure on the surrounding muscle fibres, which become more or less ischaemic, depending on the degree of pressure on the surrounding muscle fibres, caused by the parasite and the resistance of the cardiac tissues. A pedicle may then be formed, which consists of a portion of the overlying pericardial or endocardial layer. In rare cases, the cysts may extend completely through the heart wall, forming a fluctuant tumour covered only by endocardium on one side and by pericardium on the other (Goodheart, 1876; Warthin, 1902). Due to mechanical, toxic, allergic and inflammatory

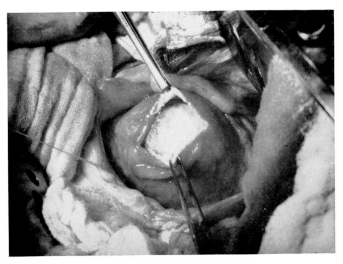

Figure 11.18.   Photograph of the exterior of a heart showing the cystic swelling of the apex of the left ventricle, the hexacanth embryo having grown slowly into a unilocular cyst. (Reproduced from Gibson (1969) by courtesy of the author and Editor of Thorax)

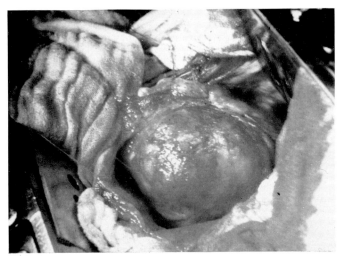

Figure 11.19.   Photograph of the inside of the hydatid cyst cavity in the wall of the left ventricle. The hydatid vesicle thins out the myocardial wall during its process of growth and exerts pressure on the surrounding muscle fibres which become more or less ischaemic. (Reproduced from Gibson (1969) by courtesy of the author and Editor of Thorax)

phenomena caused by the hydatid vesicle, the tissue reaction in the host leads to the formation of a fibrous capsule showing cellular infiltration and gradually becoming thicker with time.

The internal germinal layer of the primitive hydatid vesicle gives rise, by a process of proliferation, to multiple vesiculated structures called 'brood capsules', which may float in the capsular fluid. From these capsules scolices may develop. The size of the primary uncomplicated hydatid cyst of the heart varies from a few millimetres to 4–5 cm. During the period of intramural development of a hydatid cyst, its presence may be completely overlooked but later it may produce a localized bulge in the cardiac shape which may permit radiographic recognition of the disease.

The primary hydatid cyst of the heart has a marked tendency to rupture either into the lumen of the cardiac chamber or into the pericardial sac, depending on its primary location and on the direction of least resistance. They, however, show a marked tendency to rupture into the cavity of one of the heart chambers (Bobowicz, 1887).

The primary cyst may also rupture into the myocardium itself. While the pericardium usually reacts in front of a hydatid cyst by developing adhesions, the endocardium does not react and is, therefore, easily invaded by the cyst.

UNCOMPLICATED ECHINOCOCCAL DISEASE OF THE HEART

This may remain completely silent and latent. However, in some instances thoracic pain, palpitations, paroxysmal tachycardia, congestive heart failure or angina may be found.

DIAGNOSIS

Eosinophilia (10 per cent or more) may be of diagnostic significance but it is often absent, especially in old, altered cysts.

The intradermal (Casoni, 1911) test is only of value when positive—especially delayed positive—and is one of the most specific tests.

SEROLOGY

(1) Complement-fixation test (CFT) is by no means the most sensitive test available for diagnosis, about 70 per cent of infections giving a positive result—whilst 1–5 per cent of cases give non-specific reactions. It is, however, valuable post-operatively because it is the first to revert to negative after the successful removal of a hydatid cyst. In these post-operative cases the titre should fall in six to twelve weeks.

(2) Haemagglutination test (HA) is probably the best at present available, and is able to detect 85 per cent of cases and only gives 1–2 per cent of non-specific reactions.

(3) Beutonite flocculation test (BFT) and latex-agglutination test (L) both give more positive results than the CFT, but less than the HA and have a higher incidence of non-specific reactions.

(4) Indirect fluorescent antibody (IFA) method is giving promising results but needs more evaluation before it can be used as a routine diagnostic test.

In conclusion, the combination of HA and BFT gives a very high degree of accuracy and should be used clinically as the diagnostic tests of choice (Bull. WHO, 1968).

Complications

Primary cardiac hydatid cysts exhibit a marked tendency to rupture spontaneously in 1 of the 4 cardiac chambers, or into the pericardial sac, as a result of necrosis of the affected cardiac wall, owing to interference with the blood supply and to the continued trauma of muscular contraction.

Devé (1915) has pointed out that intracardiac rupture is the greater of the two threats, since the pericardium usually reacts to a hydatid cyst by forming dense adhesions, whereas the endocardium develops no reaction and thus is easily penetrated. Despite this fact, about 10 per cent of all primary cardiac cysts rupture into the pericardial sac (DiBello, 1955). If the cyst is viable, rupture results in the implantation in the pericardium of scolices and brood-capsules (some of which are destroyed by the ensuing inflammatory response) with resultant fibrosis and formation of dense adhesions; however, other daughter-cysts may survive and develop into multiple secondary pericardial cysts, which characteristically are all approximately of the same size.

Following its rupture, the primary cyst may undergo fibrosis and involution, but more commonly the root in the wall becomes sealed with adhesions, and the daughter-cyst formation then proceeds from the residual germinal elements (Devé, 1928; Gould, 1953). These daughter-cysts may rupture in turn, often resulting in sudden death from anaphylactic shock (Peters, Dexter and Weiss, 1945).

A foreign-body reaction, characterized by macrophages, eosinophils and numerous giant cells is frequently found in the cardiac tissue surrounding these cysts. Pseudotubercles may also be found around degenerated scolices (Gould, 1953). Reactions of this nature are believed to be caused by the development of hypersensitivity to echinococcal proteins, a condition that not only forms the basis for several skin and serological tests now used for diagnosis of echino-coccal infections, but also explains the anaphylactic reaction of an infected individual after the rupturing of a cyst into his own circu-lation (Peters, Dexter and Weiss, 1945). If, however, the adventitial membrane surrounding the cyst remains intact, leakage of hydatid fluid is prevented and sensitivity reactions do not occur.

The small cardiac echinococcal cyst may produce no symptoms (Heilbrunn, Kittle and Dunn, 1963). As the cyst enlarges myocardial compression may lead to ischaemia and even angina pectoris (Michaud et al., 1959).

The clinical manifestations of the infection are related to the size and position of the cyst, its rupture into the cardiac chambers or into the pericardium, anaphylactic reaction resulting from the entry of hydatid fluid into the circulation and peripheral embolism from ruptured distintegrating cysts.

According to Devé (1946) a primary cardiac hydatid cyst, before rupture may enlarge insidiously for as long as 10 years, followed by another latent period of 2–3 years before evidence of metastatic echinococcosis becomes apparent—and before subsequent myo-cardial rupture resulting in death.

In rare instances a cyst of the interventricular septum has given rise to conduction defects (Heimann, 1928; Corkill, 1929).

Disorders of rate or rhythm do not figure prominently in the majority of reported cases, having been noted in only 13 of the 56 cases reviewed by Peters, Dexter and Weiss (1945).

If the cyst is located in the ventricular septum, right bundle branch block or atrioventricular block may be present (DiBello, Urioste and Rubia, 1964).

However, in an additional nine cases, or 16 per cent of the total group, death was sudden, with an intact cardiac cyst constituting the only abnormality seen at autopsy. Although there is no indis-putable proof that death in these cases was caused by the pressure of the cyst, the relative frequency of its occurrence suggests the onset of fatal arrhythmias.

Ante-mortem diagnosis can be made on the basis of seeing a characteristic calcified mass—revealed by radiology. The intradermal test, since introduction by Casoni in 1911, has been used extensively for the diagnosis of human hydatidosis. However, it is clear from the literature that a high degree of non-specificity was commonly en-countered which seriously limited the usefulness of the procedure, either as a clinical test or as an epidemiological tool.

An important contribution towards overcoming non-specificity was made by Kagan et al. (1966), who were able to demonstrate an association between the nitrogen content of the antigen and the degree of non-specific reactivity in persons not having the disease. They found that the highest specificity could be obtained using an antigenic fraction prepared by chromatography of *E. granulosus* cyst fluid containing only 12–15 mg/ml of nitrogen; 15 of the 21 patients infected with *E. granulosus* gave positive results with this antigen and non-specific reactions in healthy individuals were minimal.

The results of this work have later been followed up by the studies of Williams (1972). Here the diagnostic sensitivity and specificity of the Casoni test were determined in 100 hydatidosis patients and 68 non-hydatidosis individuals, using an antigen derived from *E. granulosus* and containing only 15 mg protein N/ml. The antigen solution was shown to contain only one parasite component demonstrable by gel-diffusion, although other non-precipitating antigens may have contributed to the activity in the intradermal tests.

Eighty-six per cent of the hydatidosis patients showed reactions which were greater than the largest non-specific reactions observed in patients not having the disease. Most of the hydatidosis patients showing negative skin reactions had pulmonary infections. The degree of non-specificity observed in persons not infected with *E. granulosus* was considered to be highly satisfactory.

Cardiac echinococcal disease may also present as occasional chest pain together with an attack of dyspnoea, as in the case reported by Dodek *et al.* (1972).

References

Bobowicz, A. (1887). 'Des hydatides du coeur chez l'homme et en particulare des hydatides flottindren.' Thesis No. 287, University of Paris.

Bulletin World Health Organisation (1968). **39**, 25

Casoni, T. (1911). 'La diagnosi biologica dell'echinoccosi umana mediante l'intradermoreazione.' *Folio clin. chim. microsc.* **4**, 5

Cole, G. (1947). 'The Australasian hydatid registry; health bulletin Melbourne, 83/84: 2255, 1945.'*Trop. Dis. Bull.* **44**, 602

Corkill, N. L. (1929). 'Hydatid cyst of the heart.' *Br. med. J.* **2**, 622

D'Abreau, A. C. (1950). 'The removal of a hydatid cyst from the wall of the left ventricle.' *Thorax* **5**, 362

Devé, F. (1915). 'Sur l'écchinococcose secondaire du péricarde.' *C. r. Séanc. Soc. Biol.* **78**, 734

— (1928). 'Les kystes hydatiques du coeur et les complications.' *Algér. méd.*

— (1946). *L'échinococcose secondaire.* Paris: Masson

Dew, H. R. (1928). *Hydatid Disease.* pp. 390–397. Sydney: Medical Publishers

DiBello, R. (1955). 'El hidatidopericadio.' *An. Fac. Med. Univ. Montevideo* **40**, 244

DiBello, R., Urioste, H. A. and Rubia, P. (1964). 'Hydatid cysts of the ventricular septum of the heart. A study based on two personal cases and forty-one observations in the literature.' *Am. J. Cardiol.* **14**, 237

Diehiero, J., Canabal, E. J., Aguirre, C. V., Hazan, J. and Horjales, J. O. (1958). 'Echinococcus disease of the heart.' *Circulation* **17**, 127

Dodeck, A., Demots, H., Antonovic, J. A. and Hodman, R. P. (1972). 'Echinococcus of the heart.' *Am. J. Cardiol.* **30**, 293

Dumont, M. (1918). 'L'echinococose cerebrale metastaque.' Thesis, University Toulouse

Gibson, D. S. (1969). 'Cardiac hydatid cysts.' *Thorax* **19**, 151

Goodheart, J. E. (1876). 'Cured hydatid cyst in the wall of the heart.' *Trans. path. Soc. Lond.* **27**, 72

Gould, S. C. (1953). *Pathology of the Heart.* pp. 847–849. Springfield, Ill: Thomas

Grulee, C. G. (1905). 'Echinococcus disease of the heart with a report of a case.' *Surgery Gynec. Obstet.* **1**, 328

Heilbrunn, A., Kittle, C. F. and Dunn, M. (1963). 'Surgical management of echinococcal cysts of the heart and pericardium.' *Circulation* **27**, 219

Heimann, H. L. (1928). 'Hydatid cyst of the heart.' *Br. med. J.* **1**, 801

Jonathan, O. M. (1960). 'Hydatid disease in North Wales.' *Br. med. J.* **1**, 1246

Jorge, J. and Modre, M. (1946). 'Histodosis cardiaca. Vias de infestacion.' *Archos int. Hidatid.* **6**, 87

Kagan, I. G., Osimani, J. J., Varela, J. C. and Allain, D. S. (1966). 'Evaluation of intradermal and serologic tests for the diagnosis of hydatid disease.' *Am. J. trop. Med. Hyg.* **15**, 172

Magath, T. B. (1941). 'Hydatid disease (echinococcus) in North America.' *Penn. med. J.* **44**, 813

Michaud, M., Saubier, E., Marel, G. *et al.* (1959). 'Un cas de kyste hydatique du coeur operée et guéri.' *Lyon Chir.* **55**, 768

Peters, J. H., Dexter, L. and Weiss, S. (1945). 'Clinical and theoretical considerations of involvement of the left side of the heart with echinococcal cysts.' *Am. Heart J.* **29**, 143

Warthin, A. S. (1902). 'Heart disease: Animal parasites.' In *Reference Handbook of the Medical Sciences.* Ed. by A. H. Buck, Vol 4, p. 582. New York: Wood

Williams, J. F. (1972). 'An evaluation of the Casoni test in human hydatosis using an antigen solution of low nitrogen concentration.' *Trans. R. Soc. trop. Med. Hyg.* **66**, 160

CYSTICERCOSIS

Cysticercus cellulosae is the invasive phase of *Taenia solium*, the pig tapeworm. In man the adult tapeworm lives in the intestinal tract, the scolex or head attached to the proximal portion of the small intestine, where it may remain alive for several years. The worm consists of several hundred segments, and its presence may be detected by finding with the unaided eye maturing segments in the stools. Ova may be discharged from these segments into the intestine and faeces, but they are released irregularly.

In the event of reverse peristalsis attended by vomiting, instead of being excreted, they may produce larvae which invade the intestinal wall, and enter the circulation. The cysticercus which develops is composed of a characteristic scolex in an inverted onchosphere, and possesses a relatively large cyst wall. In man the heart is involved less often than the subcutaneous tissues, brain, eye or skeletal muscles, and then only as part of generalized disseminated visceral infection.

In contrast, in the pig (the natural intermediate host), the order of frequency for these larval cysts is striated muscle (measley pork), liver, heart and lungs.

Among the series of 284 patients with cerebral cysticercosis reported by Dixon and Hargreaves (1944) only three of the 45 who died were found to have cysts in the heart. In some parts of the world where *Taenia solium* infections are almost universal (as in the African population in Rhodesia) cardiac cysticercosis is commonly seen, although it rarely gives rise to symptoms.

PATHOLOGY

The cysts may be located within the myocardium itself, and/or may protrude in a pedunculated manner from the pericardium into the pericardial sac (*Figure 11.20*). Usually the left ventricle is most frequently affected, with the cysts being relatively few in number, their size varying from 0·5 to 3 cm in diameter. As in the case of hydatid cysts, some of them may project from the endocardial surface into the cardial cavity. They do not, however, usually project to the extent that they are merely attached to the endocardial wall by a thin pedicle.

The size of an individual lesion depends upon the age of the infection and its location. Generally speaking, following invasion by *Cysticercus cellulosae*, a comparatively slight exudative cellular response occurs in the affected organ leading to the development of a fibrous capsule. Death of the larva results in a marked allergic tissue reaction as well as increased fluid accumulation within the cyst.

As a rule the cysts tend to be of the same size, thus producing some indication as to the duration of the infection. These cysts are usually round in shape except in the interventricular septum and in the deeper portions of muscle, where they tend to be elongated and oval. There is usually macroscopic evidence of fibrosis, but, sometimes, the muscle bundles appeared to be spread apart by the growth of the cyst. The histopathological features can be studied best in those instances in which the parasite is embedded in the substance of the interventricular septum or the left ventricular wall.

Microscopically, the encapsulating reaction surrounding each parasitic cyst shows that it has three well-defined zones (*Figure 11.21*). The inner zone is characterized by dead and disintegrating

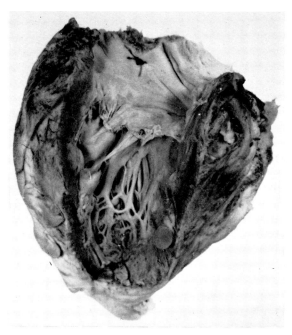

Figure 11.20. Showing several thin-walled cysticercal cysts in the myocardial wall. (Reproduced by courtesy of Dr T. G. Ashworth, Rhodesia)

leucocytes, plus foreign body giant cells. In the middle zone, fibro-plastic proliferation predominates. At the edge of the reaction are engorged capillaries, in addition to neutrophils, many lymphocytes, macrophages and plasma cells, but few eosinophils (*Figure 11.22*). Although often silent for a prolonged period, these cysts may produce cardiac decompensation if the involvement of the heart is extensive. Most writers, however, state that the clinical manifestations of cardiac cysticercosis are either totally wanting (Warthin, 1902; Devé, 1928) or at best are of a very indefinite character, such as tachycardia or abnormal heart sounds (Belding, 1958). Pulgrom

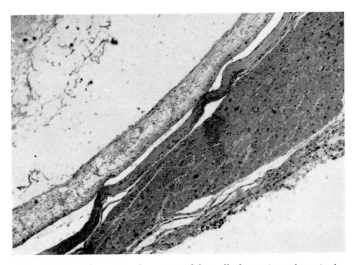

Figure 11.21. The section shows part of the wall of a cysticercal cyst in the myocardium. At the edge of the cyst a few dilated capillaries may be seen. (Haematoxylin and eosin × 80, reduced to 6/10.) (Reproduced by courtesy of Dr T. G. Ashworth, Rhodesia)

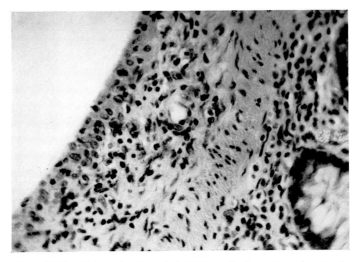

Figure 11.22. This section shows in detail the wall of a cysticercal cyst in the myocardium consisting of a main layer of dead and necrotic tissue: an intermediate layer showing fibroblastic proliferation: and an outer layer showing dilated capillaries in addition to polymorphs, plasma cells and a few fibroblasts (haematoxylin and eosin × 320, reduced to 6/10). (Reproduced by courtesy of Dr T. G. Ashworth, Rhodesia)

(1928) reported a case with lesions in the heart and brain. Austoni (1939) described severe fatal cysticercosis in a girl of 10 years of age, apparently involving the heart (electrocardiographic evidence). She had infection with a *Taenia solium* worm and at necropsy up to 20 000 parasites were estimated to be present. The abdominal organs were virtually spared. Unfortunately, the heart was not examined nor was the brain. Other reports came from Craig and Faust (1940) and Menon and Valiath (1940). A comprehensive monograph covering 450 cases of cysticercosis was compiled by Dixon and Lipscombe (1961). In 47 cases coming to necropsy, cysticerci were demonstrable, the heart being involved in 9 cases. Cysts can also interfere with the conducting system and Gotsman (1967) at the Groote Schuur Hospital in Cape Town in a communication to R. Hudson referred to two patients with complete heart block.

DIAGNOSIS

These cardiac cysts usually become evident long after the intestinal parasites have disappeared. Diagnosis, therefore, by finding *Taenia solium* in the stool is most unusual.

Late in the disseminated phase of cysticercosis, calcification of muscle may be apparent on x-ray and is practically pathognomonic. During the long intermediate phase, however, serological testing by the use of skin tests, CFTs, and precipitin tests may be found to be valuable.

These tests have the usual limitations which always exist when the antigens themselves are not standardized.

References

Austoni, M. (1939). 'Su di un caso de cisticercosi generalizzoto grave.' *Policlinie* **46**, 127

Belding, D. L. (1958). *Basic Clinical Parasitology*. New York: Appleton-Century-Crofts

Craig, C. F. and Faust, E. C. (1940). *Clinical Parasitology*. 2nd Edition London: Kimpton

Devé, F. (1928). 'Les kystes hydatiques du coeur et les complications.' *Algréie Méd.*

Dixon, H. B. F. and Hargreaves, V. H. (1944). 'Cysticercosis.' *Q. Jl. Med.* **13**, 107

Dixon, H. H. F. and Lipscombe, F. H. (1961). 'Cysticercosis: an analysis and follow-up of 450 cases.' *Spec. Rep. Ser. Med. Res. Coun.* **229**, 41

Gotsman, M. N. (1967). Personal communication to R. Hudson. *Cardiovascular Pathology*. Vol. III, pp. 514–15. London: Edward Arnold

Menon, T. B. and Valiath, G. D. (1940). 'Tissue reactions to cysticercus cellulosae in man.' *Trans. R. Soc. trop. Med. Hyg.* **33**, 537

Pulgrom, F. (1928). 'Ueber einen Fall von cysticercosis cerebri et cordis.' *Wien. klin. Wschr.* **41**, 1088

Warthin, A. S. (1902). 'Heart disease: Animal parasites.' In *Reference Handbook of the Medical Sciences.* Ed. by A. H. Buck, Vol. 4. New York: Wood

TRICHINIASIS

In most instances infections of trichiniasis are so mild as to escape clinical recognition. Trichiniasis presents one of the more interesting forms of myocarditis and one which is sometimes fatal in outcome. It is not an uncommon form of heart disease, for it has been estimated that rather more than five per cent of USA citizens are infected at some time in their lives (Kean, 1970).

The patient may have presented with a history of muscle pains and a history of progressive weakness and difficulty in walking, and often contractures of joints. On admission the patient shows pyrexia—up to 40°C—with increasing muscular pain, fluctuant contractures and eosinophilia. Myocarditis of some degree is a constant accompaniment of the infection and may constitute a serious complication, involving acute cardiac failure as the direct cause of death. The diagnosis of this condition is made by biopsy, when *Trichinella spiralis* larvae are found encysted in muscle fibres. Other laboratory findings which may be of help are a moderate degree of leucocytosis, that is with values of 15–20 000 leucocytes/mm³, absolute eosinophilia of about 15–25 per cent and a raised creatinine excretion rate which may be of the order 1500–20 000 mg/24 hr. Antibodies to *Trichinella* are frequently formed, and these are detectable by precipitin and complement-fixation tests, using an antigen prepared from the larvae. During the stage of widespread dissemination larvae enter the circulation, and are recoverable in small numbers from samples of blood.

Macroscopically, there are no constant findings. No specific macroscopic changes in the heart can be ascribed to the infection.

At autopsy the heart is not usually enlarged but the myocardium is usually flabby, pale red, soft and pliable and there may be several small haemorrhagic areas—sometimes 1–3 cm in diameter—and which are often in the left ventricle. The pericardial fluid which may be normal or increased is either clear or blood stained and may contain some trichinella larvae. The myocardial lesions follow some 4–6 weeks after infection with this parasite—usually obtained by eating partially cooked pork or sausages.

If the myocarditis preceding death has been prolonged, the heart is usually markedly dilated and soft (Fey and Mills, 1954) with pale brown flabby muscle showing fatty metamorphosis. The endocardium may be injected and be the seat of mural thrombus formation (Gould, 1943), while occasionally subendocardial haemorrhage is seen.

Microscopically, the lesion is essentially an acute interstitial myocarditis, focal in distribution and most prominent just below the endocardium or epicardium. There may be foci of necrosis of muscle fibres, with adjacent or surrounding infiltrations of acute inflammatory cells and loss of cross striations in the sarcoplasm. There is a marked interstitial round-cell infiltrate of plasma cells, mast cells, lymphocytes and eosinophils; and numerous large tissue histiocytes, resembling epitheloid cells of a type similar to those which usually have been found previously in diagnostic biopsies of skeletal muscle. Eosinophilic infiltration varies in degree but may be especially rich beneath the endocardium and in the papillary muscles (Fey and Mills, 1954). Other autopsy findings may include extensive trichinal infestation of intercostal and diaphragmatic muscle with scattered inflammatory infiltrate and extensive fibre degeneration. Chase (1957) reported a case of disseminated eosinophilic myocarditis (which was in sharp contrast to the skeletal myositis in the same case), the latter being granulomatous and containing few eosinophils.

The lesion usually develops some 4–6 weeks after the patient has been infected. An interstitial myocarditis with lymphocytes and plasma cells is seen with scattered areas of fibre necrosis. Eosinophils are usually common in the region, but very often only reflect the high level of circulating eosinophils. Sometimes the predominant cell seen in focal inflammatory areas may be a long epithelium-like connective tissue cell, as in the case described by Bell and Murphy (1956), and seems probably to have originated from a degenerating myocardial fibre. No parasites are usually seen in the myocardium.

Focal areas of myocardial necrosis are surrounded by infiltrates of polymorphs, lymphocytes, plasma cells and eosinophils in varying proportions. The myocardial fibres often show elongation or other non-specific degeneration changes. These may be scattered, small haemorrhages and occasionally a trichinella larva may be found within a focus of necrosis or leucocytic infiltration and rarely a well-formed larva may be identified; in other instances only fragments remain of one or more parasites undergoing destruction. The larvae measure from 80 to 120 μm in length and, in sections, show linear basophilic stippling. They may be found in the heart or lung as long as 54 days after infection (Stryker, 1947). Following local destruction of the larvae, or their disappearance from the circulating blood, the acute inflammatory process subsides. It is possible that minute microscopic foci of fibrosis may prove a permanent after-effect of this inflammation.

The work of Campbell and Cuckler (1962) has indicated that thiabendazole is a specific larvicide, after the use of which many of the larvae in the skeletal muscle die; thereupon an acute inflammatory reaction develops, characterized by infiltration with polymorphs and, later, lymphocytes, plasma cells, eosinophilia and giant cells. The theoretical question as to whether this larvicide will produce anaphylactic shock has apparently been assured in the negative.

Edwards, Hood and Laite (1962), as a result of their experimental studies, have concluded that the cardiac effects of trichiniasis are: 'Most likely related to the toxic effects of the larvae, or their metabolites, or to toxic products produced in the course of their final dissolution, rather than to the formation of antilarval antibodies and a subsequent antigen antibody response.'

These lesions usually show little vascular damage or ischaemic change, and marked myofibre change only in cases of local inflammation where the reaction may involve the cytoplasm, but hardly affect the myofibre nuclei. Thus, this cellular reaction may indicate a sensitivity to a component of the cell, which results in the disintegration of the myofibre but not of the whole cell or its nucleus.

The absence of parasites from the myocardium has been noted by other workers (Semple et al., 1954), who described much larger foci of inflammatory cells (up to 1–2 mm in diameter). The myocardial inflammation in trichiniasis is therefore unique in that the parasites are eventually rejected from the tissue rather than becoming encapsuled as in skeletal muscle.

The drug thiabendazole eliminates adult worms from the gastrointestinal tract and larval forms from the muscles; it is also effective in infestations by Strongyloides stercoralis. Spaeth, Adams and Soffe (1964) gave this drug to a woman aged 22 who developed trichiniasis 2 weeks after diarrhoea from eating infected raw pork. She had myalgia, headache, anorexia, pain on moving the eyes, fever, generalized oedema and a white cell count of 18 300 (13 per cent eosinophils). No parasites were found in the laked blood and no ova in the stools; the trichiniasis flocculation test became positive after four weeks and the trichiniasis skin test was markedly positive. Aspirin, Benadryl and piperazine treatment proved useless, but oral thiabendazole (500 mg) twice daily produced dramatic improvement within 36 hours.

References

Bell, R. W. and Murphy, W. M. (1967). 'Myocarditis in young military personnel. Herpes simplex, trichinosis, meningococcemia, carbon tetrachloride and idiopathic fibrous and giant cell types.' *Am. Heart J.* **74**, 309

Campbell, W. C. and Cuckler, A. C. (1962). 'The effect of thiabendazole upon experimental trichinosis in swine.' *Proc. Soc. exp. Biol. Med.* **110**, 124

Chase, G. O. (1957). 'Death due to oesinophilic myocarditis related to trichinosis.' *J. Am. med. Ass.* **165**, 1826

Edwards, J. L., Hood, C. I. and Laite, H. B. (1962). 'Studies on the pathogenesis of cardiac and cerebral lesions of experimental trichinosis in rabbits.' *Am. J. Path.* **40**, 711

Fey, L. D. and Mills, M. A. (1954). 'Fulminating trichinosis with myocarditis.' *NW Med., Seattle* **53**, 701

Gould, S. E. (1943). 'The pathology of trichinosis.' *Am. J. clin. Path.* **13**, 627

Kean, B. H. (1970). 'Parasitic diseases of the heart.' *Pathology of the Heart.* Ed. by S. E. Gould, p. 820. Springfield, Ill: Thomas

Segar, L. F., Kashtan, H. A. and Miller, P. B. (1955). 'Trichinosis with myocarditis. Report of a case treated with ACTH.' *New Engl. J. Med.* **252**, 397

Semple, A. B., Davies, J. B. M., Kershaw, W. E. and St. Hill, C. A. (1954). 'An outbreak of trichinosis in Liverpool in 1953.' *Br. med. J.* **1**, 1002

Spaeth, G. L., Adams, R. E. and Soffe, A. M. (1964). 'Treatment of trichinosis.' *Archs Ophthal.* **72**, 959

Stryker, W. A. (1947). 'The intestinal phase of human trichinosis.' *Am. J. Path.* **23**, 819

FILARIASIS

Filariasis comprises a group of diseases in which the lymphatic system or connective tissue is invaded by nematodes of Filariaidea, which produce microfilariae in blood or tissues. These are conveyed to new hosts by biting insects, especially mosquitoes. The important filariae are *Wuchereria bancrofti* and *Wuchereria malayi*, but there are also several others, notably *Loa loa* and *Onchocera volvulus*. Filariasis occurs in India, Ceylon, China, Africa, South America and many islands of the central Pacific ocean. The microfilariae reside in the victim's peripheral blood at night (when mosquitoes bite and become infected), but remain in the capillaries of the pulmonary circulation during the day.

A definite diagnosis of filarial infestation may be readily made by the microscopic examination of fresh blood, exudate or excised tissue for the presence of active microfilariae. The filaria CFT, using a group antigen, is a useful additional test, and gives positive findings in 65–75 per cent of loa and onchocerca infestations; but in the case of wuchereria parasitism the figure is significantly lower.

If the sexually mature worms can be destroyed the disease will die out, and for this, the oral drug diethylcarbamazine is now widely used and is active also against the microfilariae, although the intra-musclar arsenical drug melarsenoxide potassium dimercaptosucci-nate is more effective in killing the adult forms.

Fournier *et al.* (1961) reported on a Belgian who had filariasis which responded to treatment. Six years later, however, the patient developed dyspnoea, cardiomegaly and heart failure, with severe pulmonary hypertension and eosinophilia.

At necropsy, parietal endocardial thickening with foci of under-lying myocardial ischaemic damage was found. The author postu-lated that this was the end-result of allergic reaction to filariasis infestation.

However, the endocardial lesions produced by the obstruction of cardiac lymphatics (Miller, Pick and Katz, 1962), should be remem-bered in any study of filarial involvement of the heart, as filariae themselves may block cardiac lymphatics.

Ive and Brockington (1966) related the incidence of endomyo-cardial fibrosis to filariasis, especially to onchocerciasis. This possi-bility was denied by Shaper and Coles (1966) in Uganda, who said that most of the endomyocardial fibrosis patients belonged to the immigrant Rwanda and Burundi tribes, and that onchocerciasis was not common in these tribesmen. These authors preferred to regard filariasis in the same light as other agencies, bacterial, viral or toxic, as 'markers' of the low socio-economic status of most of the victims of endomyocardial fibrosis, rather than as directly caused by them. No relationship has been noted between filarial infections and endomyo-cardial fibrosis in Uganda or any other parts of East Africa. I have personally observed that many people in parts of East Africa with asymptomatic filarial infections (such as those due to filarial per-stans) do not develop endomyocardial fibrosis.

References

Fournier, P., Pauchant, T. M., Voicin, C. and Laduc, M. (1961). 'Con-tribution à l'étude anatomo-clinique de l'endocardite parietale fibro-plastique: SES Rapports avec la filariose.' *Archs Mal. Cœur* **54**, 869

Ive, F. A. and Brockington, I. F. (1966). 'Endomyocardial fibrosis and filariasis.' *Lancet* **1**, 212

Miller, A. J., Pick, Ruth and Katz, L. N. (1962). 'Ventricular endomyocardial changes after impairment of cardiac lymph flow in dogs.' *Br.
Heart J.* **25**, 182

Shaper, A. G. and Coles, R. M. (1966). 'Endomyofibrosis and filariasis.'
Lancet **1**, 428

ASCARIASIS

With respect to adult forms of this nematode, lodgement in the
heart has been reported in the literature on only a few occasions.
Boettiger and Werne (1929) found two adult worms in the right
ventricle of a 65 year old woman who died of congestive heart failure.
The heart was markedly hypertrophied but did not show any valvular
or endocardial lesions.

Rabinowich (1957) has reported the case of a 2 year old child
dying of pneumonia who, at autopsy, showed thrombi in the right
ventricle and atrium, each of which contained an adult ascaris,
while a third obstructed the right main pulmonary artery. In this
case the liver contained multiple abscesses, each of which contained
adult ascaris, which had evidently got to this position by ascending
the common bile duct from the intestine. The author cited three other
cases from the Russian literature, each with similar pathological
findings.

Larvae of *Ascaris lumbricoides* are not commonly found in the
myocardium but this may, of course, be accounted for by the fact that
the larvae, which reach the heart, remain there only briefly. Adelson
(1952) found coiled ascaris larvae in the myocardium of a 27 month
old male infant who died following an operation. Grossly, the heart
was dilated and a mottled, yellow-grey area was present in the
anterolateral portion of the left ventricle. Microscopically, the larvae
were surrounded by an inflammatory exudate consisting almost
entirely of eosinophils. In addition there were multiple foci of
necrosis with an adjacent granulomatous reaction. It was thought
that the larvae, after having been transported from the lungs to the
heart, were carried to the myocardium by way of a branch of the
left coronary artery. Phan Triah (1965) also reported instances in
which larvae were found in the heart. In one patient, he observed,
within a vessel of the left ventricle, lodgement of a larva of ascaris
surrounded by a granuloma consisting chiefly of histiocytes. An
unusual feature of this report is the author's belief that the larvae
develop from eggs deposited in the body by mature migrating ascaris
rather than from ingested eggs. Although this type of auto-infection

is theoretically possible, its actual occurrence remains to be substantiated.

Baar and Galindo (1965) used fluorescein-labelled anti-sera to demonstrate dead *Ascaris lumbricoides* larvae in lung sections of a case showing pulmonary ascariasis. To do this the authors prepared an antiserum by injecting rabbits with an aqueous extract of ascaris larvae, plus Freunde's adjuvant; the serum was then conjugated with fluorescein and used to prove the nature of the larvae in the lung section. This method has not to my knowledge ever been used to look for ascaris larvae in cardiac muscle, but certainly seems to be worthy of trial.

References

Adelson, L. (1952). 'Larval myocardial ascariasis: report of a case.' *Ohio St. med. J.* **48**, 723

Baar, H. S. and Galindo, J. (1965). 'Ossifying pulmonary granulomatosis due to larva of ascaris.' *J. Clin. Path.* **18**, 737

Boettiger, C. and Werne, J. (1929). 'Ascaris lumbricoides found in the cavity of the human heart.' *J. Am. med. Ass.* **93**, 32

Phan Triah (1965). 'Intracorporeal hatching of ova by migrating ascaris in a boy aged 4 years.' *Pathologica Microbiol., Basle* **28**, 443

Rabinowich, I. (1957). 'Redkii sluchai metastaticheskogo askaridoza serdtsai krupnykh sosvdov.' *Sov. Med.* **21**, 117

STRONGYLOIDIASIS

The strongyloidea parasite is rarely found in the heart as this organ is usually spared invasion of the larvae of *Strongyloides stercoralis*, even when the latter are widely disseminated during overwhelming infections (Froes, 1930).

The general rarity of cardiac involvement in this disease may be explained, however, by the small number of reports of necropsies in this disease. Undoubtedly more cases of cardiac involvement would be detected if serial electrocardiograms were taken routinely in all cases of heavy infection.

McCracken (1957), for example, has reported the case of a 25 year old white farmer, who was admitted to hospital with severe strongyloidiasis, manifested by fever, myalgia and tachycardia. An electrocardiogram taken the day after admission showed flat and diphasic T waves in the standard leads and deeply inverted in the limb leads.

The next electrocardiogram, taken after a course of gentian violet, showed a return of this tracing to normal as did the electrocardiogram taken one year subsequently.

Kyle, McKay and Sparling (1949), however, have reported finding filariform and rhabdidiform larvae of *S. stercoralis*, surrounded by accumulations of lymphocytes in the myocardium and pericardium of a 47 year old Negro.

The pathological changes in the heart consisted of scattered filariform larvae surrounded by focal accumulations of lymphocytes in the interstitial tissue of the myocardium.

No distinct evidence of cardiac damage had, however, been demonstrated during life, low T waves in the first and third standard leads of the electrocardiogram being the only clinical abnormalities, and these were of doubtful significance.

De Paola (1957), reporting on careful studies in Brazil, has repeatedly observed myocarditis at autopsy in patients dying from overwhelming *S. stercoralis* infections.

References

De Paola, D. (1957). 'Patologia da estrongyloidiasis.' Clinica de Doencas Tropicais e infectuosas da Faculdade de Medicine, p. 143. Rio de Janeiro, Brazil

Froes, H. P. (1930). 'Identification of nematodes (Strongyloides stercoralis) larvae in the exudate of a serohaemorrhagic effusion.' *J. trop. Med. Hyg.* **33**, 18

Kyle, L. H., McKay, D. G. and Sparling, H. J., Jnr (1949). 'Strongyloidiasis.' *Ann. intern. Med.* **29**, 1014

McCracken, J. P. (1957). 'Strongyloidiasis with probable cardiac involvement.' *N. Carol. med. J.* **18**, 186

VISCERAL LARVA MIGRANS

Tropical eosinophilia (Weingarten's syndrome) is characterized by a cough, exertional dyspnoea and wheezing, eosinophilia of 4000/mm³ or more, and a positive CFT with *Dirofilarial immitis* antigen.

Pulmonary eosinophilia is the systemic manifestation of helminthic disease by parasites which are unable to complete their life cycle in abnormal hosts (Beaver, 1956).

In man the most common causes of larva migrans are *Toxocara mystax* and *Toxocara canis*, but it is possible that the phenomenon is produced by infection with many other parasites as well. Apparently, the larvae, wandering throughout the body in a teleologic search for the intestinal tract in which to complete their maturation, occasionally become trapped in various organs.

Instances of myocardial damage due to non-human ascarids of the genus Toxocara have been reported.

Here they may induce focal necrosis, granulomatous formation and extensive tissue eosinophilia (Brill, Churg and Beaver, 1953), in the process of which the heart may become greatly dilated and develop congestive failure. In brief, the human is an accidental and abnormal host of these parasites.

Brill, Churg and Beaver (1953) described granulation foci in the heart of a child, and demonstrated toxocara larvae in associated pulmonary lesions. The heart was dilated and the myocardium contained small scattered nodules measuring up to 3 mm in diameter. Microscopically, the nodules were composed of dark eosinophilic material, the centres containing chromatin debris and bundles of fibrinoid collagen, surrounded by epithelioid cells and multinucleate giant cells, and at the periphery were infiltrates of eosinophils, plasma cells and polymorphonuclear leucocytes. Many of these 'allergic granulomas' were found in relation to blood vessels, frequently a small vein. Dent *et al.* (1956) encountered larvae of *T. canis* in the myocardium of a patient with an overwhelming parasitic infection. Friedman and Hervada (1960) described massive cardiac enlargement and congestive heart failure in a $2\frac{1}{2}$ year old infant with larva migrans. Diagnosis was established by finding the organism in granulomatous lesions in the liver. The electrocardiogram showed only sinus tachycardia but the patient responded well to digitalization and antibiotics.

Gelpi and Mustafa (1968) reported 108 cases, mostly in adults in Dhahran, Saudi Arabia who had a rash, followed by pyrexia, cough, sneezing, radiological infiltration of the lungs and eosinophilia. Some patients had *Ascaris lumbricoides* larvae in their sputum.

Robinson and Christian (1968) found that an antigen made from ground-up *A. lumbricoides* worms gave the same results as the routine antigen made from *D. immitis* in the CFT for tropical pulmonary eosinophilia with asthma (Weingarten's disease, 1943), of which they encountered 37 cases—mainly Indian seamen—in 6 years at the Dreadnought Hospital in Greenwich.

References

Beaver, P. C. (1956). 'Larva migrans. Parasitology reviews section.' *Expl. Parasit.* **5**, 587

Brill, R., Churg, J. and Beaver, P. C. (1953). 'Allergic granulomatosis associated with visceral larva migrans: case report with autopsy findings of Toxocara infection in a child.' *Am. J. clin. Path* **23**, 1208

Dent, J. H., Nichols, R. L., Beaver, P. C., Carrero, G. M. and Staggers, R. T. (1956). 'Visceral larva migrans with a case report.' *Am. J. Path.* **32**, 777

Friedman, S. and Hervada, A. R. (1960). 'Severe myocarditis with recovery in a child with visceral larva migrans.' *J. Pediat.* **56**, 91

Gelpi, A. P. and Mustafa, A. (1968). 'Ascaris pneumonia.' *Am. J. Med.* **44**, 377

Robinson, G. L. and Christian, Moyna (1968). 'Filarial complement-fixation test for pulmonary tropical eosinophilia with *Ascaris* antigen.' *J. clin. Path* **21**, 394

Weingarten, R. J. (1943). 'Tropical eosinophilia.' *Lancet* **1**, 103

HETEROPHYDIASIS

Organisms of the family Heterophydiae, consisting of a half dozen species, are not uncommon in the Far East. The adult flukes primarily parasitize the mucosa of the small intestine of many mammalian hosts, but seemingly are unable to ovipost normally in man, an unnatural host, in whom they wander from the mucosa to the deeper layers of the intestinal wall, where most of them become entrapped and die. In a few instances adult worms have been found in the myocardium and epicardium.

GROSS PATHOLOGY

The heart in heterophydiasis shows few specific gross alterations; it is, generally, somewhat dilated, with slight oedematous thickening of the myocardium, particularly of the right side. These are the changes on which an erroneous diagnosis of cardiac beriberi is often based.

In those hearts with sclerosis of the mitral valvular leaflets, hypertrophy is considerably more marked on the left side.

Subepicardial haemorrhages, both petechial and confluent, are frequent and conspicuous findings, particularly over the right side of the heart. The intensity and extent of the haemorrhages seem directly related to the numbers of ova present (Africa, de Leon and Garcia, 1937).

The number of eggs which reach the myocardium and the extent of the ensuing damage may be so great as to cause cardiomegaly, dilatation and decompensation—clinical manifestations which are easily confused with beriberi.

MICROSCOPIC FINDINGS

These changes may be placed under three headings.

(1) *Acute*—a generalized vascular reaction produced by the arrival of embolic showers of eggs in the myocardium; consisting of intense hyperaemia, capillary thrombosis, marked interstitial oedema and fragmentation of muscle fibres.

(2) *Chronic*

(a) *Cellular*—A diffuse infiltration of the myocardium with chronic inflammatory cells which consist chiefly of masses of deeply-staining histiocytes.

The reacting cells are not clustered about the ova to form typical tubercles, as is usually the case in other types of helminthic infections, but rather the eggs and broken shells are scattered haphazardly throughout the area of reaction. This pattern of response is considered as being specific to infections caused by heterophydiae, regardless of the organ involved.

(b) *Fibrosis*—the specific tissue reaction is replaced in the healed lesions by fibrous tissue as the cellular elements are gradually reabsorbed. The replacing connective tissue is orderly, smooth and homogeneous in appearance, lacking the contraction phenomenon which usually distorts tissue when an inflammatory process is repaired by scar formation (Africa, 1936, 1940).

More interesting, however, than the acute and chronic lesions of the myocardium, is the production of endocardial damage, with considerable destruction of the valves, especially the mitral valve. Eggs may be found within the substance of the valve, or sometimes protruding from its surface—which may be corrugated, scarred and calcified. The exact mechanism by which the eggs become attached to the surface of the valve and involve its substance is not clear. Although Africa and associates had, by 1940, uncovered a total of 14 instances of this condition, their confident prediction concerning the prevalence and importance of this condition throughout the Far East has not, at present, been substantiated.

References

Africa, C. M., De Leon, W. and Garcia, E. Y. (1937). 'Heterophydiasis: Two more cases of heart failure associated with the presence of eggs in sclerosed valves.' *J. Philipp. med. Ass.* **17**, 10

— — — (1936). 'Heterophydiasis: Lesions found in the myocardium of eleven infected hearts including three cases with valvular involvement.' *Philipp. J. publ. Hlth* **3**, 1

— — — (1940). 'Visceral complications in intestinal heterophydiasis of man.' *Acta med. philipp.* Monograph No. 1

PARAGONIMIASIS

Paragonimis westermani, the oriental lung fluke, may rarely involve the heart. Musgrave (1907) described four cases in the Philippines.

Both the visceral and parietal surfaces of the pericardium showed numerous soft, dark blue cystic areas which, on section, were revealed to contain red-brown granular material.

On the epicardial surfaces of the hearts there were many small brown irregular hard granular bodies, ranging from 1 to 4 mm in diameter. These were surrounded by zones of congestion closely following the routes of the coronary vessels in their distribution. In three of the cases the encroachment by the parasite extended a short distance into the subepicardial muscle which, on section, proved to be pale brown, coarse and very friable. None of the bodies, however, were situated within the myocardium. Numerous eggs of *P. westermani*, many in clusters, were found in the brown granular epicardial bodies noted in the pericardium.

Musgrave's observations on cardiac involvement in paragonimiasis are unique as they have not been substantiated by subsequent workers.

Reference

Musgrave, W. E. (1907). 'Paragonimiasis in the Philippine Islands.' *Philipp. J. Sci.* **2**, 15

Twelve

Collagen diseases

SYSTEMIC LUPUS ERYTHEMATOSUS

The systemic manifestations of lupus erythematosus have been known since the turn of the century. Cardiac involvement by this disease was first stressed by Libman and Sacks (1924), although the pathology of these cardiac lesions was not described in detail until the paper by Gross in 1932.

Females form the majority of patients seen with this disease. The age group most commonly involved are those in the third decade, but numerous cases are also seen in the second, fourth, fifth and sixth decades. The disease is rare under the age of ten years and in patients over sixty.

The most frequent symptoms are fever and joint dysarthria but a rash, often facial, is seen in over half the patients and ulcerative lesions of the mouth may sometimes be seen. Chest pain occurs in about half the patients and is usually pleuritic in type. About 4 per cent of patients may give a history of typical anginal pain. Loss of weight occurs in about a third of the patients, while another quarter also complain of dyspnoea. Paroxysmal nocturnal dyspnoea is only rarely seen and congestive heart failure may present separately.

Hejmancik *et al.* (1964), at the Texas Medical Branch Hospital, described the clinical, electrocardiographic and radiological findings in 142 cases of proved systemic lupus erythematosus in the years 1945–62; 58 per cent had cardiac involvement; pericarditis occurred in 17 per cent and myocardial disease in 21 per cent (7 per cent had congestive failure). Constrictive pericarditis was one of the several findings in a man aged 58 years who had syphilis at the age of 36 years, mitral valve stenosis and myocardial calcification (thought to be rheumatic). He developed a butterfly rash, pericarditis, an ESR of 20 mm/hr and positive tests for LE cells and antinuclear factor.

LABORATORY FINDINGS

The most frequent positive laboratory finding is elevation of the ESR. This exceeds 20 mm/hr in about 90 per cent of cases, while the white blood count is below 4000 cells per cubic millimetre in about half the cases.

Serum globulins are usually elevated over 3 grams per cent in 80 per cent of patients while serum albumen is below 3 grams per cent in 55 per cent. The urine shows proteinuria (1 plus or more) in about 70 per cent of patients, but this is often a transient finding. Haematuria (usually microscopic) is also found in 40 per cent of patients.

At autopsy the heart is found to be enlarged in about 30 per cent of cases. This is usually due to enlargement of the left ventricle in about half the cases. The weight of the heart may be up to 700–800 g. Half of the patients show signs of severe myocarditis. There may be marked atrophy and replacement fibrosis of cardiac muscle with an extensive infiltration of polymorphonuclear leucocytes.

Endocardial changes are frequently found (Libman–Sacks endocarditis) but a few patients may show isolated valvular involvement. Non-bacterial endocarditis may be complicated by a bacterial infection in some cases.

There is frequently coronary artery involvement and this may cause coronary infarction. The coronary arteritis may be extensive but is usually found in widely-scattered areas. An organizing thrombus may partially occlude a vessel, the wall of which shows focal degeneration, fibrin accumulation and cell infiltration.

In Hejmancik *et al.* (1964) necropsy study of 13 cases, 5 showed the changes of congestive failure, 2 had staphylococcal endocarditis, 11 pericarditis, 13 had histological evidence of myocarditis, 8 exhibited Libman–Sacks valvulitis and 6 had coronary arteritis (without cardiac infarction).

These cardiac lesions may present as pericarditis and only later do the signs of disseminated lupus erythematosus become apparent.

LUPUS-LIKE SYNDROMES

Drugs such as hydralazine can induce a systemic lupus erythematosus-like syndrome including the presence of antinuclear factors. Two theories are current: (1) that the drugs induce a syndrome which happens to resemble this disease by a toxic or allergic mechanism; in favour of this is that the disease does not involve the kidneys; it goes when the drug is stopped and, also, it can be produced in animals; (2) that the drug simply 'uncovers' true systemic lupus erythematosus: in support of this, Alarcon-Segovia *et al.* (1965) at the Mayo Clinic examined 50 patients with hydralazine-systemic lupus erythematosus and found a suggestive family (and personal) history four times more frequently than in 100 hypertensives who had not got it. This latter hypothesis would mean that a considerable proportion of hypertensive patients have a lupus diathesis and does not explain the drug-induced disease in animals. This work shows that the aetiology is still completely unknown.

Procainamide has been incriminated by Ladd (1962). Kaplan *et al.* (1965) added four examples in patients who received the drug for a month or more, for arrhythmias. They developed arthralgia, pleuritic pain, cutaneous lesions and the LE phenomenon. Withdrawing the drug cured them and relapse followed resumption of therapy. There have been several reports of lupus erythematosus following procainamide therapy (Atkins, 1969; Sheldon and Williams, 1970). McDevitt and Glasgow (1967) found 13 reported cases and added one of a woman with hypertension, cardiac infarction and paroxysmal ventricular tachycardia. She was given 500 mg of procainamide four times daily. After four months therapy she developed pleurisy, swelling of the joints of the hands, and pains in the shoulder muscles; the ESR rose to 70 mm/hr, and LE cells appeared in the blood together with rheumatic and antinuclear factor. A change to propranolol instead of procainamide cured the condition; of the total of 14 cases, 13 had heart diseases and 1 had dystrophica myotonia. None, however, developed true systemic lupus erythematosus after drug withdrawal. McDevitt and Glasgow also listed many other drugs associated with the onset of this disease— sulphonamides, anticoagulants, tridione, penicillin, phenylbutazone, tetracycline, streptomycin, isoniazid, griseofulvin and thiouracil derivatives. There is one report of procainamide therapy causing lupus erythematosus and being associated with cardiac lesions, in this case pericarditis (Swarbrick and Gray, 1972).

Bole, Friedlander and Smith (1969) reported 8 women aged between 21 and 29 years who had exacerbations of rheumatic symptoms when taking oral contraceptives; 6 had previous episodes of thrombosis. All developed serum AN antibodies and 6 showed the LE phenomenon.

References

Atkins, C. J. (1969). 'Procainamide-induced systemic lupus erythematosus.' *Proc. R. Soc. Med.* **62**, 197

Alarcon-Segovia, D., Worthington, J. W., Ward, L. E. and Wakim, K. G. (1965). 'Lupus diathesis and the hydralazine syndrome.' *New Engl. J. Med.* **272**, 462

Bole, G. C., Jnr, Friedlander, M. H. and Smith, C. K. (1969). 'Rheumatic symptoms and serologic abnormalities induced by oral contraceptives.' *Lancet* **1**, 323

Gross, L. (1932). 'The heart in a typical verrucous endocarditis (Libman-Sacks).' In *Contributions to the Medical Sciences* in honour of Dr.

Emanuel Libman by his pupils, friends and colleagues. Vol. 2. New York: International Universities Press

Hejmancik, M. R., Wright, J. C., Quint, R. and Jennings, F. I. (1964). 'The cardiovascular manifestations of systemic lupus erythematosus.' *Am. Heart J.* **68**, 119

Kaplan, J. M., Wachtel, H. L., Czarnecki, S. W. and Sampson, J. J. (1965). 'Lupus like illness produced by procaine amide hydrochloride.' *J. Am. med. Ass.* **192**, 444

Ladd, A. T. (1962). 'Procaine amide induced lupus erythematosus.' *New Engl. J. Med.* **267**, 1357

Libman, E. and Sacks, B. (1924). 'A hitherto undescribed form of valvular and mural endocarditis.' *Arch. intern. Med.* **33**, 701

McDevitt, D. G. and Glasgow, J. F. T. (1967). 'Lupus like syndrome induced by procaine amide.' *Br. med. J.* **3**, 780

Sheldon, P. J. H. S. and Williams, W. R. (1970). 'Procainamide-induced systemic lupus erythematosus.' *Ann. rheum. Dis.* **29**, 236

Swarbrick, E. T. and Gray, I. R. (1972). 'Systemic lupus erythematosus during treatment with procain amide.' *Br. Heart J.* **34**, 284

RHEUMATOID ARTHRITIS

Some cases of this disease have rheumatoid granulomata within the myocardium. These do not usually cause any ill effects but, rarely, they produce disturbances of rhythm due to deposits within the tissues of the conduction system. Inflammatory lesions are found with considerable frequency in the heart, but this interpretation has varied between rheumatic heart disease and a form of carditis specific to rheumatoid disease.

Current observations date from the studies of Baggenstoss and Rosenberg (1941, 1944) and Rosenberg, Baggenstoss and Hench (1944). These workers found lesions indistinguishable from those of rheumatic fever in the hearts of 53 per cent of 30 patients who had rheumatoid arthritis. Goehrs, Baggenstoss and Slocomb (1960) found pathological evidence of previous rheumatic injury in the hearts of 16 (44 per cent) of 36 patients who had had rheumatoid arthritis; they observed rheumatoid nodules (recent and chronic) in 7, focal collections of lymphocytes in 9, diffuse interstitial myocarditis in 4 and Aschoff bodies in 4. Lesions of the rheumatoid type were situated at the base of both the aortic and mitral valves, the walls of the left ventricle and left atrium, and the epicardium. In addition, pericarditis (42 per cent) and cardiac hypertrophy (70 per cent) were found.

From the various changes described it is possible to separate a small group of cases in which rheumatoid lesions are found. These consist of small granulomata with the same structure as subcutaneous nodules. They are usually located in the valves or endocardium but may also be found in the myocardium. These lesions were described in one case by Baggenstoss and Rosenberg (1944), and altogether Cruickshank (1958) was able to collect 13 well-described examples in the literature which he reviewed and said that rheumatoid lesions had been reported variously as occurring in from 5 to 66 per cent of patients. In general, a higher incidence of cardiac lesions has been found in autopsy studies than in clinical studies.

These pathological studies have been confirmed and extended, and several clinical and clinico-pathological reports have discussed the heart in rheumatoid arthritis (Weintraub and Zvaifler, 1963).

These studies have indicated that in some patients with rheumatoid arthritis the cardiac lesions are indistinguishable from rheumatic fever, whereas other patients have lesions (rheumatoid nodules) attributable to rheumatoid arthritis itself.

Histologically, an area of fibrinoid change is seen surrounded by a cellular zone in which fibroblasts, histiocytes, undifferentiated cells and multinucleate cells may be present. These cells frequently have a distinct radial arrangement. At the periphery there is a dense lymphocytic and plasma-cell infiltrate and various numbers of capillaries may be noted. In the later stages hyaline fibrosis or calcification may be found (*see Figure 12.1*).

Rheumatoid granulomata occur usually in patients over 40 years of age who have had the disease for over 5 years and have widespread joint involvement.

Myocarditis, usually of a non-specific type, is also found, sometimes associated with endocarditis but occasionally occurring on its own. The lesions are usually focal interstitial collections of lymphocytes, plasma cells and histiocytes and are frequently found near vessels.

As described by Cruickshank (1954), arteritis in the active form showed infiltration of all coats of small arteries with round cells. Lymphocytes predominated in the adventitia whereas histiocytes were most numerous in the other coats. In later stages fibrosis of the media and disruption of the elastica were noted. Active or healed arteritis was found in 20 per cent of cases. The arterial lesions are not, however, extensive and have to be looked for carefully.

A case of heart block caused by the presence of rheumatoid granulomata infiltrating the atrioventricular node has been reported by Gallagher and Gresham (1973) in a 65 year old woman.

Hart (1966, 1968) has said that similar heart lesions may occur in ankylosing spondylitis but that, unlike rheumatoid arthritis, there were no cardiac granulomata. Hart (1943) also said that heart block could also occur as could obliteration of large or medium-sized arteries.

Weintraub and Zvaifler (1962) described two necropsy-proved examples of rheumatoid aortitis (like that which occurs in ankylosing spondylitis), together with dilatation of the aortic root and specific myocardial granulomata.

References

Baggenstoss, A. H. and Rosenberg, E. F. (1941). 'Cardiac lesions associated with chronic infectious arthritis.' *Archs intern. Med.* **67**, 241

— — (1944). 'Unusual cardiac lesions associated with chronic multiple rheumatoid arthritis.' *Archs Path.* **37**, 54

Cruickshank, B. (1954). 'The arteritis in rheumatoid arthritis.' *Ann. rheum. Dis.* **13**, 136

— (1958). 'Heart lesions in rheumatoid disease.' *J. Path. Bact.* **76**, 223

Gallagher, P. J. and Gresham, G. A. (1973). 'Heart block with infected rheumatoid granulomas.' *Br. Heart J.* **35**, 110

Goehrs, H. R., Baggenstoss, A. H. and Slocomb, C. H. (1960). 'Cardiac lesions in rheumatoid arthritis.' *Arthritis Rheum.* **3**, 298

Hart, F. D. (1943). 'Visceral lesions associated with chronic infectious rheumatoid arthritis.' *Archs Path.* **35**, 503

— (1966). 'Lessons learnt in a 20 year study of ankylosing spondylitis.' *Proc. R. Soc. Med.* **59**, 456

— (1968). 'Ankylosing spondylitis.' *Lancet* **2**, 1340

Rosenberg, E. F., Baggenstoss, A. H. and Hench, R. S. (1944). 'The causes of death in 39 cases of rheumatoid arthritis.' *Archs intern. Med.* **20**, 903

Weintraub, A. M. and Zvaifler, N. J. (1962). 'Rheumatoid heart disease, a clinical as well as a pathological entity.' *Arthritis Rheum.* **5**, 327

— — (1963). 'The occurrence of valvular and myocardial disease in patients with chronic joint deformity, a spectrum.' *Am. J. Med.* **35**, 145

PERIARTERITIS NODOSA

The term periarteritis nodosa was proposed by Kussmaul and Maier (1866). In this disease the small and medium-sized systemic arteries are the vessels primarily affected (Ralston and Kvale, 1949), but arterioles and veins may be involved secondarily. The disorder most frequently affects males and is marked by an intermittent course which is eventually fatal—the duration being measured in months or years. Fever, malaise, weakness, loss of weight, myalgia and arthralgia are common symptoms. Involvement of the kidney in 85 per cent of cases accounts for the frequency of uraemia as a cause of death (Ralston and Kvale, 1949).

Cardiac failure is the next most common cause of death, as a consequence of hypertension or, less commonly, of ischaemia.

PATHOLOGICAL CHANGES

Vascular lesions may be seen as nodules 2–4 cm in diameter along the course of arteries, especially at points of branching. Most often they involve the mesenteric arteries near their termination but are also seen in the kidneys, pancreas, intestinal tract and in skeletal or cardiac muscle.

The lesions are focal in character with partial or complete circumferential involvement of the vessel walls. Chronologically, all the lesions seen in a heart are not of the same age.

HISTOLOGY

The affected arteries exhibit, initially, oedema and a fibrinous exudate and, subsequently, fibrinoid infiltration of the media, destruction of the media, destruction of the internal elastica lamina and a granulocytic infiltrate, sometimes eosinophilic, of the entire thickness of the artery. These changes may be accompanied by bulging of the weakened vessel wall. With chronicity, lymphocytes, plasma cells and macrophages appear in the infiltrates, the intima overlying the medial lesions proliferates and the narrowed lumen may become occluded by thrombus. Concurrently, with degenerative and inflammatory changes in the media, proliferation of fibrous tissue in the adventitia may merge with that from the intima; a scar will then replace the medial defects.

In fulminant necrotizing angiitis the diseased wall may rupture because mesenchymal proliferation does not keep pace with tissue destruction. These changes, in both early and late stages of the disease may produce infarcts, either large or small, in the myocardium.

INCIDENCE

The frequency of periarteritis nodosa appears to be increasing. Only 6 cases were observed at autopsy at the Johns Hopkins Hospital during the 20-year period ending in 1935, whereas 32 cases were identified during the subsequent 9 years (Rich, 1945).

AETIOLOGY

Some cases of periarteritis nodosa are related to drug or serum induced reaction, hypersensitivity or allergic angiitis, and are thought to be caused by these factors. Zeek (1952) has also demonstrated that the arterial lesions differ from classical periarteritis nodosa in the following ways.

The lesions are not aneurysmal, but affect smaller arteries and involve arterioles and venules as well and are frequent in the lungs and spleen. They display no predilection for points of branching and all appear to be at the same stage of development.

The frequent presence of arteritis in both periarteritis and collagen diseases suggests a relationship between them. It may be observed in both rheumatic fever and rheumatoid arthritis.

The divergent response to cortisone treatment—improvement in periarteritis but aggravative of rheumatoid arthritis (Slocomb et al., 1959)—suggests different causative mechanisms.

From the literature, Harris, Lynch and O'Hare (1939) analysed the autopsy findings in 87 cases of periarteritis nodosa and found that the heart was involved in 84 per cent of cases.

A similar high incidence was found by Ross and Spencer (1957). The latter workers found cardiac involvement in 60 per cent of cases which had lung involvement and 30 per cent in the group without lung involvement.

Holsinger, Osmundson and Edwards (1962) found involvement of the coronary arteries in 41 of 66 cases. All sizes of vessel may be involved. In the 41 cases showing an arteritis, Holsinger, Osmundson and Edwards (1962) found large vessels with lesions in 25 cases and in many of these the small vessels were also involved. In 16 cases, small arteries were affected without similar lesions in the large vessels and in 39 of the 41 cases the lesions were acute. In the large arteries small aneurysms may be clearly visible on the surface of the heart as small white beads 1–2 mm in diameter.

In the acute phases there is an acute inflammatory reaction associated with oedema and fibrinoid change in the cell wall. The elastica may be destroyed in some areas and infiltration with polymorphs, eosinophils, and plasma cells may occur. Thrombosis of the lumen, aneurysm formation or both may also be present.

The lesions may heal, leaving a fibrous scar with intimal thickening or organized thrombus. Elastic stains are useful in healed lesions to demonstrate the defects in the elastica lamina.

Myocardial infarcts are found in varying proportions of cases. Griffith and Vural (1951) found only 3 infarcts in 17 cases, while 3 others had diffuse myocardial scarring. However, only one infarct was related to periarteritis nodosa. In this series 8 of 14 cases showed myocardial arteritis, and in only one was an infarct found.

On the other hand, Holsinger, Osmundson and Edwards (1962),

found infarcts in 62 per cent of cases in their series, although some of these were small focal areas of necrosis.

Pericarditis may also be found in a variable number of cases. This is sometimes associated with infarcts and sometimes with uraemia.

References

Griffith, G. C. and Vural, I. C. (1951). 'Polyarteritis nodosa. A correlation of clinical and post mortem findings in 17 cases.' *Circulation* **3**, 481

Harris, A. W., Lynch, G. W. and O'Hare, J. P. (1939). 'Periarteritis nodosa.' *Archs intern. Med.* **63**, 1163

Holsinger, D. R., Osmundson, P. J. and Edwards, J. (1962). 'The heart in periarteritis nodosa.' *Circulation* **25**, 610

Kussmaul, A. and Maier, R. (1866). 'Ueber eine bisher nicht beschriebene eigenthümliche Arterienerkrankung (Periarteritis nodosa), die mit Morbas Brightii und rapid fortschreitender allgemeiner Muskellähmung einhergeht.' *Dt. Arch. klin. Med.* **1**, 484

Ralston, D. E. and Kvale, W. F. (1949). 'The renal lesion of periarteritis nodosa.' *Proc. Staff Meet. Mayo Clin.* **24**, 18

Rich, A. R. (1945). 'The role of hypersensitivity in pathogenesis of rheumatic fever and periarteritis nodosa.' *Proc. Inst. Med. Chicago* **15**, 270

Ross, G. A. and Spencer, H. (1957). 'Polyarteritis nodosa.' *Q. Jl. Med.* **26**, 43

Slocomb, C. H., Polley, H. F., Ward, L. E. and Henca, P. S. (1957). 'Diagnosis, treatment and prevention of chronic hypercortisonism in patients with rheumatoid arthritis.' *Ann. intern. Med.* **46**, 86

Zeek, P. M. (1952). 'Periarteritis, a critical review.' *Am. J. clin. Path.* **22**, 777

DERMATOMYOSITIS

There are only a few case reports on the pathology of the heart in dermatomyositis. It has been defined as a disease in which degeneration and inflammation of the skeletal muscles are accompanied by non-specific inflammation of the skin (Decker *et al.*, 1964). The association with neoplastic diseases is well known (15–20 per cent of all patients have visceral malignant lesions and the incidence approaches 50 per cent among patients more than 40 years old). It has been suggested that dermatomyositis may represent an autosensitivity to malignant tissue (Curtiss, Heckaman and Wheeler, 1961). As is true of other collagen diseases, the cause of dermatomyositis is unknown. It is closely related to scleroderma, indeed, in its terminal stages, sclerosis may be a prominent feature. Fibrin or fibrinoid-like change is frequently found in the lesions of dermatomyositis and, when present, is found mainly in the skin lesions affecting principally the arterial intima. Antinuclear antibodies, similar to those found in scleroderma, have been demonstrated in some patients with dermato-myositis (Kunkel and Tan, 1964).

PATHOLOGY OF THE CARDIAC LESIONS

Clinical evidence of heart disease from this cause is infrequent and when present, is not specific (Waisman, 1939; Waisman, Barwick and Walton, 1963). Morphologically, cardiac lesions are located in the myocardium and resemble the degenerative and inflammatory changes present in the affected skeletal muscles. Kinney and Maher (1940) described the findings in two cases. Both showed oedema with areas of lymphocytic infiltration and degenerative changes, mainly myocardial fibre necrosis. Oedema separating muscle fibres in focal areas together with degeneration of the fibres, including poor staining of the cytoplasm and loss of cross striations, has been observed. Interstitial inflammation with lymphocytes and histiocytes is present in these areas; usually it is of a mild degree of severity, but rarely may be severe and perivascular in distribution. In the area of muscle degeneration and oedema, mucoid changes in the collagen may be found. Only seldom, in a fatal case of dermatomyositis, are foci of fibrosis found, without other changes and without any other apparent cause; they may represent healing, at different stages, of degenerative muscle lesions.

Paget, Woolf, and Asher (1949) described oedema and focal scarring of myocardial fibres in dermatomyositis. Fibrinoid change in small coronary vessels was found in one case. These lesions, however, are not diagnostic and can only be accepted after excluding other factors (Abastade, 1962).

References

Abastade, M. (1962). 'Manifestations cardiaques des maladies dites du collagenie (dupus erythermateaux dissemine, periarterite nodease, sclerodermie, dermatomyosite).' *Bull. Mém. Soc. méd. Hôp. Paris* **113**, 1229

Barwick, D. D. and Walton, J. N. (1963). 'Polymyositis.' *Am. J. Med.* **35**, 646

Curtiss, A. C., Heckaman, J. H. and Wheeler, A. H. (1961). 'Study of the autoimmune reaction in dermatomyositis.' *J. Am. med. Ass.* **178**, 571

Decker, J. L., Bollet A. J., Duff, I. F., Shulman, L. E. and Stocklerman, G. H. (1964). 'Primer on the rheumatic diseases.' *J. Am. med. Ass.* **190**, I. 127–140; II. 425–449

Kinney, T. D. and Maher, M. M. (1940). 'Dermatomyositis: A study of five cases.' *Am. J. Path.* **16**, 561

Kunkel, H. G. and Tan, E. M. (1964). 'Autoantibodies and disease.' In: *Advances in Immunology*. Ed. by F. J. Dixon, Jnr and J. H. Humphrey, Vol. 4, pp. 351–395. New York: Academic Press

Paget, N., Woolf, A. L. and Asher, R. (1949). 'Histological observations on dermatomyositis.' *J. Path. Bact.* **61**, 403

Waisman, S. J. (1939). 'Oedema and congestion of the lungs resulting from intracranial haemorrhage.' *Surgery* **6**, 729

MYOCARDIAL INVOLVEMENT IN OTHER SYSTEMIC DISEASES

MYOCARDITIS IN MYASTHENIA GRAVIS WITH THYMOMA

Oppenheim (1900) first reported familial myasthenia gravis.

The pathology of myasthenia gravis has been well described by Russell (1953) and by Genkins *et al.* (1961). Russell described three types of striated muscle lesions.

Type I consists of acute coagulative necrosis of the muscle striations. This is accompanied by an inflammatory exudate consisting of macrophages, round cells and even polymorphs. Later this necrosis leads to fragmentation of the fibre within the sarcolemmal sheath and to removal by phagocytes. Multinucleate giant cells, sometimes seen, represent abortive attempts at regeneration. The necrosis may be limited to a single fibre or may be so extensive as to be visible on gross examination.

Type II lesion is the well-known 'lymphophage'. Here there is minimal focal necrosis with inflammatory reactions consisting of lymphocytes and mononuclear cells. Eventually the affected fibre disappears, leaving the 'lymphophage' behind.

Type III lesions consist of simple focal muscle changes with eosinophilia and swelling but no loss of striations, and no inflammatory lesions are present.

These three types of lesion, may occur singly or in any combination in a given striated muscle.

Myocardial lesions, though less common in myasthenia gravis, have been described by Rottino, Poppiti and Rao (1942), Russell (1953), Mendelow and Genkins (1954) and McCrea and Jagoe (1963). Russell described type I lesions in the myocardium in some of her cases while Mendelow and Genkins found myocardial lesions in 5 of their 12 cases, particularly those associated with thymoma. In McCrea and Jagoe's case there was a focal myocarditis and disappearance of muscle fibres which had been replaced by a cellular infiltrate consisting largely of lymphocytes and mononuclear cells, although in some areas scanty neutrophils were seen.

In the examination of the heart of a patient suffering from myasthenia gravis it is important to remember that these changes are focal and may vary in intensity in different parts of the same muscle, or even in different parts of the section under examination.

Although all the changes found in cardiac muscle are also found in striated muscle, it must be stressed that these changes are not found in smooth muscle.

The type III muscle changes are only found to a marked degree in those cases which are associated with a lymphoma.

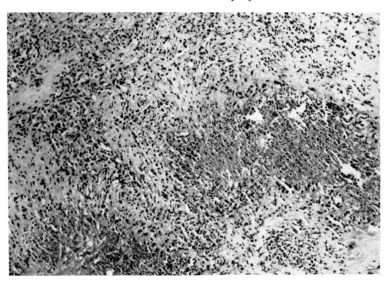

Figure 12.1. A case of rheumatoid arthritis showing a necrotic zone in the atrioventricular bundle having the structure of a rheumatoid granuloma (haematoxylin and eosin × 40). (Reproduced from Harris (1970) by courtesy of the author and Editor of the Journal of Clinical Pathology)

Death in myasthenia gravis is often sudden and unexpected. In view of the myocardial lesions found it has been suggested that a cardiac mechanism may be responsible for some cases of sudden death.

Even minor lesions in the myocardium may give rise to a vagal reflex resulting in cardiac arrest or ventricular fibrillation. The associated hypoxia of respiratory insufficiency as well, or the drug therapy being employed, may facilitate the development of this reflex (Mendelow, 1958).

MUSCLE ANTIBODIES

Complement-fixation tests have shown skeletal muscle antibodies in 40–50 per cent of cases (British Medical Journal, 1965).

Strauss *et al.* (1960) showed by direct and by fluorescein-antibody techniques, the reactivity of the A bands of skeletal muscle to the serum globulin of myasthenic patients.

Later Strauss, Kemp and Douglas (1966) extended this study further by finding that the serum gamma-globulins from myasthenic patients with thymoma also reacted with thymic epithelial cells; false positives were rare. Reciprocal studies showed that there were common reactants in the two tissues (muscle and thymus), closely related but not necessarily causal to the process producing the disease.

References

British Medical Journal (1965). 'Auto-immunity in myasthenia gravis.' **1**, 879

Genkins, G., Mendelow, H., Sobel, H. J. and Osserman, K. E. (1961). In *Myasthenia Gravis. The Second Intersectional Symposium.* Ed. by Henry R. Viets. pp. 519–530

Harris, M. (1970). 'Rheumatoid heart disease with complete heart block.' *J. clin. Path.* **23**, 623

McCrea, P. C. and Jagoe, W. S. (1963). 'Myocarditis in myasthenia gravis with thymoma.' *Ir. J. Med. Sci.* October, 453

Mendelow, H. (1958). In *Myasthenia Gravis.* Ed. by K. E. Osserman, pp. 10–43. New York: Grune & Stratton

— and Genkins, G. (1954). 'Studies in myasthenia gravis: cardiac and associated pathology.' *J. Mt. Sinai Hosp.* **21**, 218

Oppenheim, H. (1900). *Diseases of the Necrosis System.* Translated by Edward E. Mayer, 2nd Ed. p. 650. Philadelphia: Lippincott

Rottino, A., Poppiti, R. and Rao, J. (1942). 'Myocardial lesions in myasthenia gravis. Review and report of a case.' *Archs Path.* **34**, 557

Russell, D. S. (1953). 'Histological changes in the striped muscles in myasthenia gravis.' *J. Path. Bact.* **65**, 279

Strauss, A. J. L., Segeal, B. C., Hsu, K. C., Burkholder, P. M., Nastuk, W. L. and Osserman, K. E. (1960). 'Immunofluorescence demonstration of a muscle binding, complement-fixing serum globulin fraction in myasthenia gravis.' *Proc. Soc. exp. Biol. Med.* **105**, 184

— Kemp, P. G., Jnr. and Douglas, S. D. (1966). 'Myasthenia gravis.' *Lancet* **1**, 772

EOSINOPHILIA AND ENDOMYOCARDIAL DISEASE

LOEFFLER'S SYNDROME

The combination of a specific cardiac disease producing severe endocardial thickening together with eosinophilia, was first described by Loeffler (1936) when he reported a 37 year old male and a 44 year old female, both of whom died following periods of severe congestive cardiac failure. These patients also had marked eosinophilia (up to

70 per cent) and a mild leucocytosis. Necropsy in each case showed that the endocardium of both cardiac ventricles was focally or diffusely thickened by fibrous tissue over which was superimposed a

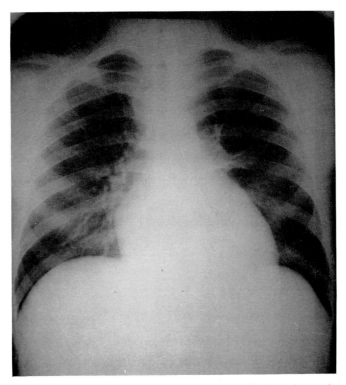

Figure 12.2.   Chest roentgenogram showing generalized cardiomegaly in Loeffler's disease (Roberts, Liegler and Carbone, 1969)

layer of thrombus. This condition was called 'fibro-plastic parietal endocarditis' by Loeffler.

Since this time, about 70 cases of this disease have been described, of which 30 have been in Europe, 7 in Africa, 3 in North America (USA) and 8 in Japan (Tajuina *et al.*, 1971). A more detailed picture of the syndrome has therefore now emerged.

Weiss-Carmine (1957), from Loeffler's department, summarized the findings in 26 necropsy patients with fibroplastic parietal endo-carditis and eosinophilia reported up to 1957. Brink and Weber (1962) 5 years later summarized the reported findings in a further 3 cases, dealing particularly with the necropsy findings. Several additional cases have been described subsequently (Andre and Duhamel, 1964; Mautner and Harris, 1966; Tajuina *et al.*, 1971).

Clinical Presentation

These patients usually present with congestive heart failure, but without any history of a previous cardiac illness or infection. On examination they are often found to have a grossly enlarged heart (*Figure 12.2*).

Age and Sex Incidence

About three-quarters of the patients are found to be men, the disease most commonly presenting in the fourth decade. Cases have been described in subjects aged between 7 and 64 years. Death usually occurs within two years of the onset of symptoms.

Pathology

At autopsy the heart is enlarged, sometimes considerably, while, in most cases, the weight of the heart is increased. In about 75 per cent of cases when the heart is opened, ante-mortem thrombi are found superimposed on the greatly thickened endocardium of either the left or right ventricle (*Figure 12.3*). The mitral and tricuspid valve leaflets are also thickened, the thickening occurring most commonly on the ventricular portions of the valve leaflets (*Figure 12.4*). There may also be a vegetative valvular endocarditis, with superimposed platelet thrombi.

The endocardium is thickened by fibrous tissue particularly at the ventricular apices and around the inflow tracts of the ventricles. The distribution of the endocardial changes is shown in the accompanying diagram (*Figure 12.5*). The endocardium is well demarcated from the underlying myocardium and is seen to be covered in most places by a fibrin thrombus from which it appears to have arisen by a process of organization.

When the myocardium is sectioned, small focal scars are in most cases seen. Large areas of the myocardium, usually subjacent to the endocardium, but separated from it by uninvolved myocardial tissue, may be found to have been replaced by fibrous tissue.

Microscopy

The endocardium and myocardium are infiltrated with eosinophils. The endocardium in some areas is thickened and replaced by fibrous tissue which covers the myocardium and, in turn, is usually covered by fibrin platelet thrombus. In this thickened endocardium there

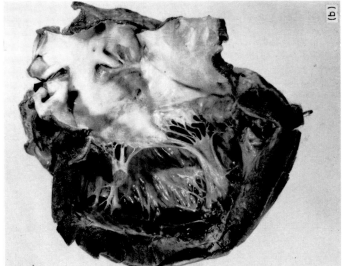

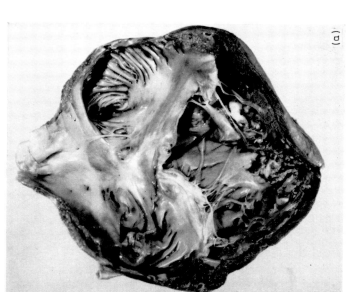

Figure 12.3. Interior of the heart. (a) Opened right atrium, tricuspid valve and right ventricle. Both chambers are dilated, and ante-mortem thrombus is present in the apex of the ventricle. The endocardium of the right ventricle is more opaque than normal. (b) Opened left atrium, mitral valve and left ventricle. Both chambers are slightly dilated. The endocardium of the left ventricle is more opaque than usual, both the anterior and posterior papillary muscles, particularly the latter, are severely scarred and atrophied and thrombus is present at the apex and behind the posterior mitral leaflet (Roberts, Liegler and Carbone, 1969)

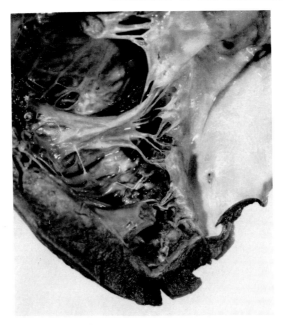

Figure 12.4. Showing marked thickening of the mitral valve cusps (by fibrosis) in Loeffler's disease (Roberts, Liegler and Carbone, 1969)

are often prominent small vascular channels, but usually this layer contains no elastic tissue. Brink and Weber (1963), however, reported cases in which hyperplasia of the elastic tissue of the endocardium was found.

Much of the myocardium itself is replaced by fibrous tissue. Many of the remaining myocardial fibres are hypertrophied while others show cytoplasmic hyaline change or are vacuolated.

The endocardium and the underlying myocardium show a diffuse infiltration with eosinophils. Both ventricles are usually affected, but either or part of one ventricle only may be involved.

The small arteries and arterioles of the heart or other organs are found to contain lesions in about half the cases which have been described. These are fibrinoid necrosis of the vessel wall, vasculitis, or intimal fibrotic thickening. In some cases, the vessel lumen is obstructed by a fibrin thrombus (*Figure 12.6*) which subsequently becomes organized. Similar vascular changes, showing fibrinous obstruction of small blood vessels, are often seen in other organs, such as the lungs (*Figure 12.7*). Some vessels later become partially

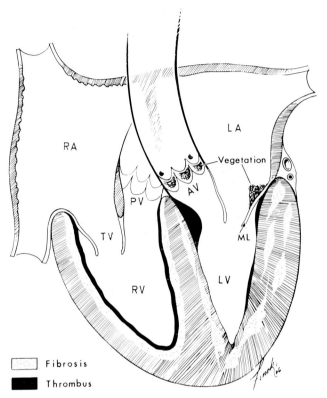

Figure 12.5. Diagrammatic representation of the cardiac lesions. All chambers are dilated and hypertrophied. The interior surface of the right ventricle (RV) is diffusely fibrotic, and the fibrous tissue is covered in most areas by fibrin-platelet thrombi. Focal mural thrombi are also present in the left ventricle (LV). Areas of replacement fibrosis are present in the deeper portions of the ventricular walls, especially the left ventricle. Vegetative material is present on the atrial aspect of the posterior mitral leaflet (PML) and on the ventricular aspect of each of the three aortic valvular (AV) cusps (Roberts, Liegler and Carbone, 1969)

recanalized so that the vessel may have as many as three or four separate lumina (*Figure 12.8*).

According to Brink and Weber (1963) the histological features vary with the state of disease. To me however, it seems possible that the cases described by these workers were actually cases of cardiomegaly of unknown origin, especially as eosinophilia is often found in the Bantu, due to the high incidence of parasitic infections in these people.

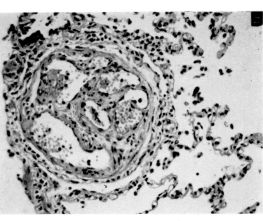

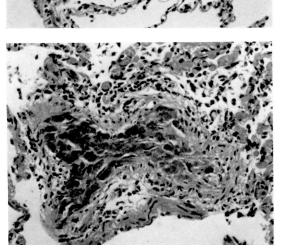

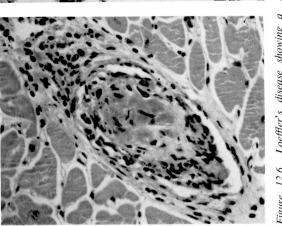

Figure 12.6. Loeffler's disease showing a small intramural coronary artery obstructed by a fibrin thrombus within its lumen. There are also some inflammatory cells in one part of its wall (haematoxylin and eosin × 400, reduced to 8/10). (Roberts, Liegler and Carbone, 1969)

Figure 12.7. Pulmonary artery occluded by a fibrin thrombus (haematoxylin and eosin × 400, reduced to 8/10). (Roberts, Liegler and Carbone, 1969)

Figure 12.8. Recanalized small pulmonary artery in Loeffler's disease (haematoxylin and eosin × 250, reduced to 8/10). (Roberts, Liegler and Carbone, 1969)

ASSOCIATION WITH EOSINOPHILIC LEUKAEMIA

The clinical and pathological features listed above are similar to those reported in patients with 'eosinophilic leukaemia'. Bousser (1957) summarized the clinical and pathological findings in 13 patients with eosinophilic leukaemia reported between 1941 and 1956; and Odeberg (1965) added observations in 12 additional necropsy patients with 'eosinophilic leukaemia' reported between 1957 and 1963.

These 25 patients ranged in age from 7 to 59 years (average age 32); 18 were males and 7 females and all had marked eosinophilia— up to 98 per cent in one case. Only 5 patients survived longer than 2 years following the onset of symptoms and death in 3 cases resulted from cardiac failure.

At necropsy over half of the subjects had extensive endomyocardial fibrosis with mural thrombosis; nearly all had infiltration of the myocardium with mature eosinophils.

Gruenwald et al. (1965) described a patient who had eosinophilia, thrombophilibitis, splenomegaly, and in whose neutrophils the Philadelphia chromosome was present and who later developed leukaemia. Other subjects with eosinophilia, who later developed leukaemia but in whom the Philadelphia chromosome could not be found, have also been described (Goh, Swisher and Risenberg, 1965).

In some of the small renal arteries, they may contain fibrin-like material in their walls (*Figure 12.9*) while some may also show a membranous glomerulonephritis (*Figure 12.10*).

In none of the patients with Loeffler's syndrome, which have been carefully studied (Roberts, Liegler and Carbone, 1969), have increased numbers of abnormal or leukaemic blast cells being found, during their illness.

I believe that the diagnosis of 'eosinophilic leukaemia' must be restricted to those patients who eventually have abnormal myelopoieses as well as eosinophilia with or without the Philadelphia chromosome.

Aetiology

The aetiology is obscure. Loeffler thought that this disease was probably due to allergy, because other allergic diseases were present in both of his two patients.

Brink and Weber (1963) agree with this opinion. The case of Tajuina et al. (1971) had also had bronchial asthma in the past and had positive skin reactions to certain other antigens.

In Loeffler's endocarditis the allergic stimulus must be present for some time (months) in order to cause such extensive cardiac scarring.

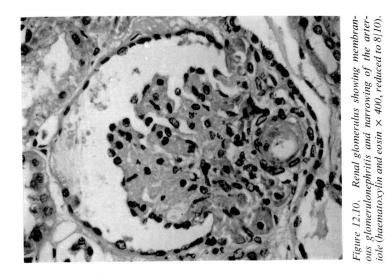

Figure 12.10. Renal glomerulus showing membranous glomerulonephritis and narrowing of the arteriole (haematoxylin and eosin × 400, reduced to 8/10). (Roberts, Liegler and Carbone, 1969)

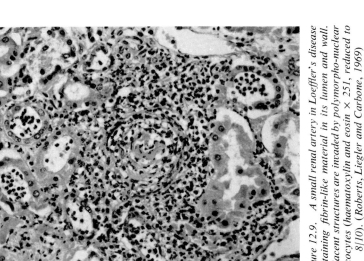

Figure 12.9. A small renal artery in Loeffler's disease containing fibrin-like material in its lumen and wall. Adjacent structures are invaded by polymorpho-nuclear leucocytes (haematoxylin and eosin × 251, reduced to 8/10). (Roberts, Liegler and Carbone, 1969)

In transient eosinophilia, for example, the result of 'tropical eosino-philia' or 'Loeffler's pneumonia', the stimulus to the production of eosinophils is transient (days) or the amount of allergin is small. Consequently, permanent damage does not occur in either of these conditions, although transient electrocardiographic abnormalities are common (Vakil, 1961).

Little anatomic information is available in patients with tropical eosinophilia or Loeffler's pneumonia since the conditions are essentially benign. One patient with Loeffler's pneumonia died accidentally, and at autopsy, extensive eosinophilic infiltration of the ventricular endocardium was found, but no endocardial scarring was present (Bayley, Lindberg and Baggenstoss, 1945).

A larger proportion of the hearts of patients who have died with eosinophilic leukaemia have more endocardial fibrosis than the amount found in any other systemic disease. From the fact the supposition may, validly, be made that the eosinophil is responsible for causing endocardial fibrosis both in eosinophilic leukaemia and in other disease states which give rise to a marked eosinophilia.

Loeffler's disease and eosinophilic leukaemia appear to be the same condition, but in view of the rarity of both these conditions no final conclusion may be drawn.

References

Andre, R. and Duhamel, G. (1964). 'Sur un cas diardocarditis de Loeffler avec étude anatomique.' *Bull. Mém. Soc. méd. Hôp. Paris* **115**, 1215

Bayley, E. C., Lindberg, D. O. N. and Baggenstoss, A. H. (1945). 'Loeffler's syndrome. Report of a case with pathologic involvement of the lung.' *Archs Path.* **40**, 376

Bousser, J. (1957). 'Eosinophilic et leucemie.' *Sang* **28**, 553

Brink, A. J. and Weber, H. O. (1963). 'Fibroplastic parietal endocarditis with eosinophilia: Loeffler's endocarditis.' *Am. J. Med.* **34**, 52

Goh, K., Swisher, S. W. and Risenberg, C. A. (1965). 'Cytogenetic studies in eosinophilic leukaemia. The relationship of eosinophilic leukaemia and chronic myelocytic leukaemia.' *Ann. intern. Med.* **62**, 80

Gruenwald, H., Kiossoglou, K., Mitus, W. J. and Dameshek, W. (1965). 'Philadelphia chromosome in eosinophilic leukaemia.' *Am. J. Med.* **39**, 103

Loeffler, W. (1936). 'Endocarditis parietalis fibroplastica mit bluteo-sinophilie.' *Schweiz. med. Wschr.* **66**, 817

Mautner, L. S. and Harris, F. (1966). 'Fibrosing endocarditis with eosinophilia, Loeffler's endocarditis parietalis fibroplastica.' *Can. med. J.* **95**, 1201

Odeberg, B. (1965). 'Eosinophilic leukemia and disseminated eosinophilic collagen disease, a disease entity?' *Acta med. scand.* **177**, 129

Roberts, W. C., Liegler, D. C. and Carbone, P. P. (1969). 'Endomyocardial fibrosis and eosinophilia. A clinical and pathological spectrum.' *Am. J. Med.* **46**, 1, 28

Tajuina, N., Hamamoto, H., Kanie, T., Mayashi, Y. and Kimula, E. (1971). 'Loeffler's parietal fibroplastic endocarditis with blood eosinophilia. Report of a case diagnosed antemorten.' *Jap. Heart J.* **12**, 581

Vakil, R. J. (1961). 'Cardio-vascular involvement in tropical eosinophilia.' *Br. Heart J.* **23**, 578

Weiss-Carmine, S. (1957). 'Die endocarditis parietalis fibroplastica (Loeffler) und ihre Stellung in Rahmey des Parietalodekact-fibrosen.' *Schweiz. med. Wschr.* **87**, 890

SCLERODERMA

In this discussion the term 'scleroderma' refers to progressive systemic sclerosis, or chronic disease of unknown aetiology with fibrous thickening of the skin and fibrosis of viscera. The disease is more common among women than men.

It has been postulated that scleroderma results from a disturbance of the autonomic nervous system, in which case much of the fibrosis could represent replacement of atrophic muscle fibres.

Another theory of its causation is concerned with the associated immunological abnormalities, based on the finding of antinuclear antibodies in 50 per cent of cases (Kunkel, 1964; Kunkel and Tan, 1964).

Although fibrinoid change is unusual, mucoid degeneration of collagen has been observed to precede the fibrotic process, and may be accompanied by a minimal lymphocytic exudation. Broadly speaking, scleroderma belongs among the collagen diseases, but immunological factors in its pathogenesis are less apparent than in other diseases of this group.

CARDIAC LESIONS

Although specific involvement of the heart in diffuse scleroderma has been reported, it may be affected indirectly by: (1) hypertension secondary to renal involvement; or (2) right ventricular hypertrophy, which may be caused by involvement of lungs and rigidity of the thoracic cage. Clinically it may be difficult or impossible to differentiate the various factors.

Myocardial scarring that cannot be attributed to any other cause is the most frequent finding (East and Oram, 1947; Rottenberg, Slocomb and Edwards, 1959).

However, according to Oram and Stokes (1961) it is relatively rare among cases of scleroderma. The scarring has no particular relationship to vessels and cannot be correlated with the presence of vascular intimal lesions, which may consist of fibrinoid degeneration of the intima. These changes are, however, found even less frequently in the heart than is fibrosis.

Weiss *et al.* (1943) reported post-mortem findings in two cases where focal scarring of the myocardium was present, which bore no relationship to blood vessels. In these cases, the scars sometimes extended to the pericardium and endocardium.

Areas of normal myocardium are interspersed between foci of myocardial fibrosis, usually consisting of seemingly normal collagen fibres. Whether or not the scarring process is a primary one, or, for unknown reasons, is secondary to the degeneration of muscle fibres, has not been established. In most cases the lesions have fibrous scars in which occasional individual muscle fibres have been detected (Piper and Helwig, 1955). Sometimes the scars contain numerous normal vessels. Although heart failure may result from these myocardial lesions, it is more frequent to find cor pulmonale secondary to sclerodermatous involvement of the lungs. Systemic hypertension may also cause left ventricular heart failure in scleroderma.

In the case reported by Mathieson and Palmer (1947), intimal thickening was noted in the vessels in the absence of hypertension.

Wegelius and Wahlberg (1957) described a case with a rapid course in which extensive mucinous oedema was present with early fibrosis and areas of degenerating muscle.

Pericarditis is often found at autopsy, sometimes with effusion and sometimes small calcific deposits are found in the epicardium. Bevans (1945) described pericarditis and focal endocardial thickening with involvement of coronary vessels by intimal fibrosis.

The interpretation of fibrous scars is difficult, but there is little doubt that the heart is involved in the same process as the skin or other organs. The cardiac manifestations may, on occasions, precede the skin changes. Significant cardiac hypertrophy is infrequent but may occur and affect either or both ventricles.

Valvular lesions have been seen only rarely in scleroderma. It is concluded that scleroderma heart disease is a fairly distinct anatomic entity that occurs infrequently, or late, in the course of progressive systemic sclerosis.

References

Bevans, M. (1945). 'Pathology of scleroderma with special reference to the changes in the gastro-intestinal tract.' *Am. J. Path.* **21**, 25

East, T. and Oram, S. (1947). 'Heart in scleroderma.' *Br. Heart J.* **9**, 167

Kunkel, H. G. (1964). 'Immunological aspects of connective tissue disorders.' *Fedn. Proc.* **23**, 623

Kunkel, H. G. and Tan, E. M. (1964). 'Autoantibodies and disease.' In *Advances in Immunology*. Ed. by F. J. Dixon and J. H. Humphrey, Vol. 4, pp. 351–395. New York: Academic Press

Mathieson, A. K. and Palmer, J. D. (1947). 'Diffuse scleroderma with involvement of the heart.' *Am. Heart J.* **33**, 366

Oram, S. and Stokes, W. (1961). 'The heart in scleroderma.' *Br. Heart J.* **23**, 243

Piper, W. N. and Helwig, E. B. (1955). 'Progressive systemic sclerosis.' *Archs Derm.* **72**, 535

Rottenberg, E. N., Slocomb, C. H. and Edwards, J. E. (1959). 'Cardiac and renal manifestations in progressive systemic scleroderma.' *Proc. Staff Meet. Mayo Clin.* **34**, 77

Wegelius, O. and Wahlberg, P. (1957). 'Early cardiac connective tissue changes in scleroderma.' *Acta. med. scand.* **156**, 487

Weiss, S., Stead, E. A. Jnr., Warren, J. V. and Bailey, O. T. (1943). 'Scleroderma heart disease.' *Archs intern. Med.* **71**, 749

Thirteen

Idiopathic diseases

AMYLOIDOSIS

Amyloidosis is a disorder of unknown aetiology characterized by the deposition of an abnormal amorphous protein complex (amyloid) in various organs and tissues of the body. This material is known to consist of one or more proteins in combination with polysaccharides but its exact chemical nature is unsettled. Amyloid involvement of the heart is usually divided into five separate subgroups: (1) senile cardiac amyloidosis; (2) primary amyloidosis—the disease is not associated with another systemic disease; (3) familial primary amyloidosis—in cases where one or more other members of the subject's family also have amyloidosis; (4) secondary amyloidosis—the disease is associated with and seems to follow the development of some chronic disease such as pulmonary tuberculosis; (5) amyloidosis associated with multiple myeloma and a few other neoplastic diseases.

Cases of cardiac amyloidosis may also be divided into: (1) isolated amyloidosis—the deposits being present only in the heart; and (2) systemic amyloidosis—where amyloid deposits are found in many other organs of the body.

The general features found in cardiac amyloidosis are described below and then specific studies carried out in each of the subgroups 1–5 will be listed. At the end of 1971 some 339 cases of cardiac amyloidosis had been reported in 15 separate studies (Buja *et al.*, 1971).

CLINICAL FEATURES

The majority of cases reported are of men and the average age is 56. Many of these patients present with congestive heart failure, the length of which may vary from a few days to 9–10 years. About a third of the patients studied have complained, at some time, of attacks of angina pectoris. Patients very rarely have cardiac enlargement of sufficient size to be demonstrated clinically, though a small peri-cardial effusion is often present and sometimes may be found at autopsy to be large—over 500 ml. These patients often present with a history of diarrhoea or, less commonly, with a peripheral neuro-pathy. Sometimes the patient may present with findings suggesting constrictive pericarditis, the clinical effect being due to the rigidity of the ventricular walls by amyloid.

Death usually results from congestive cardiac failure or, less commonly, from a pulmonary embolism but some patients die suddenly, without any obvious cause being found at autopsy; and it is thought that in these patients cardiac arrest is due to the develop-ment of an arrhythmia or ventricular asystole.

PATHOLOGY

The heart is usually only slightly enlarged so that it will weigh something between 450 and 500 g on average but sometimes may be much larger—up to 700 g (Coelho and Pimental, 1961) and the ventricles are not commonly dilated. In the majority of hearts examined it has been found that the left ventricular wall may be up to 1·5 cm or more in thickness. On cutting, the ventricular myo-cardium is found to be firm, rubbery and non-compliant.

Histologically amyloid is found to be present between many myo-cardial cells (*Figure 13.1*); this change may be found to be present throughout the entire myocardium but in some cases this change may occur only focally (*Figure 13.2*). Both of the left ventricular papillary muscles are found to contain extensive deposits of amyloid.

Sections of the sinus node or atrioventricular node commonly show extensive deposits of amyloid; deposits of amyloid extending to the conduction tissue are found in about 25 per cent of these patients.

The endocardium has a tan, waxy appearance. Focal deposits of amyloid are often grossly visible in the atrial and ventricular endo-cardium in about two-thirds of the cases reported (*Figure 13.3*). Thrombi are sometimes found in the atria and in these areas the under-lying endocardium may be heavily infiltrated with amyloid.

In the cardiac valves small deposits of amyloid are sometimes seen in the valve cusps which are usually flat, but a few are focally thickened. In the coronary vessels amyloid is usually found in the adventitia and media of intramyocardial arteries and veins of most of the patients who have been studied; and sometimes the lumen of these intramyocardial arteries and veins may be narrowed by intimal deposits of amyloid.

The lumen of the extramyocardial arteries is not diminished by deposits of amyloid although atherosclerotic changes may be present in these vessels. The extent to which cardiac amyloidosis may mimic coronary heart disease has been emphasized rarely in the past, although Brigden (1964) reported two patients, seen at autopsy, who had had cardiac amyloidosis. Langsch (1961) reported another

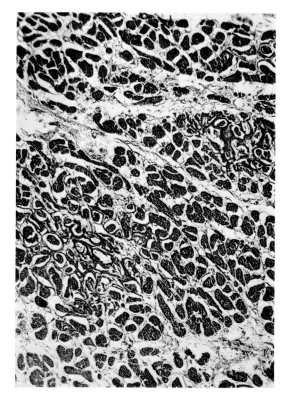

Figure 13.1. Photomicrograph of left ventricular myo-cardium showing two areas of moderately heavy amyloid deposition around the muscle fibres (methyl violet × 83, reduced to 2/3). (Pomerance, 1965)

two patients with cardiac pain and extensive luminal narrowing of intramyocardial arteries by amyloid deposits while Brandt, Cathcart and Cohen (1968) reported a further two patients with angina pectoris, who had 'widely patent coronary vessels' and extensive deposits of amyloid within the myocardium and intra-myocardial arterioles.

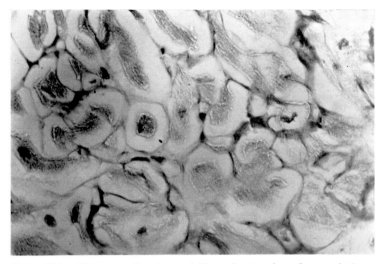

Figure 13.2.   The myocardium in amyloidosis showing that often amyloid may only partially surround muscle fibres (alkaline Congo red × 290, reduced to 2/3)

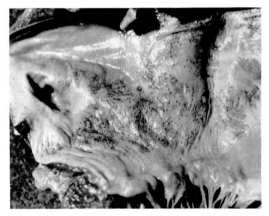

Figure 13.3.   Heart opened to show part of left atrium with multiple small dark foci of amyloid in the atrial endocardium (formol saline fixed specimen) (× 1 approx).
(Pomerance, 1965)

SENILE CARDIAC AMYLOIDOSIS

Baerger and Braunstein (1960) have described the clinicopathological features of this form of amyloidosis, distinguished from all other forms by the prevailing age of the patients, and the character-

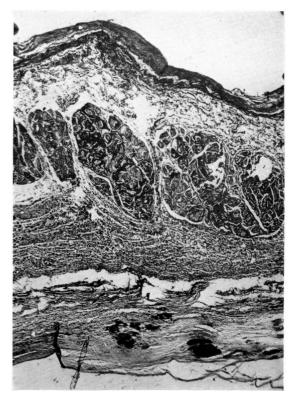

Figure 13.4. Photomicrograph of atrial septum, showing nodular masses of amyloid in the endocardium of the left atrium, and heavy deposition of amyloid around the myocardial fibres (methyl violet × 45, reduced to 2/3).
(*Pomerance, 1965*)

istic distribution of the amyloid deposits. The amyloid is largely restricted to the cardiovascular system. The patients, predominantly males, are almost invariably 70 years of age or older. Despite the increase in incidence with progressive age, deposition does not seem to be cumulative. Apparently no single feature of a group's clinical findings serves to establish the clinical diagnosis. Most patients, especially those having only minor degrees of amyloid deposition, are asymptomatic. Cardiomegaly, although infrequent, may result from co-existent hypertensive disease; while changes in serum proteins are not characteristic, usually the levels of total serum proteins and of alpha II and gamma-globulin are moderately elevated, whereas the concentration of albumin is normal or decreased. Low voltage in the electrocardiogram has been emphasized but is an inconstant finding. In senile amyloidosis the deposits are encountered interstitially, within the myocardium, beneath the epicardium and endocardium and in the heart valves. If amyloid is abundant the heart has a waxy appearance.

Even though the major coronary arteries are rarely involved, the deposition in the wall of the myocardial arterioles may be so great as to occlude their lumen. The deposition of amyloid, either in the form of multiple, small and patchy masses in the interstitium of the heart or as small or large areas, results in varying degrees of myocardial atrophy. The aetiology of this disorder is unknown and hypotheses so far offered in explanation of its pathogenesis are inadequate. Amyloid deposits in the heart, barring their massive accumulation, are deemed unlikely to be the cause of death in patients so afflicted.

Pomerance (1966) reported on 21 cases of senile cardiac amyloidosis in 1965 and a further 45 cases in 1966. The ages ranged from 73 to 98 years, males predominating. Deposition was found in 23 per cent of the over 80s and in 50 per cent of the over 90s, appearing as a peppering of small translucent nodules in the atrial endocardium, better seen after fixation; microscopy also showed amyloid networks around individual myocardial cells (*Figure 13.4*). Extra-cardiac deposits occurred in 38·5 per cent especially in the lungs, vessel walls and alveoli; cardiac failure occurred in 58·6 per cent of cases, and, in some cases, seemed to be directly due to the amyloidosis; cardiomegaly was uncommon. The only constant features were advanced age and the distribution of the deposits; it resembled the spontaneous amyloidosis sometimes seen in elderly mice susceptible to amyloidosis, suggesting a genetic determination.

Schwartz (1969) made extensive studies of senile amyloidosis using 0·1 per cent aqueous thioflavine T in a study of 400 cases of senile dementia, and in the heart found it in coronary arteries and in the interstitium of the myocardium.

PRIMARY SYSTEMIC AMYLOIDOSIS

Clinical justifications for regarding the primary form of amyloidosis as a separate disease entity are based on the following reasons: (1) the cardiac disorder attending primary systemic amyloidosis is much more serious in nature; (2) it occurs among much younger persons; (3) there is a tendency for amyloid to invade all types of muscles—those of the heart, alimentary tract, voluntary muscles including the tongue and the media of small arteries. In primary amyloidosis the heaviest involvement is usually in the mesenchymal organs, heart, muscle, skin and lungs. In these cases the staining reactions for amyloid tend to be variable. Amyloidosis is localized to the heart which is involved in 90 per cent of cases to a variable extent.

Clinical Manifestations

Most patients appear healthy and can provide no history of antecedent cardiac disease; some suffer from congestive heart failure without adequate explanation of its aetiology.

Primary amyloidosis often presents with weakness, fatigue, ankle oedema, dyspnoea and loss of weight. Less common are periorbital purpura, and macroglossia with submaxillary lymphadenopathy. Hepatomegaly occurs in 50 per cent of cases but splenomegaly is less common. Refractory heart failure, the nephrotic syndrome, Bence–Jones protein, raised ESR or hypoalbuminaemia may also be seen (Kyle, Kattke and Schirger, 1966). Occasionally purpura is an outstanding feature as in the 79 year old man reported by Roma (1961); the lesions were mainly on the face and neck and occurred in the terminal illness. Physical examination or cardiac catheterization may produce findings indistinguishable from those observed in constrictive pericarditis. The electrocardiographic findings of low QRS voltage are not very specific. Biopsy of the skin, muscle, nerve or rectal mucosa may reveal the presence of amyloid.

Macroscopic Changes

The myocardium is involved more often than the pericardium or epicardium; both the atria and the ventricles may be either diffusely or locally involved.

The deposits of amyloid occur in a nodular or a diffuse form, although both types may co-exist. The nodular form is the most common type and can be recognized as small greyish or yellowish nodules in all parts of the heart. If diffusely affected the atrial and ventricular walls are likely to be thick and leathery; usually the muscle is firm and pale grey-tan or brown, and has a waxy-translucent homogeneous appearance. The deposits in the endocardium occur mainly in the atria and valves but may also be found in the ventricles. They vary in size and sometimes occur as linear streaks. Any or all of the valve cusps may show nodules at their bases or in their free edges and, in a few cases, may be uniformly thickened by a layer of amyloid which gives rigidity to the cusps and interferes with valve function (Koletsky and Stecher, 1939).

On cutting the myocardium, the resistance is increased and when the heart is opened the chambers do not collapse, but retain their globular shape. Irregular pearly-grey streaks or flecks may be scattered diffusely throughout the pericardium, particularly in the region of the atrioventricular sinus. Sometimes occasional cases show extensive thickening of the pericardium with amyloid which also occur in the endocardium and may extend deeply into the underlying tissues, especially in the atria, where the full thickness of the myocardium may be involved. Gross infarction of the myocardium may result from obstruction of a coronary artery by a nodular deposit of amyloid.

Microscopic Changes

There are two types of involvement, both of which follow a characteristic pattern. In the *first type*, amyloid is found in blood vessels, including the main coronary arteries, arterioles, capillaries and veins. All the blood vessels and all layers of their walls may be involved. In the *second type*, the interstitial tissue of the myocardium is diffusely infiltrated and the compressed myocardial fibres may undergo extensive necrosis or atrophy. Should atrophy develop, the sarcoplasm is vacuolated and contains deposits of lipid or pigment; nuclear degeneration and necrosis frequently supervene. Extensive deposition destroys the muscle cells leaving empty amyloid lined cell walls or solid sheets of amyloid. Fragmentation of myocardial fibres is frequent. Jones and Frazier (1950) believe that the amyloid is deposited in and about altered reticulum. Teilum (1956) has presented evidence that the reticulo-endothelial cells, containing polysaccharide substance, stainable by the PAS technique, may participate directly in the synthesis of amyloid and related substances.

Microscopically, the amyloid in the endocardium usually occurs in homogeneous masses but it may, sometimes, have a stratified appearance. These deposits usually occupy the deeper layer of the endocardium and are most commonly seen in the atria; of 43 cases of primary systemic amyloidosis (Lindsay, 1946) amyloid deposits were present in the heart valves. Valvular involvement is usually slight and may be demonstrated only in microscopic sections: in a few cases, however, discrete nodules measuring from 1 to 3 mm are visible on the valves either in the cusps or in the annulus. Sometimes, however, the infiltrate is diffuse leading to thick rigid cusps and stenotic surfaces. It is reported that all four valves are affected with almost equal frequency (Lindsay, 1946), and should the amyloid infiltrate into the chordae tendinae it is usually first deposited in the valvular endocardium, extending next into the substance of the chordae.

Although the large coronary arteries may be so extensively infiltrated as to produce occlusion and myocardial infarction, more often the medium-sized and small arteries are involved; the arterioles, capillaries and veins may be infiltrated. Involvement of the epicardium may be nodular or diffuse. In the nodular form the deposits may be few or many and may range from 1 to 4 cm in diameter; they are usually pearly-grey and translucent, occasionally yellow-grey and they occur frequently in the ventricular wall.

The lesions in the pericardium may show similar appearances but, in addition, amyloid rings may be found in the epicardium and around fat cells. In the myocardium the nodules often have a laminated appearance and are sometimes related to blood vessels. Should amyloidosis be diffuse, the epicardium and pericardium become thick, grey-yellow and semi-translucent; microscopically the blood vessels of the pericardium as well as the interstitial myocardial tissue are involved. Often rings of amyloid surround the fat cells of the pericardium.

James (1966) demonstrated an abundance of amyloid material in all areas of the conduction system in five patients with amyloidosis and conduction defects. Microscopic examinations disclosed amyloidosis of the conduction system. That the conducting system may also be involved was also reported by Lamb and Shacklet (1960). Electron microscopy of the heart of a Pakistani male with primary amyloidosis of three years duration (Husband and Lannigan, 1968) showed amyloid in relation to basement membrane of muscle cells, around capillaries and in connective tissues as fine fibrils 140–450 Å wide, in bundles and in haphazard arrangement, and some fibrils appeared to be beaded. None was found inside muscle cells, although it was present between them. Extensive deposits were also present in the thyroid, kidney and tongue.

FAMILIAL AMYLOIDOSIS

Various cases of primary generalized amyloidosis have been reported with a familial basis (Maxwell and Kimball, 1936; Andrade, 1952; Rukavina, Block and Jackson, 1956). The case of amyloidosis described by Rukavina, Block and Jackson (1956) showed that the inheritance was by a Mendelian dominant.

In this form of the disease the deposits appear chiefly in the kidneys, heart, peripheral nerves or ganglia, causing clinical symptoms with predominant nephropathic, cardiopathic or neuropathic presentation. The cardiopathic form is manifested in patients in their late thirties or early forties, causing dyspnoea, exertional fatigues and right-sided heart failure, followed by death 2–5 years after its onset.

The concentration of glucosamine in the serum has been found to be increased in non-familial primary amyloidosis but of a normal level in the familial type.

SECONDARY AMYLOIDOSIS

In most of these cases the amyloid is deposited mainly in the paradiaphragmatic organs, liver, kidney, spleen, adrenal and, to a lesser extent in mesenchymal tissues, muscle, heart and lungs. In secondary amyloidosis Dahlin (1949) reported involvement of the heart in up to 43 per cent of cases. Most frequent during the first three decades of life, it is invariably associated with preceding chronic suppurative disease or protein abnormalities; the myocardial deposits are usually small and perivascular.

Heart involvement occurs in over half the patients with secondary amyloidosis. Myelomatosis is usually associated with IgA globulinaemia, but Shenfield (1969) reported it associated with IgG myeloma in a 62 year old woman who had congestive heart failure, with non-specific low voltage and T wave inversion in the electrocardiogram.

AMYLOIDOSIS ASSOCIATED WITH MYELOMATOSIS AND OTHER
NEOPLASTIC CONDITIONS

In approximately 10–15 per cent of patients with myeloma, amyloid is deposited in the myocardium, usually in close proximity to myeloma cells and is similar to that found in primary systemic amyloidosis. Azzopardi and Lehner (1966) reported that 14 of 93 cases of systemic amyloidosis were associated with a malignancy such as myelomatosis, Hodgkin's disease, carcinoma (especially renal), or lymphosarcoma.

CONSEQUENCES OF CARDIAC AMYLOID DEPOSITS

Amyloid deposits initially surround myocardial cells and capillaries. After the initial deposition of amyloid fibrils, the myocardial cells are gradually replaced by amyloid; this deposition may account for large areas of the myocardium. Later degeneration of cardiac muscle cells may result from ischaemia and other metabolic abnormalities caused by this thick layer of amyloid surrounding the muscle cells and capillaries.

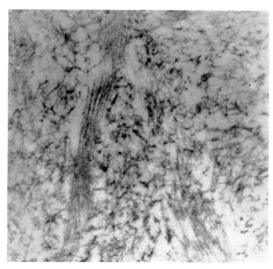

Figure 13.5.   Collagen fibrils with well-defined characteristics, periodically together with amyloid fibrils in connective tissue (× 33 000, reduced to 2/3). (Husband and Lannigan, 1968)

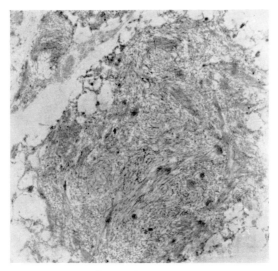

Figure 13.6.   Amyloid fibrils partly arranged haphazardly and partly arranged in bundles (× 27 000, reduced to 2/3). (Husband and Lannigan, 1968)

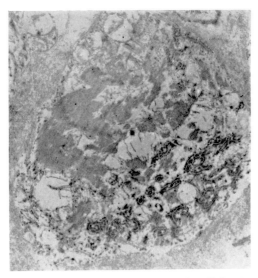

Figure 13.7. Oblique section of muscle cell showing preserved myofibrils and intercalated disc surrounded by amyloid. The basement membrane can be recognized in places. The mitochondria are swollen and show fragmentation of the cristae (× 3700, reduced to 2/3).
(Husband and Lannigan, 1968)

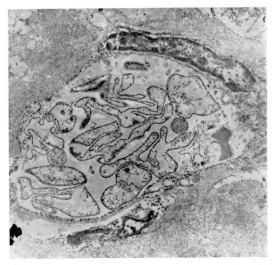

Figure 13.8. Capillary surrounded by amyloid. The nuclei of two pericytes are prominent. The basement membrane can be seen at some areas (× 2700, reduced to 2/3).
(Husband and Lannigan, 1968)

ELECTRON-MICROSCOPY OF AMYLOID

Cohen and Calkins (1959) showed that the basic and diagnostic structure of amyloid was fibrillary each fibril being 5–30 μm wide. Sometimes these fibres are arranged regularly (*Figure 13.6*) but at other times in a haphazard fashion (*Figure 13.6*). In a further report Shirahama and Cohen (1965) showed that the fibril comprised up to 8 laterally aggregated filaments, each about 7·5 μm wide with a periodicity of 10 μm. Lehner, Nunn and Pearse (1966) studied amyloid in various forms, primary, secondary, experimental and that in familial Mediterranean fever. Sections of cardiac muscle cell usually show preserved muscle fibrils and intercalated discs surrounded by amyloid (*Figure 13.7*); capillaries are sometimes seen to be surrounded by amyloid while their basement membrane may be completely replaced by amyloid (*Figure 13.8*). All forms resisted formalin fixation, paraffin embedding, and pepsin digestion. Buja *et al.* (1971) in studying by electron microscopy amyloid obtained from a cardiac case noted that it consisted of non-branching, non-periodic but occasionally beaded fibrils 80–130 Å (average 100) in diameter.

EFFECT ON THE HEART

In view of the widespread nature of amyloid deposition the clinical features of amyloidosis may be very variable. When the heart is heavily involved it usually gives rise to congestive cardiac failure; sometimes in severe amyloidosis the clinical picture may be that of constrictive pericarditis, this being attributed to rigidity of the ventricular walls (Findlay and Adams, 1948).

Sometimes, as mentioned previously, amyloidosis may present as an arrhythmia, due to involvement of conduction tissue or sometimes due to the development of a myocardial infarct.

References

Andrade, C. (1952). 'Peculiar form of peripheral neuropathy: Familiar atypical generalized amyloidosis with special involvement of peripheral nerves.' *Brain* **75**, 408

Azzopardi, J. G. and Lehner, T. (1966). 'Systemic amyloidosis and malignant disease.' *J. clin. Path.* **19**, 539

Baerger, L. and Braunstein, H. (1960). 'Senile cardiac amyloidosis.' *Am. J. Med.* **28**, 357

Brandt, K., Cathcart, E. S. and Cohen, A. S. (1968). 'A clinical analysis of the course and prognosis of forty-two patients with amyloidosis.' *Am. J. Med.* **44**, 955

Brigden, W. (1964). 'Cardiac amyloidosis.' *Prog. cardiovasc. Dis.* **7**, 142

Buja, L. M., Ba Khoi, Nguyen and Roberts, W. C. (1971). 'Clinically significant cardiac amyloidosis.' *Am. J. Cardiol.* **26**, 394

Coelho, E. and Pimental, J. C. (1961). 'Cardiac involvement in a peculiar form of paramyloidosis.' *Am. J. Cardiol.* **8**, 624

Cohen, A. S. and Calkins, E. (1959). 'Electronmicrographic observations on a fibrous component in amyloid of diverse origins.' *Nature Lond.* **183**, 1202

Dahlin, D. C. (1950). 'Classification and general aspects of amyloidosis.' *Med. Clins N. Am.* **34**, 1107

Findlay, J. and Adams, W. (1948). 'Primary systemic amyloidosis simulating constrictive pericarditis with steatorrhoea and hyperesthesia.' *Archs intern. Med.* **81**, 342

Husband, E. M. and Lannigan, R. (1968). 'Electron microscopy of the heart in a case of primary cardiac amyloidosis.' *Br. Heart J.* **30**, 265

James, T. N. (1966). 'Pathology of cardiac conduction system in amyloidosis.' *Ann. intern. Med.* **65**, 28

Jones, R. S. and Frazier, D. E. (1950). 'Primary cardiovascular amyloidosis.' *Archs Path.* **50**, 366

Koletsky, S. and Stecher, R. M. (1939). 'Primary systemic amyloidosis involvement of cardiac valves, joints and bones, with pathologic fracture of the femur.' *Archs Path.* **50**, 366

Kyle, R. A., Kattke, B. A. and Schirger, A. (1966). 'Orthostalic hypotension or a clue to primary systemic amyloidosis.' *Circulation* **34**, 883

Lamb, G. and Shacklet, R. G. (1960). 'Human cardiac conduction tissue lesions.' *Am. J. Path.* **36**, 411

Langsch, H. G. (1961). 'Primare atypsche Amyloidose als exzeptionelle Erkrankung der Coronararterien.' *Beitr. path. anat.* **125**, 123

Lehner, T., Nunn, E. R. and Pearse, A. G. E. (1966). 'Electronmicroscopy of paraffin embedded sections in amyloidosis.' *J. Path. Bact.* **91**, 297

Lindsay, S. (1946). 'The heart in primary systemic amyloidosis.' *Am. Heart J.* **32**, 419

Maxwell, E. S. and Kimball, I. (1936). 'Familial amyloidosis with case reports.' *Med. Bull. Veterans' Adm.* **12**, 365

Pomerance, A. (1965). 'Senile cardiac amyloidosis.' *Br. Heart J.* **27**, 711

Rona, G. (1961). 'Primary systemic amyloidosis associated with purpura.' *Can. med. Ass. J.* **84**, 1386

Rukavina, J. G., Block, W. D. and Jackson, C. E. (1956). 'Primary systemic amyloidosis: a review and an experimental, genetic and clinical study of 29 cases with particular emphasis on the familial form.' *Medicine, Baltimore* **35**, 239

Schwartz, P. (1969). 'Cardiovascular involvement in the aged.' *Geriatrics* **24**, 81

Shenfield, G. M. (1969). 'Congestive cardiac failure due to secondary amyloidosis.' *Proc. R. Soc. Med.* **62**, 265

Shirahama, T. and Cohen, A. S. (1965). 'Structure of amyloid fibrils after negative staining and high resolution electronmicroscopy.' *Nature Lond.* **206**, 737

Teilum, G. (1956). 'Per-iodic acid-Schiff positive reticulo-endothelial cells producing glycoprotein. Functional significance during formation of amyloid.' *Am. J. Path.* **32**, 945

MYOCARDIAL SARCOIDOSIS

Sarcoidosis is a multisystem, granulomatous disorder of unknown aetiology, predominantly affecting the lungs, reticulo-endothelial system, eyes and skin.

The central nervous system, heart, bones and salivary glands are only occasionally affected in fewer than 10 per cent of patients (James *et al.*, 1969).

Sarcoid lesions of the epicardium and superficial layers of the myocardium were first observed by Bernstein, Konzelmann and Sidlick (1929) while the first death attributable to myocardial sarcoidosis was reported by Gentzen (1937). Subsequent sporadic case reports have appeared in the literature while Forbes and Usher (1962) published the first well-documented fatal case of myocardial sarcoidosis in the British Isles.

In 1967 Scadding noticed clinical features suggesting myocardial sarcoidosis in only 2 out of a series of 275 cases which he had studied.

Fatal myocardial sarcoidosis is relatively uncommon, the necropsy incidence, however, being higher than that detected clinically. Ricker and Clark (1949) found sarcoid involvement of the myocardium in 2 out of 22 cases whereas none of Scadding's (1967) 11 fatal cases, where a complete necropsy was done, had any *myocardial* involvement. Maycock *et al.* (1963) analysed 145 patients with a review of 9 series from the literature and found 19 (13 per cent) had some kind of cardiac abnormality. Longcope and Freiman (1952) mentioned the involvement of the heart in 20 per cent of their necropsy series which is certainly higher than in the clinical series of Maycock *et al.* (1963). Siltzbach (1968) believes that myocardial localization produces significant symptoms in less than 5 per cent of patients, although at necropsy cardiac lesions are found in as many as 20 per cent of cases. This discrepancy stems from the difficulty in recognizing myocardial sarcoidosis in life. Heart involvement is suspected when a patient with pulmonary, ocular or cutaneous sarcoidosis develops a cardiac arrhythmia or bundle branch block.

Although this evidence is only circumstantial, it is an indication for a therapeutic trial of cortico-steroids to see if the arrhythmia or electrocardiographic abnormality can be corrected.

Sarcoidosis is often symptomless but usually presents itself in one of three ways as shown by Douglas (1967) in his report on 450 cases:

(1) it usually occurs in the third or fourth decades as bilateral hilar node enlargement with erythema nodosum (39 per cent); (2) as pulmonary opacities in 179; or (3) by fleeting polyarthralgia of the knees, elbows or wrists, while a skin rash may sometimes occur.

Invasion of the myocardium by sarcoid granulomas, with ensuing myocardial fibrosis, has been considered to be responsible for the clinical manifestation of sarcoid heart disease (Longcope and Fisher, 1942; Longcope and Freimen, 1952; Peacock, Lippachuts and Lukes, 1957; Porter, 1960; Maycock et al., 1963).

The sex incidence in cases of sarcoidosis showing myocardial involvement is equal but there seems to be an increased incidence in Negroes as judged by reports from the American literature (Rajasenan and Cooper, 1969).

Clinically myocardial sarcoidosis may present as (a) an arrhythmia, (b) congestive cardiac failure with or without cardiomegaly, (c) by sudden death, (d) as an atypical electrocardiogram, or (e) as involvement of the valves or pericardium. Both Stein et al. (1973) in New York and Mikhail, Mitchell and Ball (1973) in London have both surveyed their sarcoidosis patients by electrocardiography and have noted a surprisingly high incidence of abnormalities.

During a three month period at the Mount Sinai Hospital, 80 patients with histologically confirmed sarcoidosis, but without cardiac symptoms, had routine electrocardiography of which half were found to be abnormal (Siltzbach et al., 1971). At the Central Middlesex Hospital, London, 14 of 27 patients with histologically confirmed sarcoidosis were found to have abnormal electrocardiograms (Mikhail, Mitchell and Ball, 1973).

Sudden or unexpected death is common in myocardial sarcoidosis and has been reported in about 50 per cent of cases. Thus, Forbes and Usher (1962) in reviewing the literature found that 19 out of 25 cases had sudden or unexpected deaths. Ghosh et al. (1972) have analysed lately a series in which four of their six patients died suddenly and unexpectedly, usually with no suspicion of myocardial involvement clinically. This paper emphasizes the fact that very often myocardial sarcoidosis may be completely asymptomatic, the disease only being found at autopsy following the sudden death of the patient.

DIAGNOSIS

The Kveim-Siltzbach intradermal test is used in diagnosing this disease. In recent years it has, however, been asserted that the Kveim-Siltzbach test is not specific as a test for the diagnosis of sarcoidosis. For the past 25 years L. E. Siltzbach has studied the

Kveim test at the Mount Sinai Hospital, New York, where Crohn has likewise been studying regional ileitis. It is not therefore surprising that Kveim reactivity in Crohn's disease has been carefully analysed and documented. Siltzbach *et al.* (1971) found this test to be negative in Crohn's disease. James (1971) and Selroos (1972) in Helsinki have not found positive skin tests in any other diseases than sarcoidosis and Jones Williams (1971) observed a positive skin test in only one of 32 patients, who did not have sarcoidosis. Chapman, Gleeson and Taylor (1971) had similar findings in 32 patients with Crohn's disease. If the test is inconclusive, biopsy of a lymph node particularly of the superior mediastinum is useful and often diagnostic.

These results are in sharp contrast with those of other workers; Mitchell *et al.* (1971) and Karlish *et al.* (1972) recorded positive Kveim-Siltzbach tests in half of their patients with Crohn's disease.

This loss of specificity was not restricted to Britain, as Israel and Goldstein (1971) were claiming complete lack of specificity in leukaemia, tuberculosis and infectious mononucleosis.

The explanation for these conflicting results has now been solved as a result of the work of Tzumi in Kyoto and Siltzbach in New York. These workers have shown that only certain batches of the Melbourne antigen are seemingly responsible for the non-specific results although, at present, the reason for this is not known.

PATHOLOGY

Macroscopic Findings

The heart is usually normal in size and weight but there may be many fibrous adhesions between the epicardium and the pericardium. The coronary arteries are normal and the ventricular walls are usually slightly thickened, but the cardiac valves and the endocardium are usually normal.

Numerous, confluent and grey-white areas may be seen on the surface of the ventricular endocardium (*Figure 13.9*) while similar but smaller areas may be seen in the free walls of both ventricles (*Figure 13.10*). Sometimes a papillary muscle, usually the anterior of the left ventricle is partially replaced by this grey-white tissue.

Sometimes cardiac sarcoidosis may present as a ventricular aneurysm as in the two cases reported by Clark and Blount (1966) and Hines and Sancetta (1963), both of these patients dying of their cardiac lesions. Lull *et al.* (1972) reported another case of cardiac ventricular aneurysm due to sarcoidosis and presenting as refractory ventricular tachycardia. This case was successfully treated by excision of the aneurysm.

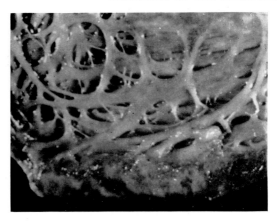

*Figure 13.9. Numerous confluent and grey-white areas
may be seen on the surface of the ventricular endocardium*

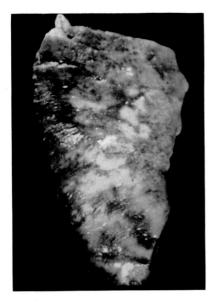

*Figure 13.10. Mid section
through the left ventricular wall
parallel to the endocardial surface
emphasizes the extent of the myocardial replacement by sarcoid
infiltrates. (Reproduced from
Krakówka, Gunnar and Greenfield
(1965) by courtesy of the authors
and Editor of the* American Heart
Journal)

Myocardial sarcoidosis can easily be overlooked because the lesions may, mistakenly, be attributed to ischaemaic fibrosis. This should not happen because the areas of sarcoidosis are often haphazardly distributed in a pattern which does not follow any distribution of a major coronary vessel. Furthermore, a diligent search may reveal lesions in the right ventricle and atria as well.

Microscopic Findings

A microscopic examination of the heart reveals the presence of multiple areas of non-caseous granulomatous inflammation; giant cells of the Langhans type are present in many of the granulomas (*Figure 13.11*).

The changes observed are very similar to those found in other granulomatous reactions.

Sarcoid granuloma of the heart are not always as sharply defined as those found in other organs. They tend to be more diffuse and giant cells may not be present, but the presence of such cardiac lesions in association with more characteristic ones elsewhere, however, is enough to establish a diagnosis of sarcoidosis.

Areas of dense myocardial fibrosis, which vary considerably in size, together with large numbers of chronic inflammatory cells are found both within the interventricular septum and in the walls of the ventricles (*Figure 13.12*). Some isolated myocardial fibres may appear to be trapped in these areas (*Figure 13.13*).

Evidence of muscle cell damage in the form of loss of striations and hyalinization of myocardial fibres may be observed in the heart muscle immediately surrounding the granulomata (*Figure 13.14*). The myocardium not involved in, or adjacent to, this infiltrative and fibrotic process appears to be normal and shows very little evidence of fibre hypertrophy.

Numerous mast cells are often found in the myocardium bordering the sarcoid granulomata but their role is not known (*Figure 13.15*).

A multiplicity of small lesions may also be found. These lesions do not always occur in the endocardium but may be pericardial or occur deep within the myocardium (*Figure 13.16*).

HISTOCHEMISTRY

The amount of lipofuscin observed is considered to be normal for the age of the patient. Study of the endocardium reveals a normal amount of elastic tissue fibres.

Ferrans *et al.* (1965) have found very little glycogen in the myocardium—as estimated by the PAS stain before and after digestion

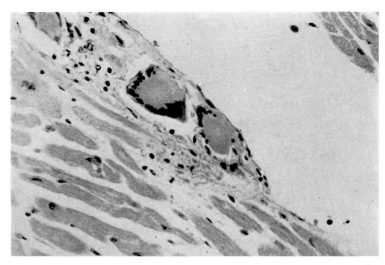

Figure 13.11.   Sub-endocardial giant-cell granuloma in sarcoidosis (haematoxylin and eosin × 600, reduced to 2/3). (Reproduced by courtesy of Dr Hayes, Jamaica)

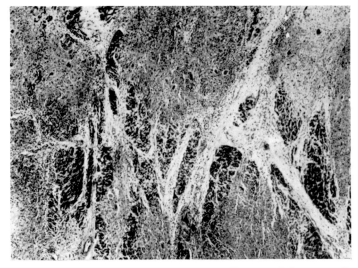

Figure 13.12.   Microscopic view of myocardial infiltration of the myocardium. Most of the infiltrate is of cellular fibrillar collagenous character. Dispersed giant cells are seen. Plump epithelioid cells are sparse. There is a little lymphoid infiltration accompanying the infiltrate (haematoxylin and eosin × 80, reduced to 2/3). (Reproduced from Krakówka, Gunnar and Greenfield (1965) by courtesy of the authors and the Editor of American Heart Journal)

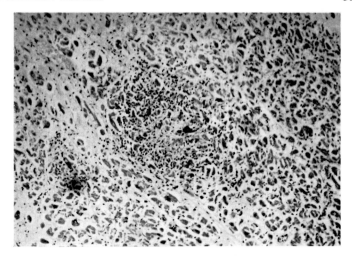

Figure 13.13. Some isolated myocardial fibres may appear to be trapped in these areas of myocardial fibrosis and inflammatory cell infiltrate (haematoxylin and eosin × 100, reduced to 6/10). (Reproduced by courtesy of Dr G. A. Gresham)

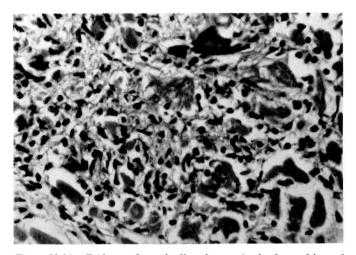

Figure 13.14. Evidence of muscle fibre damage in the form of loss of striations and hyalization of muscle fibres, which may be observed in the cardiac muscle immediately surrounding the granuloma (haematoxylin and eosin × 100, reduced to 6/10). (Reproduced by courtesy of Dr G. A. Gresham)

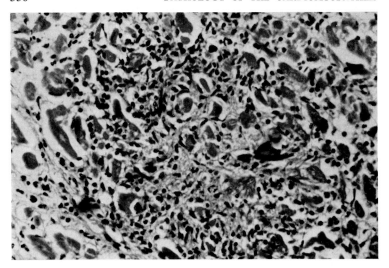

Figure 13.15.   Numerous mast cells are often found in the myocardium bordering
the sarcoid granuloma but their role is unknown (haematoxylin and eosin × 250,
reduced to 2/3). (Reproduced by courtesy of Dr G. A. Gresham)

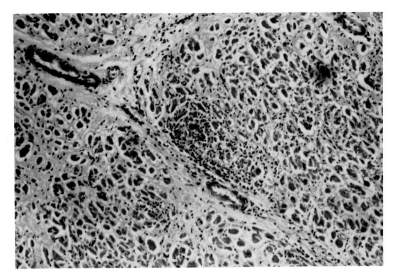

Figure 13.16.   Showing the multiplicity of small fibrotic and cellular lesions
which may be found in the myocardium is sarcoidosis (haematoxylin and eosin
× 100, reduced to 2/3). (Reproduced by courtesy of Dr G. A. Gresham)

with amylase. No accumulation of PAS-positive substances has been observed by these workers.

Numerous mast cells are often demonstrated in sections by the use of cresyl violet or toluidine blue staining methods. These cells, usually in groups of two or three, are located at the border zones between the myocardium and the areas of granulomas and fibrosis.

No mast cells are seen in the centres of the granulomatous lesions and only a few are seen in the normal parts of the myocardium.

Using fluorescent lipid stains, numerous lipid droplets can be seen to be present in the inflammatory cells in those areas of granulomatous invasion and fibrosis. These lipid droplets are also present in the cytoplasm of the endothelial cells in the myocardial capillaries.

In those parts of the myocardium bordering on the edges of granulomata some myocardial cells contain a normal amount of succinic dehydrogenase and cytochrome oxidase. In other cells the amount of these enzymes was found to be markedly decreased or completely absent. Only the giant cells within the granulomatous areas gave positive reaction for these enzymes. In the rest of the myocardium these enzymes were present in normal amounts.

ELECTRON MICROSCOPY

Sections taken from grossly normal areas of myocardium often contain muscle fibres which show various degrees of degeneration, as well as others which appear essentially normal.

The earliest electron-microscopic evidence of myocardial degeneration consists of swelling of the mitochondria. The swollen mitochondria are evenly distributed within a given cell, although adjacent cells are sometimes affected in differing degrees. In many cells small foci of increased electron density are present in some of the myofibrils. At these points the myofilaments are obscured and sometimes appear to be disrupted.

The myocardial cells found in sections taken from the periphery of the granulomatous lesions are found to be more severely diseased, and contain many vacuoles, and swollen and fragmented mitochondria. The total number of mitochondria is markedly reduced in these cells. The overall size of such muscle fibres is also markedly reduced.

The interstitial cells are found sometimes singly, sometimes in small clusters. Cytoplasmic vacuoles, some of which are almost as large as the nucleus, are present in large numbers. Myelin figures and lipid droplets are not uncommon. Mast cell granules have a normal appearance.

Capillaries are frequently found in the interstitial spaces. The endocardial cells of these capillaries differ from those of the normal myocardium in two respects. Pinocytotic vesicles are present through-out the cytoplasm in much greater number than in normal areas. Lipid droplets are also present in the cytoplasm of the endothelial cells, sometimes in great numbers. It is also not uncommon to en-counter lipid droplets of comparable size in the lumen of some capillaries.

AETIOLOGY

The relationship between sarcoidosis and tuberculosis is still un-settled. A study by Sutherland, Mitchell and Hart (1965) did not support a tuberculous aetiology for sarcoidosis. In a trial study by the Medical Research Council of children about 14 years of age who received antituberculous vaccination (BCG or vole bacillus vaccine) and who were later followed up annually by chest x-ray, tuberculin testing, postal enquiry or home visiting for 10 years, 52 developed sarcoidosis. (This incidence was similar to that in children in whom vaccinations were not done and in those who had previously been tuberculin positive.) Sarcoidosis was thus neither promoted nor inhibited by antituberculous vaccinations. The attack rate rose with age to a peak of 1149 per 10 000 as $20-22\frac{1}{2}$ years. The average incidence was three times as high in females. Fewer positive tuber-culin tests were found shortly after the sarcoidosis started, but BCG 'converted' the Mantoux reaction.

Hyperglobinaemia has been known since it was reported by Salvesen (1935) and is usually thought to be almost constantly present in this disease. James and his colleagues, however (Greenberg et al., 1964) have studied a series of 246 patients with proven sarcoidosis but found only 85 (34 per cent) with abnormal globulin patterns.

References

Bernstein, M., Konzelmann, F. W. and Sidlick, D. M. (1929). 'Boeck's sarcoid: report of a case with visceral involvement.' *Archs intern Med.* **44**, 721

Chapman, J. A., Gleeson, M. H. and Taylor, G. (1971). 'Kviem tests in Crohn's disease.' *Lancet* **2**, 1097

Clark, E. J. and Blount, A. W. (1966). 'A fatal case of myocardial sar-coidosis.' *Lancet* **86**, 568

Douglas, A. C. (1967). 'The clinical features of thoracic sarcoidosis.' *Proc. R. Soc. Med.* **60**, 983

Ferrans, V. J., Hibbs, R. E., Black, H. C., Walsh, J. T. and Burch, G. E. (1965). 'Myocardial degeneration in cardiac sarcoidosis. Histochemical and electron microscopic studies.' *Am. Heart J.* **69**, 159

Forbes, G. and Usher, A. (1962). 'Fatal myocardial sarcoidosis.' *Br. med. J.* **2**, 771

Gentzen, G. (1937). 'Über Riesenzellengranulome bei zwei Fällen von Endocardfibrose.' *Beitr. path. Anat.* **98**, 375

Ghosh, P., Fleming, H. A., Graham, G. A., Stovin, P. G. I. (1972). 'Myocardial sarcoidosis.' *Br. Heart J.* **34**, 769

Greenberg, G., Feizi, T., James, D. G. and Bird, R. (1964). 'Serum proteins in sarcoidosis.' *Lancet* **2**, 1313

Hines, J. D. and Sancetta, S. M. (1963). 'Myocardial sarcoidosis simulating healed myocardial infarction.' *Ohio med. J.* **59**, 689

Israel, H. L. and Goldstein, R. A. (1971). 'Relation of Kviem-antigen reaction to lymphadenopathy. Study of sarcoidosis and other diseases.' *New Engl. J. Med.* **284**, 345

James, D. G. (1971). Proceedings of the Symposium Européen sur la Surcoidose, Geneva.

— Siltzbach, L. E., Sharma, O. P. and Carstairs, L. S. (1969). 'A tale of two cities: a comparison of sarcoidosis in London and New York.' *Archs intern. Med.* (Chicago) **123**, 187

Jones Williams, W. (1971). 'The Kviem controversy.' *Lancet* **2**, 926

Karlish, A. J., Cox, E. V., Hampson, F. and Hemstead, E. A. (1972). 'Kviem test.' *Lancet* **1**, 438

Krakówka, C. A., Gunnar, R. M. and Greenfield, G. B. (1965). 'Clinical pathologic conference.' *Am. Heart J.* **70**, 526

Longcope, W. T. and Fisher, A. M. (1942). 'Involvement of heart in sarcoidosis on Beshier's Boech-Schaumann's disease.' *J. Mt Sinai Hosp.* **8**, 784

— and Freiman, D. G. (1952). 'A study of sarcoidosis based on a combined investigation of 160 cases including 30 autopsies from the Johns Hopkins Hospital and Massachusetts General Hospital.' *Medicine* **31**, 1

Lull, R. J., Dunn, B. E., Gregoratos, G., Cox, W. A. and Fisher, G. W. (1972). 'Ventricular aneurysm due to cardiac sarcoidosis with surgical cure of refractory ventricular tachycardia.' *Am. J. Cardiol.* **30**, 282

Maycock, R. L., Bertrand, P., Morrison, C. B. and Scott, J. R. (1963). 'Manifestations of sarcoidosis analysis of 145 patients with a review of nine series selected from the literature.' *Am. J. Med.* **35**, 67

Mikhail, T. L., Mitchell, D. N. and Ball, K. P. (1973). *Transactions of the Sixth International Conference on Sarcoidosis.* Ed. by Dr Yataka Hosoda. Tokyo: Tokyo University Press

Mitchell, D. N., Cannon, P., Dyer, N. H., Hinsen, K. F. W. and Willoughby, J. M. T. (1971). 'Kviem test.' *Lancet* **1**, 907

Peacock, R. A., Lippachuts, E. J. and Lukes, A. (1957). 'Myocardial sarcoidosis.' *Circulation* **16**, 67

Porter, G. H. (1960). 'Sarcoid heart disease.' *New Engl. J. Med.* **263**, 1350

Rajasenan, V. and Cooper, E. S. (1969). 'Myocardial sarcoidosis, bouts of ventricular tachycardia, psychiatric manifestations and sudden death. A case report.' *J. natn. med. Ass.* **61**, 306

Ricker, W. and Clark, M. (1949). 'Sarcoidosis a clinicopathologic review of three hundred cases, including twenty-two autopsies.' *Am. J. clin. Path.* **19**, 725

Salvesen, H. A. (1935). 'The sarcoid of Boeck, a disease of importance to internal medicine.' *Acta med. scand.* **86**, 127

Scadding, J. G. (1967). *Sarcoidosis.* p. 291. London: Eyre and Spottiswood

Selroos, D. (1971). Proceedings of the Symposium Européen sur la Surcoidose, Geneva

— (1973). *Transactions of the Sixth International Conference on Sarcoidosis.* Ed. by Dr Yataka Hosoda. Tokyo: Tokyo University Press

Siltzbach, L. E. (1968). *Current Diagnosis.* Ed. by H. and R. Conn, p. 935. Philadelphia: Saunders

— Vieira, L. O. B. D., Topilsky, M. and Janowitz, H. D. (1971). 'Is there Kviem responsiveness in Crohn's disease?' *Lancet* **2**, 634

Stein, E., Jacklen, I., Stein, W., Stimmal, B. and Siltzbach, L. E. (1973). *Transactions of the Sixth International Conference on Sarcoidosis.* Ed. by Dr Yakata Hosoda. Tokyo: Tokyo University Press

Sutherland, I., Mitchell, D. N. and Hart, P. d'Arcy (1965). 'Incidence of intrathoracic sarcoidosis among young adults participating in a trial of tuberculous vaccines.' *Br. med. J.* **2**, 497

Williams, W. J. (1967). 'The pathology of pulmonary sarcoidosis.' *Proc. R. Soc. Med.* **60**, 986

GIANT-CELL MYOCARDITIS

Giant-cell myocarditis is the term used to describe a myocarditis of unknown origin, consisting of necrosis and degeneration of myocardial fibres, with granuloma formation and the presence of multinucleate giant cells. Saphir (1941) in his review of myocarditis stressed the differences between granulomatous myocarditis and the idiopathic myocarditis associated with a diffuse inflammatory reaction without giant cells (isolated or Fiedler's myocarditis). However, it has been suggested that the term, granulomatous myocarditis, as used by Saphir, should only be used when referring to myocarditis with true tubercles (Tesluk, 1956).

Alternate names are given to giant-cell myocarditis, the most common being shown in Table 13.1, together with the author who first used the term.

TABLE 13.1

Condition	Author
Giant-cell granulomatous myocarditis	O'Donnell and Mann (1966)
Diffuse giant-cell myocarditis	
Idiopathic primary myocarditis	Whitehead (1965)
Fiedler's myocarditis	Parrish (1965)
Acute isolated myocarditis	Covey (1942)

Giant-cell myocarditis may present in several different ways, as was shown by Whitehead (1965) in his study of 18 cases. In 10 the history was less than 3 weeks, and in most of the remainder was under 3 years. Two patients were found dead in bed; 4 died of acute heart failure; 2 of Stokes–Adams attacks and 2 of pulmonary embolism. Of 7 more chronic cases, 5 died from congestive heart failure (2 also with pulmonary embolism) and one each from acute heart failure and a Stokes–Adams attack. Sudden death may sometimes occur. Rapid progressive heart failure often occurs and is associated with cardiac arrhythmias, while non-specific ST depression or T wave inversion (Gubbay, 1961; Palmer and Michael, 1965) may be seen in the electrocardiogram.

In some parts of the tropics, cases of granulomatous (giant-cell) myocarditis are sometimes seen and may only be found at autopsy, when investigating a sudden death, such as the case of an African woman in Kenya reported by Hudson (1970). I have seen a similar case in a 38 year old African male in Tanzania.

AGE AND SEX DISTRIBUTION

All the reports in the literature of this type of myocarditis have been in children or adults, with the exception of the case of Goldberg (1955), who described giant-cell myocarditis in a six week old infant. Males appear to be more commonly affected. Whitehead (1965) in his series of 18 cases described 12 males and 6 females who were aged between 11 months and 88 years. This disease has been described in Caucasians and Negroes, but to my knowledge there is, as yet, no description of this condition in Mongoloid peoples, that is in the Chinese or Japanese.

PATHOLOGY

Macroscopic Changes

The heart is usually found to be enlarged, often weighing 500 g or more. There may be a small pericardial effusion, while the epicardial surface of the heart is dull with patchy scattered areas of grey discoloration. The walls of all the cardiac chambers are usually thin, while the myocardium, often appearing translucent, contains scattered dark-grey foci. Intracardiac mural thrombi are also often present.

The myocardium of both ventricles usually reveals scattered diffuse and patchy areas of dull whitish-grey discoloration with foci of haemorrhage.

Microscopic Changes

The myocardium shows interstitial oedema on examination and many scattered diffuse and patchy areas of granulomatous tissue with varying degrees of fibrous tissue. These areas consist of groups of multinucleate giant cells, plasma cells, lymphocytes, neutrophils, histiocytes and fragments of degenerated or necrotic cardiac muscle cells (*Figure 13.17*).

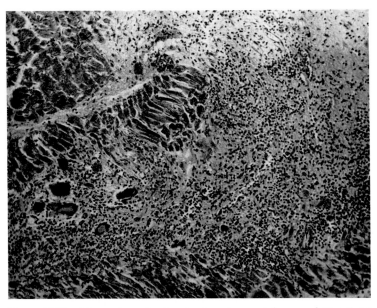

Figure 13.17. Myocardium showing focal replacement by granulation tissue, inflammatory cells and necrotic muscle fibres. The giant cells are scattered throughout the inflammatory tissue (haematoxylin and eosin × 100, reduced to 3/4). (O'Donnell and Mann, 1966)

Occasionally areas of diffuse or local myocardial necrosis with neutrophil infiltration are also seen and in these areas there are no giant cells. According to Whitehead (1965) three types of lesions may be found: (1) the acute cases showed diffuse or patchy infiltration by plasma cells and eosinophils, with relatively normal adjacent muscle cells; while phosphotungstic acid and haematoxylin staining showed loss of striations, granular disintegration and dark clumps of cells with pyknosis and lysis of nuclei and aggregation of sarcoplasma and nuclei to form early giant cells. (2) These giant cells showed subacute inflammatory changes and fibrosis of the myocardium, while (3) they showed giant cells containing lipofuscin granules in fibrous scars in the myocardium. These lesions were sometimes 2–4 cm long, in the long axis of the heart, and were seen only in areas of muscle necrosis in those severe cases who survived for several days.

Giant cells are seen in almost all areas of fibrosis and usually show marked pleomorphism (*Figure 13.18*), their cytoplasm staining slightly more basophilic than the surrounding myocardial fibres. Some of these cells contain brown or faintly eosinophilic round- or oval-shaped granules within their cytoplasm.

The nuclei of the giant cells are usually oval- or spindle-shaped and vesicular or hyperchromatic, with or without prominent nucleoli. The nuclei vary in number from 3 to 50 and are arranged in many different patterns while the cells themselves contain varying amounts of cytoplasm (*Figure 13.19*).

ORIGIN OF GIANT CELLS

The giant cells have been considered to represent: (1) an attempt at regeneration of muscle cells (Goldberg, 1955; Tesluk, 1956); (2) are derived from degenerated muscle fibres—the giant cells are thought by some as being sarcolemmal in origin and analogous to the giant cells found sometimes in muscle, being seen frequently in skeletal muscle; (3) other writers (Long, 1961; Burke *et al.*, 1969) have disputed the two previous interpretations and think that these giant cells are foreign body in type and phagocytic in nature.

Sometimes elongated giant cells can be seen lying parallel to muscle fibres. Dilling (1956) believes that the giant cells should not be identified as originating from muscle unless their origin can be clearly established, e.g., as by an established continuity with recognizable muscle fibres.

The inflammatory exudate forms an intimate association with surrounding myocardial fibres, and since many of the giant cells appear to be in continuity with or close proximity to degenerated or necrotic myocardial fibres, it has been suggested that the giant cells are myocardial in origin and represent abortive attempts at regeneration (Miller, Senhauser and Marlt, 1966).

In some cases of giant-cell myocarditis there may be a considerable amount of fibrosis. There may also be considerable thickening of the endocardium by new fibrous tissue, with, in a few cases, small overlying deposits of fibrin or thrombus. The endocardium may also be involved in the inflammatory process, the cell infiltrate consisting of lymphocytes, eosinophils and plasma cells, but no giant cells are usually seen.

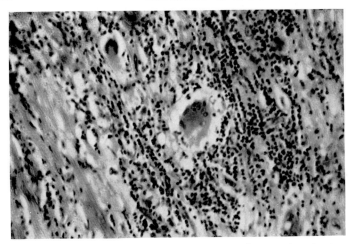

Figure 13.18. Myocardium from a case of giant-cell myocarditis showing only a few hyaline and necrotic myocardial fibres together with a very marked infiltration with chronic inflammatory cells—which are mostly lymphocytes and a few plasma cells in an area of fibrosis (haematoxylin and eosin × 50, reduced to 6/10). (Reproduced by courtesy of Dr McCrea)

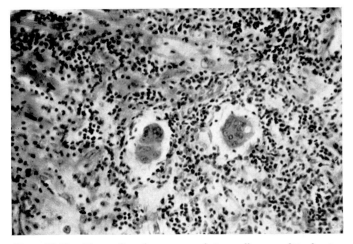

Figure 13.19. Myocardium from a case of giant-cell myocarditis showing that the nuclei of the giant cells are oval or spindle-shaped and some have prominent nucleoli. There is also a marked infiltration with chronic inflammatory cells, mostly lymphocytes and a few plasma cells. All the remaining myocardial cells have lost their normal striations and have become hyaline in appearance (haematoxyline and eosin × 50, reduced to 6/10). (Reproduced by courtesy of Dr McCrea)

INVOLVEMENT OF OTHER ORGANS

In the majority of cases of giant-cell myocarditis other organs are not involved, this being an isolated myocardial disease.

In those cases which show a giant-cell and lymphocytic infiltration of other organs, the lungs (*Figure 13.20*) and kidney (*Figure 13.21*) are most commonly involved.

In some cases of giant-cell myocarditis an associated myositis is also found. In these cases, particularly in the larger muscles, such as the deltoid, areas of massive necrosis of muscle cells—with a replacement by a dense mononuclear infiltrate composed of lymphocytes, eosinophils, plasma cells and many giant cells, similar to those found in the heart—are seen. This most commonly occurs in those cases where a thymoma is also present.

ASSOCIATED DISEASES

The three diseases which are known to have a close association with giant-cell myocarditis are (1) Wegener's syndrome; (2) thymoma and (3) chronic cardiac valve disease.

(1) *Wegener's syndrome.*—Walton (1958), in reviewing 54 cases of Wegener's syndrome, found granulomas of the heart on 6 occasions and focal necrotizing cardiac arterial lesions in a further 15 cases. McCrea and Childers (1969) reported another case of giant-cell myocarditis associated with Wegener's syndrome, pulmonary granulomas and vascular renal lesions.

(2) *Thymoma.*—Several instances have been reported of thymoma co-existent with myositis and giant-cell myocarditis (Langston, Wagman and Dickenman, 1959; Funkhouser, 1961; McCrea and Jagoe, 1963).

Since many workers regard the arterial lesions of Wegener's syndrome as aetiologically related to peri-arteritis, it would seem that giant-cell arteritis might fall within this group of diseases.

(3) *Chronic cardiac valve disease.*—Husband and Lannigan (1965) found three examples of giant-cell myocarditis in left atrial appendage biopsies from women of 41, 42 and 54 years, who had mitral stenosis. The three cases came from a series of 465 biopsies taken since valvulotomies started (58 per cent of the first 175 had Aschoff nodules and 6 per cent had non-specific lesions). The three appendages showed extensive focal and diffuse infiltration with lymphocytes, plasma cells, giant cells and occasional eosinophils and mononuclear cells. The giant cells were associated with necrotic muscle cells and were of Langhans type with 2–40 nuclei; no Aschoff nodules, tubercles, areas of caseation, or acid-fast bacilli were seen.

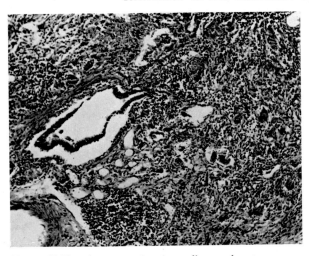

Figure 13.20. Asymptomatic giant-cell granulomatous myo-carditis showing nodular proliferation of fibroblasts in the lung. Giant cells and lymphocytes are also seen as part of the cellular exudate (haematoxylin and eosin × 75, reduced to 6/10). (O'Donnell and Mann, 1966)

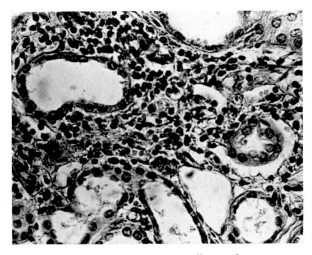

Figure 13.21. Asymptomatic giant-cell granulomatous myo-carditis showing interstitial mononuclear cell infiltration between the tubules of the kidney. The exudate also consists of a few plasma cells and eosinophils (haematoxylin and eosin × 75, reduced to 6/10). (O'Donnell and Mann, 1966)

Similar cases have been reported by McCrea and Childers (1969) and Thorbjarnarson and Glenn (1956), the latter authors finding giant-cell myocarditis in the heart of a patient who died at surgery for chronic valve disease, while Zschoch (1961) reported rheumatic mitral and aortic valve disease co-existent with widespread giant-cell myocarditis confined solely to the left atrium in a woman of 60 years. In this case there were no Aschoff nodules.

Rheumatic heart disease is *not* therefore associated with giant-cell myocarditis. Aschoff nodules may be found in some of the affected hearts but are no more frequent than in other unaffected subjects.

In making a diagnosis of giant-cell myocarditis the following conditions should always be considered: (1) tuberculosis; (2) sarcoidosis; (3) Chagas' disease; (4) syphilis (Kean and Hoekenga, 1952).

AETIOLOGY

Nothing is known of the aetiology of giant cell myocarditis and it is unlikely that it is a single disease entity.

Many cases formerly classified in this category in children are now known to be tubercular in origin. Many causative agents have, however, been suggested, the most common being: (1) viral infection (Covey, 1942; Tesluk, 1956); (2) fungal infections (Collyns, 1959; McCrea and Childers, 1969); (3) isolated examples of sarcoidosis; (4) hypersensitivity or auto-immune reaction (Palmer and Michael, 1965; O'Donnell and Mann, 1966); (5) drug therapy.

(1) Viral infections have been postulated on the basis of clinical histories and non-specific light microscopic findings. Intracytoplasmic granules have sometimes been found in giant cells and degenerated myocardial fibres by electron microscopy; these granules, however, lack sufficient internal structure and organization to allow them to be identified as virus particles.

Tesluk (1956) attempted to demonstrate a virus by cytopathic studies with tissue cultures but failed to do so. A similar finding was reported at a case conference at the Massachusetts General Hospital (1959).

(2) In no case has a fungus been demonstrated histologically or cultured from the myocardium.

(3) The possibility of isolated myocardial sarcoidosis has been considered in several reported cases (Rab, Chondhury and Chondhury, 1963).

The histological features of giant-cell myocarditis differ from a sarcoid lesion in many details. The lesions are more diffuse and there are few, if any, epithelioid cells, while the cellular composition of the associated inflammatory cells is much more pleomorphic. Asteroid bodies, however, have been observed in the giant cells by other writers (Gubbay, 1961). However, it is well known that the finding of asteriod bodies is not diagnostic of sarcoidosis.

(4) Hypersensitivity or auto-immune reactions as a cause of the disease has been postulated by Palmer and Michael (1965). This suggestion has been supported by other authors (Parrish, 1965; Miller, Senhauser and Marlt, 1966) because of the histological findings and absence of obvious aetiological agents, but is not otherwise substantiated.

That allergy is an aetiological factor is also largely discounted by the studies of Dilling (1956) who collected 13 reported cases in which no allergic manifestations were noted.

Drug therapy is also sometimes suggested as an aetiological agent. Hudson (1970) described giant-cell myocarditis in a 46 year old woman with Graves' disease following neomercazole therapy.

It is not clear whether the association of giant-cell myocarditis with thymoma and myositis is incidental or related.

References

Burke, J. S., Medline, N. M. and Katz, A. (1969). 'Giant cell myocarditis and myositis associated with thymoma and myasthenia gravis.' *Archs Path.* **88**, 359

Collyns, J. A. H. (1959). 'Isolated granulomatous myocarditis.' *Am. Heart J.* **58**, 630

Covey, G. M. (1942). 'Isolated granulomatous myocarditis (Fiedler's myocarditis).' *Am. J. clin. Path.* **12**, 160

Dilling, Nancy V. (1956). 'Giant cell myocarditis.' *J. Path. Bact.* **71**, 295

Funkhouser, J. W. (1961). 'Thymoma associated with myocarditis and the L.E. cell phenomenon.' *New Engl. J. Med.* **264**, 34

Gillie, L. and Fox, H. (1968). 'Mitral stenosis together with a giant-cell myocarditis limited to the left atrium.' *Am. J. clin. Path.* **21**, 756

Goldberg, G. M. (1955). 'Myocarditis of giant cell type in an infant.' *Am. J. clin. Path.* **25**, 510

Gubbay, E. R. (1961). 'Giant cell myocarditis.' *Can. med. Ass. J.* **85**, 349

Hudson, R. E. B. (1970). 'Giant cell myocarditis.' In *Cardiovascular Pathology* Vol. 3, p. 498. London: Edward Arnold

— (1970). 'Granulomatous myocarditis in an African woman.' In *Cardiovascular Pathology* Vol. 3, p. 483. London: Edward Arnold

Husband, E. M. and Lannigan, R. (1965). 'Unusual giant cell lesions in biopsy specimens of the left atrial appendage in mitral stenosis.' *Br. Heart J.* **27**, 269

Kean, B. H. and Hoekenga, N. T. (1952). 'Giant cell myocarditis.' *Am. J. Path.* **28**, 1995

Langston, J. D., Wagman, G. F. and Dickenman, R. C. (1959). 'Granulomatous myocarditis and myositis associated with thymoma.' *Archs Path.* **68**, 367

Long, W. H. (1961). 'Granulomatous (Fiedler's) myocarditis with extracardiac involvement.' *J. Am. med. Ass.* **177**, 184

Massachusetts General Hospital (Case Report) (1959). *New Engl. J. Med.* **261**, 1283

McCrea, P. C. and Jagoe, W. S. (1963). 'Myocarditis in myasthenia gravis associated with thymoma.' *Ir. J. med. Sci.* **454**, 453

— and Childers, R. W. (1969). 'Two unusual cases of giant cell myocarditis associated with mitral stenosis and with Wegener's syndrome.' *Br. Heart J.* **26**, 490

Miller, W. V., Senhauser, D. A. and Marlt, J. M. (1966). 'An inquiry into the nature of myocardial giant cells.' *Missouri Med.* **63**, 811

O'Donnell, W. M. and Mann, R. H. (1966). 'A symptomatic granulomatous myocarditis.' *Am. Heart J.* **76**, 686

Palmer, H. P. and Michael, I. E. (1965). 'Giant cell myocarditis with multiple organ involvement.' *Archs intern. Med.* **116**, 444

Parrish, J. A. (1965). 'Fielder's myocarditis.' *Br. Heart J.* **27**, 458

Pyun, K. S., Ye A. Kim, Kotzenstein, R. E. and Kikkawa, Y. (1970). 'Giant cell myocarditis. Light and electromicroscopic study.' *Archs Path.* **90**, 181

Rab, S. M., Chondhury, G. M. and Chondhury, R. (1963). 'Giant cell myocarditis.' *Lancet* **2**, 172

Saphir, O. (1941). 'Isolated myocarditis.' *Am. Heart J.* **24**, 167

Tesluk, H. (1956). 'Giant-cell versus granulomatous myocarditis.' *Am. J. clin. Path.* **26**, 1326

Thorbjarnarson, B. and Glenn, F. (1956). 'Sarcoidosis associated with sudden death during mitral valvotomy.' *Archs Surg., Chicago* **73**, 862

Walton, E. W. (1958). 'Giant cell granuloma of the respiratory tract (Wegener's granulomatosis).' *Br. med. J.* **2**, 265

Whitehead, R. (1965). 'Isolated myocarditis.' *Br. Heart J.* **27**, 230

Zschoch, H. (1961). 'Beitrag zur Pathogenese der granulomatosen Reisenzellmyocarditis.' *Zentbl. allg. Path. Anat.* **102**, 132

Fourteen

Metabolic diseases

ENDOCRINE ABNORMALITIES

HYPERTHYROIDISM

Although clinically there is marked evidence of disturbance in cardiac function in primary and secondary thyrotoxicosis, there is still considerable doubt as to the pathological changes in the heart.

Although it has been disputed that thyrotoxicosis can produce cardiac failure (Friedberg and Sohval, 1937), there is little doubt that in a proportion of these cases no other cause of cardiac failure can be found post mortem (Kepler and Barnes, 1932); in others this has been denied (Weller *et al.*, 1932; Friedberg and Sohval, 1937).

Saphir (1942) and Sandler and Wilson (1959) reviewed the association of heart disease and thyrotoxicosis. Tachycardia, ectopic beats, fibrillation or other permanent cardiac arrhythmias are common, but heart failure is rare. The increase in metabolic rate is associated with an increase in cardiac output, tachycardia and increased pulse pressure. Auricular fibrillation later occurs in a fairly high proportion of patients; the incidence increasing with advancing age.

It is well recognized that heart disease may coexist with thyrotoxicosis but not universally accepted that it alone can cause heart failure. It is evident that age and its corresponding lesions are decisive factors in determining the frequency with which cardiovascular disease accompanies hyperthyroidism (McPhedran, 1942). 'Pure heart disease', which can be attributed solely to thyrotoxicosis, is found only in one-third to one-sixth of hyperthyroid patients reported to have cardiovascular disease.

McDevitt *et al.* (1968) showed that the difference between the heart rate in hypo- and hyperthyroidism was due to the direct action of thyroxine itself and not to potentiation of catecholamines by thyroxine.

Sandler and Wilson (1959) found evidence of heart disease in 151 of 462 thyrotoxic patients treated with radio-active iodine; 86 patients had associated ischaemic, hypertensive, pulmonary or congenital heart disease. In the remaining 65 patients, atrial fibrillation, congestive heart failure, or cardiomegaly in the absence of any other evidence of co-existing heart disease was present. Neither the incidence of goitre, the severity of duration of thyrotoxicosis, nor sex of the patient appeared to be related to the incidence of involvement of the cardiovascular system. In approximately a third of patients manifesting atrial fibrillation, the rhythm of the heart reverted spontaneously to a normal rate after radio-active iodine therapy.

PATHOLOGY

There are no characteristic lesions produced in the human heart by thyrotoxicosis (Weller *et al.*, 1932; White, 1951), although periodically reports have appeared which describe changes in the myocardium.

In a few instances necrosis of the myocardium (more abundant lipid and fat changes, and interstitial myocarditis) have been found. Lesions of the myocardium in animals with experimental hyperthyroidism were first described by Farrant (1913). These lesions showed haemorrhages, degenerative necrosis of muscle, inflammatory cell infiltrates of small round cells and, if survival was long enough, a fibroblastic reaction. Weller *et al.* (1932) described focal areas of fibrosis in the myocardium together with a lymphocytic infiltrate. Such alterations have not been conclusively demonstrated to have been caused by thyroid disease. Other pathologists (Friedberg and Sohval, 1937; Sandler and Wilson, 1959) have been unable to show any consistent histological changes.

While it may be true that thyrotoxicosis induces a shift from a preponderant carbohydrate substrate to a preponderant fat substrate as a source of myocardial energy, there is no evidence of any significant biochemical disturbance in thyrotoxicosis which can explain its deleterious effect on the function of the myocardium.

Experimental studies support the concept of pure thyrotoxic heart disease. Thyroid over-dosage is known to produce cardiac hypertrophy (Herring, 1917; Hashimoto, 1921), and also focal myocarditis (Goodpasture, 1921; Zalka, 1935). Hashimoto (1921) also described focal lymphocytic infiltrates and myocardial degeneration in rats. Hoet and Marks (1926) found absence of glycogen in experimental hyperthyroidism. Nora and Flaxman (1943) have found that experimentally-induced thyrotoxicosis produces fraying and splitting of myocardial fibres, cellular infiltration and fibrosis. Diametrically opposed experimental results have been obtained by Rake and McEachern (1931), who concluded that thyrotoxicosis was produced in animals, by the injection of thyroxine, but did not produce pathological changes.

Susin and Herdson (1967) have shown experimentally that when sodium L-thyroxine is administered to young male rats at a daily dose of approximately 100 mg/kg at least 50 per cent of the animals die within three weeks. Mean relative heart weights are twice those of controls—apparently due to myocardial cell hypertrophy. These workers also found occasional foci of myocardial cell necrosis and inflammation, together with extensive mitochondrial alterations. There was also swelling of sarcoplasmic reticulin and separation of some intercalated discs. A magnesium-deficient diet produced less-marked histological and fine structural myocardial changes, whereas rats receiving L-thyroxine in addition to a magnesium deficient diet show similar but more conspicuous changes to those receiving L-thyroxine alone.

References

Farrant, R. (1913). 'Hyperthyroidism: its experimental production in animals.' *Br. med. J.* **2**, 1363

Friedberg, C. K. and Sohval, A. R. (1937). 'The occurrence and the pathogenesis of cardiac hypertrophy in Graves' disease.' *Am. Heart J.* **13**, 599

Goodpasture, E. W. (1921). 'The influence of thyroid products on the production of myocardial necrosis.' *J. exp. Med.* **35**, 407

Hashimoto, H. (1921). 'The heart in experimental hyperthyroidism with special reference to its histology.' *Endocrinology* **5**, 579

Herring, P. T. (1917). 'The action of thyroid upon the growth of the body and organs of the white rat.' *Q. Jl. exp. Physiol.* **11**, 231

Hoet, J. P. and Marks, H. P. (1926). 'Observations on the onset of rigor mortis.' *Proc. R. Soc.*, Series B, **100**, 72

Kepler, E. J. and Barnes, A. R. (1932). 'Congestive cardiac failure and hypertrophy in hyperthyroidism. A clinical and pathological study of 178 fatal cases.' *Am. Heart J.* **8**, 102

McDevitt, D. G., Shanks R. G., Hadden, D. R., Montgomery, D. R. D. and Weaver, J. A. (1968). 'The role of the thyroid in the control of heart-rate.' *Lancet* **1**, 998

McPhedran, H. (1942). 'Cardiovascular changes in toxic goitre.' *Can. med. Ass. J.* **46**, 471

Nora, E. D. and Flaxman, N. (1943). 'The heart in experimental thyrotoxicosis.' *J. Lab. clin. Med.* **28**, 797

Rake, G. and McEachern, D. (1931). 'Experimental hyperthyroidism and its effect upon myocardium in guinea pigs and rabbits.' *J. exp. Med.* **54**, 23

Sandler, G. and Wilson, G. M. (1959). 'The nature and prognosis of heart disease in thyrotoxicosis. A review of 150 patients treated with I 131.' *Q. J. Med.* **28**, 347

Saphir, O. (1942). 'Myocarditis; general review, with analysis of 240 cases.' *Archs Path.* **33**, 88

Susin, M. and Herdson, P. B. (1967). 'Fine structural changes in rat myocardium induced by thyroxine and by magnesium deficiency.' *Archs Path.* **83**, 86

Weller, C. V., Wanstron, R. G., Gordon, H. and Bucher, J. C. (1932). 'Cardiac histopathology in thyroid diseases. Preliminary report.' *Am. Heart J.* **8**, 8

White, P. D. (1951). *Heart Diseases.* 4th Edition. New York: Macmillan

Zalka, E. von (1935). 'Über das Vorkommen und Entstehen der Silber-gebilde im Plexusepithel.' *Beitr. path. Anat.* **94**, 404

HYPOTHYROIDISM (MYXOEDEMA)

The clinical features of hypothyroidism include bradycardia (low cardiac output), radiological enlargement of the cardiac shadow and electrocardiographic changes. All of these changes are usually reversible on thyroid hormone therapy.

Zondek (1918) first described the clinical features of heart involvement in myxoedema and since then considerable controversy has prevailed regarding the ability of myxoedema to produce heart failure. In 1936, Higgins thought that the role of hypothyroidism is questionable and in an excellent review 25 years later, Hamolsky, Kurland and Freedburg (1961) commented on the confusion in the literature concerning the significance of certain cardiac lesions in the presence of myxoedema.

The underlying pathological changes are not well documented, in view of the absence of detailed examinations of large enough series of untreated cases.

These changes are largely non-specific and their clinicopathological evaluation is most difficult, since they are almost always attended by the complications of ageing, diabetes mellitus, atherosclerosis, hypertension, or other cardiovascular disease. Furthermore since most cause-and-effect correlations have been made in patients with severe long-standing myxoedema, it is imperative to recognize and assess the effects of the other endocrine glands on the cardiovascular system in such patients. To most cardiologists, however, the condition has become well known, but its causes remain disputed. Zondek (1965) still believes that the basic cause is myocardial oedema by myxoedema fluid, which also manifests as pericardial effusion; although the latter is not the cause of heart failure.

Characteristically, there is a low cardiac output, slow peripheral circulation, bradycardia, heart enlargement and sometimes pericardial effusion. The accumulation of fluid is usually slow, but it may be rapid and cause tamponade as in the case recorded by Martin and Spathis (1965), in a woman aged 52 from whom 1500 ml of fluid was aspirated.

In severe myxoedema the heart is, radiologically, usually markedly enlarged and all chambers are dilated, but the ventricular walls exhibit little, if any, hypertrophy. Most of the published material consists of individual cases or small numbers of cases, and it is difficult to give a single explanation for the enlargement. However, in the series of 10 cases (reported by Douglass and Jacobson, 1957) none had pericardial effusions.

The enlarged cardiac shadow has also been attributed to pericardial effusion, but this is not a common finding.

The size of the heart, in relation to a direct effect by myxoedema, could not be established in the latter series, since most of the patients had severe coronary artery disease.

Microscopical changes found in the myocardium are similar to those occurring in the subcutaneous tissue and skeletal muscle (Douglass and Jacobson, 1957). Specific myocardial changes warranting a diagnosis of either 'myocarditis' or 'myxoedema heart disease' are lacking. The histological changes most often encountered are swelling of the muscle cells, some of which are pale, while others are deeply stained and contain small pyknotic nuclei; vacuolization; degeneration of fibres, with a relative loss of the transverse striations; and occasionally fatty infiltration and interstitial oedema. The presence of interstitial fibrosis is difficult to evaluate in view of the average age of subjects suffering from this disease, and the frequent occurrence of coronary artery disease.

Brilliantly PAS-positive material (similar to that demonstrated by Webster and Cooke (1936) in rabbits made hypothyroid) may also accumulate in the human heart. The precise chemical nature of this material is unknown, but it is believed to be related to the mucopolysaccharides of ground substance and to contain a high concentration of protein and nitrogen.

The basophilic degeneration of myocardial fibres has been described but is not specific to myxoedema, although it is much more widespread than in other conditions (Fisher and Mulligan, 1943; Doerr and Holldack, 1948).

Basophilic degeneration of myocardial fibres which differs from the material found in the connective tissues (Brewer, 1951) may also be seen. Brewer found deposits of two different types of mucoid material in histochemical studies of tissues from a patient with myxoedema. He concluded that the skin and tongue were infiltrated with a mixture of mucoprotein containing hyaluronic acid and chondrotin-sulphuric acid, but that the heart was infiltrated with a histologically distinct mucoprotein that was only weakly acid. The material in the heart did not exhibit metachromasia with toluidine blue, nor did it have an affinity for methylene blue, at a pH with an acid content higher than five. Histological evidence of pericardial alterations has not been recorded, even though instances have been reported in which more than a litre of protein rich fluid (6·8 g/100 ml of fluid) may accumulate in the pericardial cavity.

Myocardial infarction has been precipitated by over rapid therapy in myxoedema.

Experimentally, the changes described in cardiac muscle have varied in different experiments. The presence of brilliantly PAS-positive material in the myocardium of animals made hypothyroid has been described by Webster and Cooke (1935) but these changes are not consistently found. The other degenerative changes described are also not consistently found.

Hypothyroidism usually shows low voltage and abnormal T waves on an electrocardiogram, but ventricular fibrillation may occur (Marcuson, 1965).

References

Brewer, D. B. (1951). 'Myxoedema: autopsy report with histochemical observations on the nature of the mucoid infiltrations.' *J. Path. Bact.* **63**, 503

Doerr, W. and Holldack, K. (1948). 'Über das Myxödemhertz.' *Virchows Arch. path. Anat. Physiol.* **315**, 653

Douglass, R. C. and Jacobson, S. D. (1957). 'Pathologic changes in adult myxoedema: a survey of 10 necropsies.' *J. clin. Endocrinol. Metab.* **17**, 1354

Fisher, C. E. and Mulligan, R. M. (1943). 'Qualitative study of correlation between basophilic degeneration of myocardium and atrophy of thyroid gland.' *Archs Path.* **36**, 206

Hamolsky, M. W., Kurland, G. S. and Freedburg, A. S. (1961). 'The heart in hypothyroidism.' *J. chron. Dis.* **14**, 558

Higgins, W. H. (1936). 'The heart in myxoedema: correlation of physical and postmortem findings.' *Am. J. med. Sci.* **191**, 80

Marcuson, R. W. (1965). 'Ventricular fibrillation with myxoedema heart disease with spontaneous reversion.' *Br. Heart J.* **27**, 455

Martin, L. and Spathis, G. S. (1965). 'Case of myxoedema with a huge pericardial effusion and cardiac tamponade.' *Br. med. J.* **2**, 83

Webster, B. and Cooke, C. (1936). 'Morphologic changes in the heart in experimental myxoedema.' *Archs intern. Med.* **58**, 269

Zondek, A. (1965). 'Pathogenesis of myxoedema heart.' *Lancet* **2**, 694

Zondek, H. (1918). 'Das Myxödemherz.' *München med. Wschr.* **65**, 1180

ACROMEGALY

Acromegaly is caused by the continued production of human growth hormone after that age when it is normally produced. Hartog *et al.* (1964) reported that the fasting levels of human growth hormone in five patients with acromegaly were 24–74 μg/ml and remained high during a glucose tolerance test.

The patient with acromegaly suffers from headache, diabetes mellitus, constricted vision or blindness and premature death from cardiovascular disease or hypopituitarism.

The cause of the acromegaly is usually a pituitary tumour which has to be removed surgically or can be treated by irradiation, or the implantation of radio-active implants. Most of these pituitary tumours are found, on histological examination, to consist of mixed eosinophilic, chromophobic adenomas while only a few consist of eosinophilic adenomas (Gordon, Hill and Ezrin, 1962).

The adenoma may be quite small. If it is functioning the results depend on the patient's age; if the epiphyses have not yet closed gigantism may result. In some cases the proliferation of adenoma cells may be diffuse or multifocal. In the adult the hands and feet are enlarged; the nose, lips and tongue are enlarged and thick; the bones are enlarged, especially the mandible (causing projection of the lower jaw) and also the bones of the thorax. The skin is coarse and hair growth may be excessive. Goitre, due to multiple colloid adenomata may occur and glycosuria is common. The hearts of these patients may be enlarged, but this enlargement may be due to aortic regurgitation because of aortic valve insufficiency caused by thickening of the cusps, which may also be fenestrated or because of hypertension.

Cardiomegaly is part of the syndrome, and is usually attributed to the excess of growth hormone. However, the heart enlargement (*Figure 14.1*) may or may not be associated with hypertension, and this was first reported by Amsler in 1912. Courville and Mason (1938) considered that the size of the heart was disproportionate to the general muscular development and that the histological appearances were variable, some of the myocardial fibres actually being smaller than normal (*Figure 14.2*). Usually, however, the myocardial fibres are hypertrophied (*Figure 14.3*).

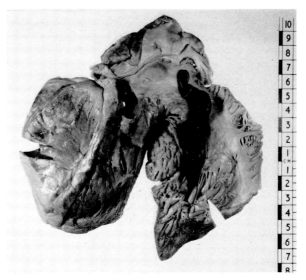

Figure 14.1. The heart of a 50 year old man who has had acromegaly since the age of 18

Hejmancik, Bradfield and Herrmann (1951) in the most detailed study of acromegaly heart disease made so far, showed in a clinical study of 21 patients, that 13 of the patients had evidence of heart disease; 5 were in heart failure and 2 had episodes of left ventricular failure. Nine of 15 patients who had electrocardiogram examinations, showed abnormalities such as left ventricular hypertrophy and impaired intraventricular conduction; 6 had hypertension which was badly tolerated; 4 had elevated basal metabolic rates and 5 had diabetes. Four autopsies were performed and, in all, the heart was found to be much enlarged; in one case it weighed 1140 g; histology showed hypertrophy of the cardiac muscle fibres and in two cases there was a diffuse increase of the fibrous interstitial tissue. Some patients with acromegaly have thyrotoxicosis, presumably due to thyroid hypertrophy caused by excessive production of TSH. It is uncertain therefore if the auricular fibrillation which is sometimes found is due to acromegaly or thyrotoxic heart disease.

References

Amsler, C. (1912). 'Zur Lehre der Splanchnomegalie bei Acromegalie.' *Berl. klin. Wschr.* **49**, 1600

Courville, C. and Mason, V. R. (1938). 'The heart in acromegaly.' *Arch. intern. Med.* **61**, 704

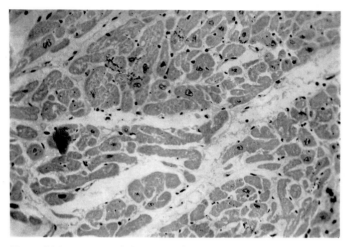

Figure 14.2. Section of the myocardium from a 50 year old man with acromegaly. There is considerable variation in the size of many of the muscle fibres, some being actually smaller than normal (haematoxylin and eosin × 240, reduced to 6/10)

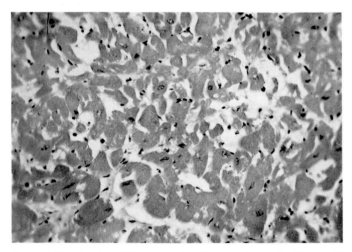

Figure 14.3. Section of the myocardium from the heart of a 50 year old man who had acromegaly from the age of 18. The majority of the muscle fibres are hypertrophied (haematoxylin and eosin × 240, reduced to 6/10)

Gordon, D. A., Hill, F. M. and Ezrin, C. (1962). 'Acromegaly: a review of 100 cases.' *Can. med. Ass. J.* **87**, 1106

Hartog, M., Doyle, F., Fraser, R. and Joplin, G. (1965). 'Partial pituitary ablation with implants of gold-198 and yttrium-90 for acromegaly.' *Br. med. J.* **2**, 396

Hejmancik, M. R., Bradfield, J. Y. and Herrmann, G. R. (1951). 'Acromegaly and heart: a clinical and pathological study.' *Ann. intern. Med.* **34**, 1445

CARDIAC CALCIFICATION

Cardiac calcification is nearly always dystrophic, i.e., due to deposition of calcium in previously degenerate, devitalized or dead tissue. It may also occur in the thickened endocardium, being commonly seen in cases of fibro-elastosis or endomyocardial fibrosis, but is especially seen in association with infective processes— particularly parasitic infections such as trichuris infections or in association with old infarcts.

Hamne and Ranstrom (1957) described two cases in children associated with necrosis of muscle fibres, but in some cases of Coxsackie virus infection calcification is found in necrotic muscle fibres. Less commonly, calcification may be metastatic, i.e., due to deposits of calcium in previously normal tissue. An example of this is the case reported by Hudson (1965). This was an elderly woman with constrictive pericarditis who was found, at autopsy, to have marked metastatic calcification throughout the right atrium, and two foci of calcification within the right ventricle and over the posterior left ventricle, with spreading into the posterior mitral valve ring. Other cases of massive myocardial calcification, of unknown origin, have also been reported (Duke, 1957).

AGE DISTRIBUTION

Idiopathic calcification of the myocardium may occur at any age. It is sometimes seen in the newborn (van Buchem, 1946) and even in the premature infant (Diamond, 1932).

AETIOLOGY

Gore and Arons (1949) described thirteen examples of microscopic myocardial calcification; all were associated with myocardial necrosis as in ischaemia or myocarditis, but in four cases the cause was obscure. A special feature in eleven cases was advanced renal disease, but their suggestion that anaemia-produced focal necrosis in myocardial fibres was not confirmed by Langendorf and Pirani (1947). In one case hypervitaminosis D was implicated. The calcification occurred in the muscle fibres rather than in the interstitium. They believed that small focal areas of necrosis occurred and that calcification took place rapidly because of the increase in calcium metabolism. They concluded that this process was not strictly speaking metastatic calcification, and suggested that it was accelerated dystrophic calcification.

Vitamin D fed to dogs produced calcification in the endocardium, especially in relation to elastic tissue, but not in the myocardial fibres (Mulligan and Stricker, 1948). However, it appears that in some cases true metastatic calcification can occur, especially in hypervitaminosis D.

Hypokalaemia has been suggested as an aetiological factor in massive myocardial necrosis with calcification. Littman and Meadows (1963) reported two possible examples: (1) a man 32 years of age with large areas of yellowish calcification in the inner third of the left ventricle and electrocardiographic evidence of hypokalaemia; and (2) a Negro 41 years of age with oesophageal carcinoma and scattered myocardial calcification lesion. The deposition was in the sarcoplasm only, not involving sarcolemmal sheaths, interstitial tissue or vessels. The appearances closely resembled those of experimental potassium deficiency in rats, in which degenerative muscle fibre lesions appear in the sarcoplasm and nuclei of the papillary muscles and columnae carneae, later involving the inner half of the myocardium, especially the right wall of the right ventricle, and eventually healing by fibrosis (Cannon, Frazier and Hughes, 1952; French, 1952).

The concept that, in most cases of metastatic calcification, necrosis of myocardial fibres precedes the deposition of calcium receives some support from experimental studies. Injection of parathyroid extracts in rats has shown necrosis of muscle fibres preceding calcification (Cantarow, Stewart and Housel, 1938). Shohl, Goldblatt and Brown (1930) produced calcification in the myocardium by feeding irradiated ergosterol to rats, but although the calcification was associated with necrosis (calciphylaxia) they were unable to determine if necrosis always preceded calcification. Selye and de Salcedo (1958) showed that if calcium salts are used as 'conditioners' of the myocardium in animals subjected to stress, calcification occurred in the 'infarctoid cardiopathy' so produced. High calcium diets fed to rats had produced myocardial calcifications, but the calcium was deposited in the interstitial tissue and was surrounded by necrotic muscle fibres (Stephens and Barr, 1933).

PAGET'S DISEASE

Calcification of heart valves and myocardium sometimes occurs in Paget's disease, and involvement of the conducting system, causing heart block, has been reported (Windholz and Grayson, 1947). This is not surprising, since the bundle of His and its main branches are in the area adjacent to the membranous septum, which is one of the earliest regions involved in ring calcification of the cardiac valves. Thus, Pomerance (1970), in a study of 258 cases of mitral valve calcification, found it to occur in 8·5 per cent of patients over 50 years of age, but in none of the cases was an association with deposits of calcium in the myocardium to be found.

References

Cannon, P. R., Frazier, L. E. and Hughes, R. H. (1952). 'Influence of potassium on tissue protein synthesis.' *Metabolism* **1**, 49

Cantarow, A., Stewart, H. L. and Housel, E. L. (1938). 'Experimental acute hyperparathyroidism; morphologic changes.' *Endocrinology* **22**, 13

Diamond, M. (1932). 'Calcification of the myocardium in premature infant.' *Archs Path.* **14**, 137

Duke, M. (1957). 'Massive calcification of the myocardium of unknown origin.' *Archs Path.* **64**, 34

French, J. E. (1952). 'A histological study of the heart lesions in potassium deficient rats.' *Archs Path.* **53**, 485

Gore, I. and Arons, W. (1949). 'Calcification of the myocardium; a pathologic study of thirteen cases.' *Archs Path.* **48**, 1

Hamne, B. and Ranstrom, S. (1957). 'Calcification of heart muscle in infants.' *Acta. path. microbiol. scand.* **41**, 111

Hudson, R. E. B. (1965). 'Cardiac calcification.' In *Cardiovascular Pathology.* Vol. I, pp. 1316–21. London: Edward Arnold

Langendorf, A. and Pirani, C. L. (1947). 'The heart in uremia; an electrocardiographic and pathologic study.' *Am. Heart J.* **33**, 282

Littman, M. S. and Meadows, W. R. (1963). 'Massive myocardial necrosis with calcification. Report of two cases of possible hypokalemic etiology.' *Circulation* **28**, 938

Mulligan, R. M. and Stricker, F. L. (1948). 'Metastatic calcification produced in dogs by hypervitaminosis D and haliphagia.' *Am. J. Path.* **24**, 451

Pomerance, Ariela (1970). 'Pathological and clinical study of calcification of the mitral valve ring.' *J. clin. Path.* **23**, 354

Selye, H. and de Salcedo, I. (1958). 'Infarctoid cardiopathy produced by hydrocortisone and monobasic sodium phosphate.' *Archs intern. Med.* **102**, 551

Shohl, A. T., Goldblatt, H. and Brown, H. B. (1930). 'The pathological effects upon rats of excess irradiated ergosterol.' *J. clin. Invest.* **8**, 505

Stephens, D. J. and Barr, D. P. (1933). 'Influence of acid and phosphate on metastatic calcification.' *Proc. Soc. exp. Biol. Med.* **30**, 93

Van Buchem, F. S. (1946). 'Extensive calcification of the heart at an early age.' *Acta med. scand.* **125**, 182

Windholz, F. and Grayson, C. (1947). 'Roentgen demonstration of calcifications in the interventricular septum in cases of heart block.' *Am. J. Roentg.* **58**, 411

HAEMOCHROMATOSIS AND HAEMOSIDEROSIS

Patients with refractory chronic anaemias—particularly aplastic anaemia—who receive repeated multiple transfusions over a long period of time, or who have been given excessive iron therapy may develop, in time, a condition that is almost indistinguishable from the cardiac lesions which are sometimes found in idiopathic haemochromatosis.

The patients with both haemochromatosis and haemosiderosis have speckled bronze or grey pigmentation of the whole body, particularly the hands and neck, which is due to melanosis or iron pigment. Those patients with haemochromatosis usually have enlarged livers and spleens and often also have cirrhosis, diabetes mellitus and gonadal atrophy. In children adolescence is delayed and only about half of these patients live to adulthood.

The age and sex distributions of patients with acquired haemochromatosis from congenital haemolytic anaemia is different from that in idiopathic haemochromatosis (Althausen *et al.*, 1951; Lewis, 1954; Finch and Finch, 1955), in which the peak incidence is between 45 and 55 years, with the male sex predominantly affected, and for transfusional haemochromatosis, in which most patients are over 30 years of age (Schwartz and Blumenthals, 1948; Dubin, 1955).

Common to all three groups, however, is the excessive absorption and deposition of iron with destruction and fibrosis in the tissues. In all three congestive cardiac failure is the leading cause of death.

This massive iron overload may lead eventually to recurrent benign pericarditis and to congestive heart failure with arrhythmias (*Figure 14.4*). Pericarditis occurs in about half the patients with haemochromatosis, but is not usually fatal. It starts with pericardial pain and a pericardial friction rub, but has usually cleared in 2–3 weeks. In one fatal case the pericardial space was obliterated by adhesions (Engel, Erlandson and Smith, 1964).

Pericarditis, however, is not a prominent feature in idiopathic or transfusional haemochromatosis. Its prevalence in cases of chronic anaemia which have been transfused repeatedly may represent an increased susceptibility to infections in this group. It is possible that iron deposition in the myocardium may render the epicardial layer

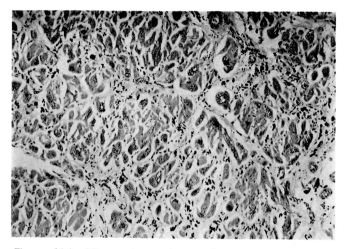

Figures 14.4. Microscopic examination shows iron granules within myocardial cells which vary greatly in size and preservations of architecture. Interstitial fibrosis and extensive scarring are also present (Masson's trichrome stain × 80, reduced to 6/10). (Engel, Erlandson and Smith, 1964)

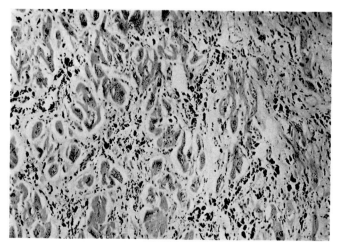

Figure 14.5. Haemosiderosis as a result of very many blood transfusions for aplastic anaemia. Many of the myocardial fibres have become filled with iron pigment. Also note the increase in fibrous tissue and that some myocardial fibres contain no iron (haematoxylin and eosin × 80, reduced to 6/10)

liable to inflammation in the presence of a virus or other agent capable of causing pericarditis.

Congestive heart failure usually starts about the age of ten years, in haemochromatosis, or after something less than 10 years in acquired haemosiderosis, and usually ends fatally.

The cardiac involvement usually starts with cardiac enlargement. At necropsy the heart is dilated and up to twice normal size from

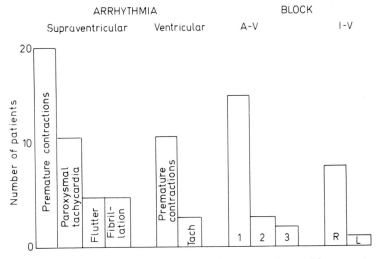

Figure 14.6. Electrocardiographic abnormalities in patients with congestive cardiac failure, in late cardiac complications of chronic, severe, refractory anaemia with haemochromatosis (Engel, Erlandson and Smith, 1964)

hypertrophy. It is deep brown from iron deposits in the cardiac muscle. Microscopy will show deposits of iron both within muscle cells and histiocytes (*Figure 14.4*), while surrounding these myocytes there are usually extensive areas of fibrosis and focal degeneration (*Figure 14.5*).

Some muscle cells may be two-thirds filled with iron, while others show poor staining with nuclear damage or destruction. The muscle cells are often vacuolated and have lost their striations. Similar changes are seen in haemosiderosis.

Arrhythmias are thought to be due to similar changes taking place in the cardiac condition system but this is not certain as the conduction system is often spared the changes seen in the general myocardium. Other changes in cardiac rate or rhythm may also be observed (*Figure 14.6*).

James (1964) studied the hearts from five patients—dying of haemochromatosis—one 66 year old woman and four men aged between 66 and 83 years with various disorders of rhythm or conduction: atrial flutter or fibrillation, sinus tachycardia, varying degrees of heart block and syncope. In all five, iron deposition was found in the AV node and myocardium but not in the SA node; the reason for this was obscure but possibly, being a periarterial structure, the SA node was spared, as were the walls of the coronary arteries. Alternatively, the metabolism of the two nodes was different, as were the glycogen content and the xanthine oxidase activity which Ayvazian (1964) has shown in haemochromatosis.

Schellhammer, Engel, and Hagstrom (1966, 1967) obtained different results in their study of iron deposits in the conducting system of the hearts of six patients with acquired iron storage disease. In 5, deposition was uniform; 2 had suffered no abnormality of conduction; 2 had done so and also had rhythm disturbance and 1 had supraventricular arrhythmias. Moderate to heavy deposits were found throughout the AV system and ordinary myocardium, but the autonomic nerves and ganglia were generally spared. Three of the five patients had deposits in the SA node. In the one patient with minimal deposition anywhere, supraventricular arrhythmia was present. Scarring was heavier in the SA node and myocardium than in the AV system. The authors thus found no correlation between the iron deposits and the conducting system disturbances nor between scarring and the density of the iron deposits. They credited Trousseau (1865) with the description of iron saturation of the tissues and Von Recklinghausen with the term 'haemochromatosis' to describe the triad of hepatic cirrhosis, fibrosis of the pancreas and bronzing of the skin.

ABNORMAL HAEM BIOSYNTHESIS IN THE MYOCARDIUM

Watt, Lochhead and Goldberg (1967) studied new haem formation in myoglobin in the myocardium of man and pig by using radioactive iron ^{59}Fe and ^{14}C protoporphyrin. The addition of normal amounts of iron potentiated the action of haemsynthetase and ALA-dehydrase; the addition of amounts of iron as in haemochromatosis inhibited ALA-dehydrase but not haemsynthetase. This could possibly underlie the cardiac complications of haemochromatosis.

References

Althausen, I. L., Doil, R. K., Weiden, S., Mottenhan, R., Turner, C. N. and Moore, A. (1951). 'Hemochromatosis: investigation of twenty-three cases with special reference to etiology, nutrition, iron metabolism, and studies of hepatic and pancreatic functions.' *Archs intern. Med.* **88**, 553

Ayvazian, J. H. (1964). 'Xanthinuria and hemochromatosis.' *New Engl. J. Med.* **270**, 18

Dubin, I. N. (1955). 'Idiopathic hemochromatosis and transfusion siderosis; a review.' *Am. J. clin. Path.* **25**, 514

Engel, Mary A., Erlandson, Marion and Smith, C. H. (1964). 'Late cardiac complications of chronic, severe refractory anaemia with haemochromatosis.' *Circulation* **30**, 698

Finch, S. C. and Finch, C. A. (1955). 'Idiopathic hemochromatosis, iron storage disease; Iron metabolism in hemochromatosis.' *Medicine, Baltimore* **34**, 381

James, T. N. (1964). 'Pathology of the cardiac conduction system in hemochromatosis.' *New Engl. J. Med.* **271**, 92

Lewis, H. P. (1954). 'Cardiac involvement in hemochromatosis.' *Am. J. med. Sci.* **227**, 554

Recklinghausen, F. von (1889). 'Ueber Hemochromatosis.' *Beitr. klin. Wschr.* **26**, 925

Schellhammer, P. F., Engel, Mary A. and Hagstrom, J. W. C. (1966). 'Arrhythmias, conduction defects and cardiac lesions in acquired iron storage disease.' *Circulation* **34**, Suppl. III 208

— — — (1967). 'Histologic studies of the myocardium and conduction system in acquired iron-storage disease.' *Circulation* **35**, 631

Schwartz, S. O. and Blumenthals, L. A. (1948). 'Exogenous hemochromatosis resulting from blood transfusion.' *Blood,* 3, 617

Trousseau, A. (1865). *Clinique médicale de L'Hotel-Dieu de Paris.* 2nd Ed. Paris: Bailliere

Watt, D. A., Lochhead, A. C. and Goldberg, A. (1967). 'Haem biosynthesis: in the heart muscle of man and the pig.' *Panminerva Med.* **8**, 303

NUTRITIONAL CAUSES

NUTRITIONAL DEFICIENCY STATES

The role of nutritional factors in the production of cardiac disease is difficult to assess.

The areas of the world where nutritional diseases are likely to occur are also those areas where parasitic infestation and other similar diseases are likely. In addition deficiency of one dietary factor is unusual and it is difficult to assess the role of individual types of deficiency or malnutrition.

UNDERNUTRITION AND STARVATION

Starvation or extreme undernutrition usually decreases the size of the heart. Whether acute or prolonged, it results in a reduction in the size of the heart corresponding to the loss of weight of the body as a whole. Although reduction in epicardial fat is conspicuous, the major portion in the loss of cardiac tissue is in the muscle of all chambers.

Data compiled during World War II and in the post-war period have yielded considerable information regarding the size and percentage of decrease among persons subjected to malnutrition and starvation (Follis, 1958). In prison camps the average cardiac weight of starved persons was 200–220 g, a decrease of 25–30 per cent of normal. Follis recorded studies of 492 patients who died in the Warsaw Ghetto. Heart weight in the 'select' population varied only from 220–275 g, an average decrease of 20 per cent in weight. In extreme degrees of malnutrition the outstanding feature is 'brown atrophy'. Follis also stated that caloric restriction, as in starvation, leads to no dramatic morphological changes other than atrophy.

CLINICAL MANIFESTATIONS

The atrophy from starvation appeared to coincide with the functional changes of bradycardia, hypotension, weak pulse, decreased cardiac output, increased circulation time and decrease in venous pressure. The cardiac state does not seem to be an important factor in the appearance of oedema in starvation and physical exertion may possibly increase the venous return beyond the capacity of the atrophic heart. If this be so, then famine oedema may be essentially similar to the oedema in congestive heart failure from other causes. However, the possible contribution of hypoproteinaemia should not be overlooked. It is noted that starved persons may first suffer cardiac failure after abrupt resumption of feeding. This is said to be due to the response of the heart which may then become inadequate to meet the increased metabolic load, and that incipient or overt circulatory factors may then supervene. The 'flooding syndrome', described by Lamy, Lamotte and Lamotte-Barallon (1946) among undernourished prisoners in concentration camps, refers to rapid pulmonary oedema which often developed following plasma infusions. 'Brown atrophy' may also be seen in undernourished persons who are otherwise healthy but are deprived of adequate food or who restrict their intake as in 'anorexia nervosa'; it is also induced by chronic debilitating diseases such as cancer or tuberculosis and endocrine disease such as Addison's or Simmond's.

PATHOLOGICAL CHANGES

In starvation the heart is reduced in weight with loss of epicardial fat and shrinkage of the muscle.

All hearts in severe states of calorie deficiency or starvation are severely underweight, the weights often varying from 60 to 100 g. A pericardial effusion of between 100–500 ml is often present. There is an extreme loss of epicardial fat and this has usually vanished completely from the atrioventricular and interventricular grooves bearing the coronary artery system which then stands out in bold relief. This loss of fat and the accompanying myocardial atrophy may render the coronaries tortuous, and at places the focal prominence of the vessels may give an impression of aneurysmal dilatation.

In some cases there may be a gelatinous transformation of the subepicardial fat (Ramalingaswami, 1958).

The myocardium of the ventricles and atria may be reduced almost to paper thinness, most markedly so on the right side, and the myocardium, on sectioning, is brown, soft and atrophic and crumbles under pressure.

The endocardium is normal except for slight opacification along the outflow tracts. There are usually no overlying thrombi but they may be seen in the region of the mitral and tricuspid valves.

MICROSCOPIC EXAMINATION

Microscopic examination usually reveals an extreme degree of reduction in size of myocardial muscle fibres with marked nuclear overcrowding. Cross striations become inconspicuous and muscle fibres exhibit cytoplasmic homogenization, the nuclei of muscle cells in places showing abnormal shapes, and include Anitschkow myocytes. Lipochrome (wear and tear) pigment is present in muscle cells in a paranuclear position but is not conspicuous. The loss of subepicardial fat is striking and in this area a focal basophilic change in the stroma is evident.

Later there may be evidence of cloudy swelling, myocardial cell degeneration, vacuolization and occasionally fatty degeneration (Keys, 1948). Uehlinger (1958) found 'brown atrophy' with no evidence of fatty degeneration or fibrosis in inmates of concentration camps. Before leaving the subject of the heart in starvation, the history of an error as narrated by Keys et al. (1950) may be mentioned.

Voit, an outstanding nineteenth century investigator in a paper written in 1866 and dealing with other problems, cited the heart weights of two cats, one of which was starved for 13 days and the other well fed. At the end of the experiment the heart of the starved cat weighed only 2·3 per cent less than that of the other. This unfortunate experiment on a single cat, lasting for 13 days, has formed the basis for the belief, handed down from textbook to textbook, that the heart resists starvation.

References

Follis, R. H. (1958). *Deficiency Disease.* p. 577. Springfield, Ill: Thomas

Keys, A. B. (1948). 'Cardiovascular effects of undernutrition and starvation.' *Mod. Concepts cardiovasc. Dis.* **17**, 21

— Brozer, J., Hanschel, A., Mickelsen, O. and Taylor, H. L. (1950). *The Biology of Human Starvation.* Vol. 1. p. 763. Minneapolis: University of Minnesota Press

Lamy, M., Lamotte, M. and Lamotte-Barallon, S. (1946). Quoted by McCance, R. A. (1951). In 'Studies in under-nutrition, Wappertal 1946–49.' *Spec. Rep. Ser. med. Res. Coun.* **275**, 74

Ramalingaswami, V. (1958). 'Nutritional disease.' *Fedn. Proc.* **17**, Suppl. No. 2, 43

Uehlinger, E. H. (1958). 'Beri-beri.' *Fedn. Proc.* **17**, Suppl. 2

KWASHIORKOR

Kwashiorkor, first described by Cicely Williams, in 1933, is a syndrome usually consisting of a variable degree of oedema, diarrhoea, hepatomegaly, lassitude and psychic abberrations, retardation of growth, loss of weight, muscular wasting and changes in the hair.

The term kwashiorkor is derived from the Bantu 'Ga' and means 'red boy', denoting the pigmentary changes usually seen in the hair or skin. This is a nutritional disease which damages the liver, pancreas, and to a lesser extent, all the internal organs. Although regarded as a form of protein malnutrition occurring in infancy, it apparently is caused by multiple deficiencies. It affects chiefly ill-nourished children during the periods of late breast feeding, weaning and post-weaning. (In Africa, the Bantu often breast feed their children until they are two to three years old.)

Sometimes fatal cardiac failure is a serious problem on occasions in the early stages of recovery during the treatment of kwashiorkor, and has been reported occasionally from Mexico (Gómez *et al.*, 1958); Jamaica (Garrow, Picou and Waterlow, 1962); and Guatemala (Viteri *et al.*, 1964). Wharton *et al.* (1969) in Kampala, Uganda, found that it was more common in those with anaemia, and also a large sodium intake, leading to fluid retention and haemodilution; fewer cases occurred if sodium intake was restricted to 1 mEq/kg/day.

Smythe, Swanepoel and Campbell (1962) in Cape Town have also implicated the heart as a cause of sudden death in kwashiorkor. It seems that the heart failure is due to myocardial damage as described below.

PATHOLOGICAL CHANGES

The wasting of skeletal muscle and atrophy of the heart are often conspicuous features (Smythe, Swanepoel and Campbell, 1962;

Swanepoel, Smythe and Campbell, 1964). The cardiothoracic ratio is significantly reduced, but upon recovery returns to normal. Myocardial lesions in kwashiorkor were originally described by Bablet and Normet (1937), who first suspected that the myocardium might be seriously disturbed. Microscopic examination of the heart has not disclosed the nature of the wasting and has failed to establish whether it consists only of shrinkage in size of muscle fibres, or if there is also a reduction in the number of individual fibres present. In some instances post-mortem examination has demonstrated oedema of the myocardium, capillary dilatation and congestion and vacuolization, fragmentation and hyalinization of muscle fibres (Trowell, Davies and Dean, 1954).

In a detailed study of the hearts of five children who died from kwashiorkor (Wharton *et al.*, 1969), one heart was noted to be flabby but otherwise no abnormality was seen. Microscopically all the hearts showed some abnormality, mainly in the papillary muscles and subendocardial region of the left ventricle. There were always small fibres with poorly-staining areas of myocardium and indistinct striations, many of them with intracellular vacuolization, and others with deformed nuclei and classical Anitschkow myocytes were sometimes seen. In one case, vacuolization was so extreme as to make it difficult to recognize heart muscle fibres at all. Two others, from children with anaemia, had extreme fatty infiltration of the myocardium. Two cases showed occasional patchy necrosis of fibres with a scanty cellular reaction around them, and in one of these cases fibrous tissue scars of previous necrosis were present. Two cases showed separation of the fibres by interstitial oedema and in one inflammatory cells were noted in the subpericardial connective tissue. These workers then compared the changes found with those in the hearts of 100 children who had died of any cause between the ages of three months and three years. The cases with kwashiorkor showed significantly more fibre vacuolization and had more intercellular oedema.

In the single post-mortem reported by Wharton *et al.* (1969) in a patient with kwashiorkor who died, apparently from cardiac failure, the heart appeared pale but in all other respects seemed macroscopically normal. Microscopically, the heart muscle fibres were smaller than normal and were separated from each other by an oedematous stroma. The fibres in the papillary muscles and in the subendocardial zone were vacuolated; the material was not fat and was not stained in paraffin sections. The cytoplasm of the fibres was stained with varying degrees of intensity (*Figure 14.7*). A few fibres were necrotic and surrounded by lymphocytes and macrophages (*Figure 14.8*). The nuclei showed all graduations of change between normality and the formation of Anitschkow myocytes (*Figure 14.9*). There were a few lymphocytes present in the subpericardial connective tissue. The extent of change in the heart appears to be correlated with the duration of the disease and with complicating phenomena such as infection, anaemia and imbalance of electrolytes.

From a consideration of these facts it will be seen that the heart in kwashiorkor is almost always abnormal. The cardiac changes found in the myocardium vary only in degree from those in the hearts of other children in those areas where kwashiorkor is commonly found. It seems, apparently, that the lesions are non-specific and are probably due to the combined effects of anaemia, malnutrition and other unknown traumas.

Electron microscopic and histochemical studies by Cat *et al.* (1963) suggests that the clinical and histological findings in the disease cannot be explained by a functional deficit of the mitochondria of the sarcosomas. Sudden death of severely affected children is not infrequent and, paradoxically, may occur during apparent recovery.

Experimental protein malnutrition in 29 rhesus monkeys, deprived of this foodstuff for 12 weeks, was studied by Chauhan, Nayak and Ramalingaswami (1965). Electrocardiography showed sinus tachycardia, with flattened or inverted T waves. At necropsy the heart weights averaged 10·4 g (controls 12·2 g). In the early stages myocardial fibres showed cytoplasmic coagulation, fragmentation and hydropic degeneration and the interstitium showed foci of cell infiltration producing a histological picture similar to a myocarditis. Later the myocardial fibres became atrophic and the interstitium fibrotic. Areas of fat necrosis occurred in the epicardium and these were associated with lymphocytes and giant-cell granulomas.

I have found very similar changes (*Figure 14.10*) in the hearts of Macacus monkeys which have been kept for prolonged periods— up to two years—on low protein diets. These diets, consisting largely of plantain or maize, were similar to those normally eaten by the indigenous inhabitants of Uganda. I differed, however, in finding none with areas of myocardial fatty infiltration as described by Wharton *et al.* (1969).

No endocardial lesions were produced, so that there was no support for the view that malnutrition is an important factor in the pathogenesis of EMF. Indeed, the appearances were similar to those described for kwashiorkor and adult protein malnutrition. Skeletal muscle showed similar but more severe changes.

Sims (1972) examined the conducting tissue of the heart histologically in seven cases of kwashiorkor. Atrophic changes were found,

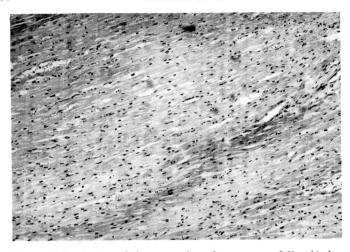

Figure 14.7. Section of the myocardium from a case of Kwashiorkor showing marked variations in the intensity of cytoplasmic staining with eosin (haematoxylin and eosin × 80, reduced to 6/10). (Reproduced by courtesy of Dr Waterston)

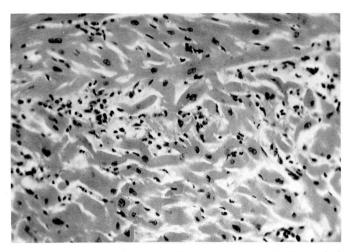

Figure 14.8. Kwashiorkor myocardium showing necrotic fibres which have been surrounded by macrophages and lymphocytes (haematoxylin and eosin × 430, reduced to 6/10)

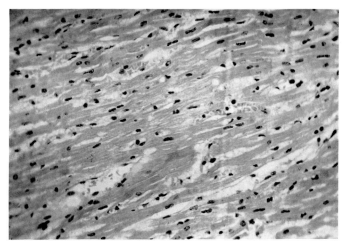

Figure 14.9. The nuclei in Kwashiorkor myocardium showing marked variations in size and shape (haematoxylin and eosin × 430, reduced to 6/10)

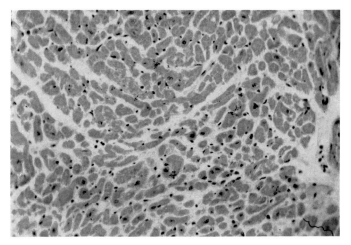

Figure 14.10. Gross variations in nuclear size and shape in the myocardium of a Macacus monkey which had been kept on a low protein diet for two years (haematoxylin and eosin × 180, reduced to 6/10)

and in five myocytolysis was present. No cellular reaction or fibrous repair was found in relation to the areas of myocytolysis. These findings may be associated with a disturbance of atrioventricular conduction during life, perhaps accounting for some of the unexplained sudden deaths occurring in children with kwashiorkor.

Deo, Sood and Ramalingaswami (1965) in studying the kwashiorkor syndrome in young rhesus monkeys found similar changes but stressed that they increased in severity with the duration of the deficiency. At first the changes were patchy, consisting of swelling and hydropic change in the sarcoplasm of muscle fibres, eosinophilic coagulation and fragmentation of the sarcoplasm, hazy striations, small foci of necrosis and infiltration with lymphocytes. As the deficiency progressed, atrophy of muscle fibres was a prominent and consistent change. The muscle fibres were thin and strap-like with marked reduction of cytoplasmic mass. In some areas atrophy was so marked as to leave thin eosinophilic streaks as remnants of the original muscle fibres. The number of muscle fibres per square inch of projected area in camera lucida drawings showed a proportionate crowding and increase in the deficient animals. This finding demonstrates that the small heart size is due to all the muscle fibres becoming smaller and *not* to a diminution in the number of the cardiac muscle fibres present in the heart.

The changes in the skeletal muscle were more severe than in the heart. Higginson, Gillanders and Murray (1952) have studied the ultrastructural changes in cells in experimentally-induced protein deficiency in rhesus monkeys. In the myocardial fibres in deficient animals they observed patchy defects in the form of deficiency of myofilaments, finely granular cytoplasm containing dilated vesicles, reduction in the number and a moth-eaten appearance of mitochondria suggesting lysis of their membranes (Racela *et al.*, 1966).

It is clear that protein malnutrition, naturally-occurring in man or experimentally-induced in monkeys does result in significant cardiac abnormalities of which atrophy seems to be the most dominant.

It is believed that death, in these cases, may occur from the predisposition of an atrophic heart to sudden cardiac arrest or fibrillation (Smythe, Swanepoel and Campbell, 1962).

The concept that damage done in childhood due to malnutrition may be clinically manifest years later is attractive but difficult to prove. Follow-up studies have been carried out in Cape Town (Smythe, Swanepoel and Campbell, 1962), Jamaica (Garrow and Pike, 1967) and in Kampala, Uganda (Cook and Hutt, 1967), on children treated successfully for kwashiorkor some two to ten years previously, and in none of these studies has there been any evidence of cardiac sequelae.

References

Bablet, J. and Normet, L. (1937). 'Les lésions histopathologiques de la bouffissure d'Annan.' *Bull. Acad. Med.* **117**, 242

Cat, I., Campello, A. P., Voss, D. O., Braga, H. and Bacila, M. (1963). 'Respiration-rates and oxidative phosphorylation of heart sarcosomes in kwashiorkor.' *Lancet* **2**, 415

Chauhan, Sushila, Nayak, N. C. and Ramalingaswami, V. (1965). 'The heart and skeletal muscle in experimental protein malnutrition in rhesus monkeys.' *J. Path. Bact.* **90**, 301

Cook, G. C. and Hutt, M. S. (1967). 'The liver after kwashiorkor.' *Br. med. J.* **3**, 454

Deo, M. G., Sood, S. K. and Ramalingaswami, V. (1965). 'Experimental protein deficiency: pathological features in the rhesus monkey.' *Archs Path.* **80**, 14

Garrow, J. S. and Pike, M. C. (1967). 'The long-term prognosis of severe infantile malnutrition.' *Lancet* **1**, 1

Garrow, J. W., Picou, D. and Waterlow, J. C. (1962). 'The treatment and prognosis of infantile malnutrition in Jamaican children.' *W. Ind. Med. J.* **11**, 217

Gómez, F., Ramos-Galván, R., Cravioto, J. and Frenk, S. (1958). 'Prevention and treatment of chronic severe infantile malnutrition (Kwashiorkor).' *Ann. N.Y. Acad. Sci.* **69**, 969

Higginson, J., Gillanders, A. D. and Murray, J. F. (1952). 'The heart in chronic malnutrition.' *Br. Heart J.* **14**, 213

Racela, A. S., Grady, H. J., Higginson, J. and Svoboda, D. J. (1966). 'Protein deficiency in rhesus monkeys.' *Am. J. Path.* **49**, 419

Sims, B. A. (1972). 'Conducting tissue of the heart in Kwashiorkor.' *Br. Heart J.* **34**, 828

Smythe, P. M., Swanepoel, A. and Campbell, J. A. J. (1962). 'The heart in kwashiorkor.' *Br. med. J.* **1**, 67

Swanepoel, A., Smythe, P. M. and Campbell, J. A. (1964). 'The heart in kwashiorkor.' *Am. Heart J.* **67**, 1

Trowell, H. C., Davies, J. N. P. and Dean, R. F. A. (1954). *Kwashiorkor.* London: Arnolds

Viteri, E., Béhar, M., Arroyave, G. and Scrimshaw, N. S. (1964). 'Clinical aspects of protein malnutrition.' In *Mammalian Protein Metabolism.* Ed. by H. N. Munro and J. B. Allison, Vol. 2, p. 523. New York: Academic Press

Wharton, B. A., Howells, G. R. and McCance, R. A. (1967). 'Cardiac failure in kwashiorkor.' *Lancet* **2**, 384

— Balmer, Susan E., Somers, K. and Templeton, A. C. (1969). 'The myocardium in kwashiorkor.' *Q. Jl. Med.* **38**, 107

Williams, Cicely D. (1933). 'A nutritional disease of childhood associated with a maize diet.' *Archs Dis. Child.* **8**, 423

VITAMIN DEFICIENCY STATES

Decreased intake of various vitamins or interference with their utilization may produce both biochemical and morphological alterations in the myocardium (Follis, 1958). The following discussions describe only those vitamin deficiencies with produce, or are directly implicated in, structural changes in the heart.

DEFICIENCY OF VITAMIN C (ASCORBIC ACID)

Only a few detailed reports are available on the heart in scurvy. Serious deficiencies of this vitamin can still be seen in this country, but usually only occur in old people or single men living alone. Humans lack the enzyme which converts gulonolactone to ascorbic acid, so this vitamin must be taken in the diet. It is essential in the body for the synthesis of the hydroxyproline of collagen; deficiency leads to the development of a thin watery, ground substance in which poorly-supported blood vessels may bleed, producing petechiae and ecchymoses. The available evidence, though incomplete, indicates that sudden death may be associated with cardiac hypertrophy, especially of the right ventricle. In 1918 Erdheim observed hypertrophy of the right ventricle to be present in about two-thirds of children who died of scurvy and that in severe disease both ventricles might be enlarged. No further histological studies have been reported concerning this evidence.

Crandon, Lund and Dill (1940) reported hypotension in experimental scurvy; this became normal again in three weeks of vitamin therapy but two patients died and, at necropsy, nothing could be found in the heart or elsewhere in the body and no cause of death was apparent.

Follis (1942) described the cardiac findings in three infants who had died suddenly of severe scurvy. At necropsy two of them displayed hypertrophy of the right ventricle but a careful histological study revealed nothing additional of note. Sudden death may occur but the nature of the cardiac disease is obscure.

Bartley, Krebs and O'Brien (1953) reported on two volunteers deprived of the vitamin; one developed severe lower chest pain, dyspnoea, cyanosis, and ST elevation in the electrocardiogram; the other had constricting chest pain, a systolic murmur and prolonged PR interval. Smart (1966) said that the chest pain could result from haemorrhage into the myocardium or pericardial sac. Various other lesions have been attributed to ascorbic-acid deficiency and in the guinea-pig, non-specific valvulitis (Winsor and Burch, 1945; Taylor, 1957), myocarditis and pericarditis (Taylor, 1957); and when the deficiency is combined with beta-haemolytic streptococcus infections Aschoff-like nodes may be produced in the myocardium and heart valves (Rinehart and Mettier, 1934). The anaemia frequently associated with scurvy may affect the heart indirectly.

DEFICIENCY OF VITAMIN E

Although the precise locus of action for alpha-tocopherol is not known, it is necessary for the *in vitro* maintenance of metabolism of striated and cardiac muscle. Its deficiency leads to a marked disturbance of respiration in muscle and increased oxygen consumption. In rats that have been on a deficient diet for more than 12 months, necrosis of cardiac muscle fibres and healing by fibrosis have been observed.

Bragdon and Levine (1949) and Mason and Emmel (1945) have demonstrated the evolution of changes in the myocardium, slow but progressive destruction of muscle fibres, a most conspicuous change consisting of the presence of abundant connective tissue accompanied by the separation and disappearance of muscle fibres, presence of ceroid in fibres and in the macrophages of the connective tissue, and no observed alteration in the lipid or cholesterol content of the heart.

Binder *et al.* (1965), in an extensive study, established that there were three stages of deficiency; the first a latent period of nine months before the second stage in which red blood cell membranes became unduly haemolysable by hydrogen peroxide because there is not enough anti-oxidant vitamin E to protect them from peroxidases. Hyperbaric oxygen administered to such a patient could cause a haemolytic attack.

In the third stage ceroid granules appeared in the muscle coats of the intestine ('brown bowel' syndrome); the ceroid pigment was formed from oxidation of unsaturated fats and reacted with PAS reagent. Ceroid could also be seen in skeletal muscles, producing histological dystrophic changes. However, it took years of deprivation to cause a subnormal level of serum vitamin E.

DEFICIENCY OF VITAMIN D

Vitamin D increases the absorption, mobilization and renal excretion of calcium and phosphorus. The effect of dosage is delayed for several weeks and overdosage (1 mg or more daily) may cause irreversible hypercalcaemia and renal failure, with lassitude, anorexia, thirst, nausea, vomiting, psychoses, convulsions and coma.

Although deranged vitamin D metabolism is concerned in idiopathic infantile hypoglycaemia, the part played by excess of vitamin D in supravalvar stenosis is uncertain; in animals it can produce subendothelial oedema or even calcification, especially just above the aortic valve.

References

Bartley, W., Krebs, H. A. and O'Brien, J. R. P. (1953). 'Vitamin C requirements of human adults.' *Spec. Rep. Ser. med. Res. Coun.* **280**

Binder, H. J., Herting, D. C., Hurst, V., Finch, S. C. and Spiro, H. M. (1965). 'Tocopheral deficiency in man.' *New Engl. J. Med.* **273**, 1289

Bragdon, J. H. and Levine, H. D. (1949). 'Myocarditis in Vitamin E deficient rabbits.' *Am. J. Path.* **25**, 265

Crandon, J. H., Lund, C. C. and Dill, D. B. (1940). 'Experimental human scurvy.' *New Engl. J. Med.* **223**, 353

Erdheim, J. E. (1918). 'Ueber das Barlow-Herz.' *Wien. klin. Wschr.* **31**, 1293

Follis, R. H. (1942). 'Sudden death in infants with scurvy.' *J. Pediat.* **20**, 347
— (1958). *Deficiency Diseases.* p. 577. Springfield Ill: Thomas

Mason, K. E. and Emmel, A. F. (1945). 'Vitamin E and muscle pigment in the rat.' *Anat. Rec.* **92**, 33

Rinehart, J. F. and Mettier, S. R. (1934). 'Heart valves and muscle in experimental scurvy with superimposed infection, with notes on similarity of lesions to those of rheumatic fever.' *Am. J. Path.* **10**, 61

Smart, G. A. (1966). 'Scurvy.' In *Price's Textbook of the Practice of Medicine.* Ed. by Sir R. Bodley Scott, p. 400. London: OUP

Taylor, S. (1937). 'Scurvy and carditis.' *Lancet* **1**, 973

Winsor, T. and Burch, G. E. (1945). 'Electrocardiogram and cardiac state in active sickle-cell anaemia.' *Am. Heart J.* **29**, 685

ANAEMIA

CHRONIC HYPOCHROMIC OR MEGALOBLASTIC ANAEMIA

Haemoglobin levels below eight gram per cent and of three months' duration produce cardiac hypertrophy in man as a direct result of anaemia; and this effect is not related to age, sex, or aetiology of the anaemia (Sanghvi, Misra and Banerjee 1960). The heart may also become dilated. Cardiac hypertrophy has been produced in rats and dogs by experimentally-induced anaemia (Norman and Mc-Broom, 1958; Paplanus, Zbar and Hays, 1958).

In severe chronic anaemia the myocardium is flabby. Fatty degeneration of the myocardium is commonly found, but this may not be visualized macroscopically, although often the endocardium covering the ventricular myocardium has a typical 'thrush's breast' appearance.

Histologically, small fat globules can be demonstrated in the cytoplasm, and sometimes the whole fibre appears to be filled with numerous droplets of varying size. According to Freidberg and

Horn (1939) focal myocardial necrosis may be prominent in young persons who die of severe anaemia following gastro-intestinal haemorrhage. The muscle fibres between affected fibres may be normal in appearance but in severe anaemia practically every fibre is involved. The factors which may produce lesions are diminished oxygen supply to the heart, and possibly cardiac overwork. While it is certain that anoxia is an important factor, the significance of overwork is uncertain. Anaemia rarely causes congestive cardiac failure and it is doubtful if it is ever the sole cause of fatal heart disease. It may, however, be an important contributory cause.

The work of Dible and associates (Dible, 1934; Dible and Gerrard, 1938) has shown that the fat is mainly ordinary transport fat which has been brought to the cardiac cells from a storage depot and has not been metabolized correctly. The significance of this fatty degeneration is difficult to evaluate. It occurs so frequently, in association with other factors, that the actual part played by the fatty degeneration cannot be elucidated. In most cases it probably represents a mild degree of damage to the cells from which recovery is possible.

In patients with pre-existing heart disease, the development of anaemia may precipitate myocardial failure, whereas treatment of anaemia may alleviate the failure. Kinney and Mallory (1945) reported cases in which acute anaemia following haemorrhage from peptic ulcers induced congestive heart failure and myocardial infarction. Angina pectoris has also been precipitated by anaemia.

References

Dible, J. A. (1934). 'Is fatty degeneration of heart muscle a phanerosis?' *J. Path. Bact.* **39**, 197
— and Gerrard, W. W. (1938). 'Source of fat in experimentally produced fatty degeneration of the heart.' *J. Path. Bact.* **46**, 77
Freidberg, C. K. and Horn, H. (1939). 'Acute myocardial infarction not due to coronary arteries.' *J. Am. med. Ass.* **112**, 1675
Kinney, T. D. and Mallory, G. K. (1945). 'Cardiac failure associated with acute anemia.' *New Engl. J. Med.* **232**, 215
Norman, T. D. and McBroom, R. D. (1958). 'Cardiac hypertrophy in rats with phenylhydrazine anaemia.' *Circulation Res.* **6**, 765
Paplanus, S. H., Zbar, M. J. and Hays, J. W. (1958). 'Cardiac hypertrophy as a manifestation of chronic anemia.' *Am. J. Path.* **34**, 149
Sanghvi, L. M., Misra, S. N. and Banerjee, K. (1960). 'Cardiac enlargement in chronic severe anaemia.' *Circulation* **22**, 412

SICKLE-CELL ANAEMIA

About 70 per cent of patients with sickle-cell anaemia show electrocardiogram abnormalities, although about 50 per cent of the patients with clinical heart disease have normal electrocardiograms (Uzsoy, 1964).

Sickling has long been recognized as a severe and frequently lethal genetic variant, but heterozygous sickel-cell states have usually been considered benign or even protective.

Radiology of the chest reveals definite cardiomegaly in 80 per cent of patients and 70 per cent of the patients have a globular-shaped heart.

The sudden death of a previously asymptomatic young Negro, heterozygous for sickle haemaglobin, was first reported by Brugge and Diggs (1951). Since then, several other reports of morbidity and mortality in the sickle-cell trait have been reported (Smith and Conley, 1955; McCormick, 1961; Diggs, 1965). Oliviera and Gomez-Patino (1963) first reported a case of fatal thrombus formation in a 29 year old Negro, who presented with symptoms which closely resembled rheumatic fever. He had cardiac enlargement and the electrocardiogram demonstrated diffuse progressive myocardial changes, but anaemia was never present. At autopsy, the coronary arteries were filled with sickle cells and there was extensive fibrosis with an interstitial infiltrate of macrophages and lymphocytes. Since this date, two further papers by Fleischer and Rubler (1968) and Rubler and Fleischer (1967) have been published and the cardiac pathology of these diseases is now fairly well demonstrated.

Clinical History

The patients are usually relatively young. Negroes and Africans can often be shown to have a sickling trait; they are found to have cardiac enlargement and later develop congestive heart failure. Later the patients most commonly die from pulmonary infarction. The patients have been previously in good health without a history of symptoms associated with sickle-cell disease and never manifest any symptoms of anaemia.

The relationship between sickle-cell anaemia and rheumatic fever was first reported by Plachta and Speer (1952). These diseases have much in common, including tachycardia, heart enlargement, abnormalities in AV conduction, anaemia and a positive C-reactive protein test.

Pertinent Autopsy Findings

At autopsy the heart is often enlarged up to 500 or 600 g although it may be much smaller than is normally found, even down to a weight of 120 g. Sometimes this is very marked. One of the patients in Rubler and Fleischer's series had a heart weighing 800 g.

Most of the cardiac enlargement is due to biventricular hypertrophy and dilatation. Definite dilatation of both ventricles is found in about 50 per cent of cases, but sometimes the dilatation is related to only one ventricle. The myocardium is usually seen to be pale and flabby. The endocardium and valves are normal in the majority of cases, but in some of the other cases the appearance of the endocardium is suggestive of endocarditis. There is usually a considerable amount of endocardial thickening extending up to the level of the atrioventricular valve leaflets from the apex of the ventricles. Large ante-mortem thrombi are very commonly seen in the heart, particularly in the dilated atria. The lungs are congested and the pulmonary arteries contain old and recent thrombi.

Microscopic examination of the heart demonstrated hypertrophied muscle fibres in the ventricles (*Figure 14.11*), especially in those involving papillary muscles. There is usually basophilic degeneration and vacuolization of the cytoplasm (*Figure 14.12*) with sometimes calcific deposits in some of the areas of hypertrophy, as well as extensive interstitial fibrosis and fragmentation of muscle fibres (*Figure 14.13*). Some of the myofibrils also show loss of striations (*Figure 14.14*). There is also a considerable amount of endocardial fibrosis and interstitial fibrosis between the muscle fibres (*Figure 14.15*); and some of the intracardiac arterioles and capillaries are seen to be occluded with sickle-shaped erythrocytes.

The patients may be found to have other signs of sickle-cell anaemia such as splenic infarcts, occlusion of arterioles in the finger tips or pulmonary infarcts. The coronary arteries are widely patent and not obstructed by thrombi or other occlusive processes.

Lisker *et al.* (1965) reported the case of a 14 year old Negro girl with sickle-cell-C anaemia who developed acute rheumatic fever. She died in hospital on day 48, following two days of severe haematemesis. At necropsy the heart weighed 430 g, there were nodules on the valves and Aschoff nodes in the myocardium. The capillaries of all organs showed sickle cells. The authors found seven cases reported in the literature, but theirs was the only one with haemaglobin-C disease.

Cardiomyopathy and Pulmonary Infarction

It is well known that patients with cardiomyopathy have an increased incidence of pulmonary infarction due to emboli arising from endocardial mural thrombi, but the marked association of these two conditions is most frequently observed in Negro populations where a strong sickle-cell trait is also seen. Indeed Moser and Shea (1957) and McCormick (1951) have stated that a relationship

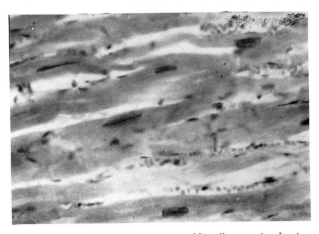

Figure 14.11. The myocardium in sickle-cell anaemia showing hypertrophy and squaring of nuclei (haematoxylin and eosin × 640, reduced to 3/4). (Fleischer and Rubler, 1968)

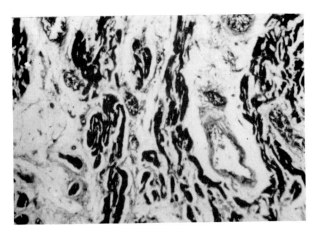

Figure 14.12. The myocardium showing interstitial fibrosis, smudging, loss of striations and vacuolization of the myofibrils and clumped sickle cells within the arterioles and capillaries (Masson's trichrome strain × 120, reduced to 6/10). (Fleischer and Rubler, 1968)

METABOLIC DISEASES 377

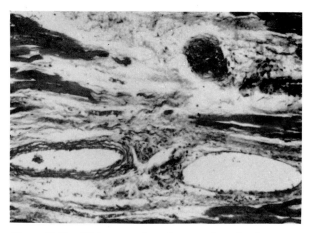

Figure 14.13. High-power view of myocardium showing extensive interstitial fibrosis, fragmentation of the myofibrils and small vessels filled with clumped red cells (Masson's trichrome stain × 320, reduced to 3/4). (Rubler and Fleischer, 1967)

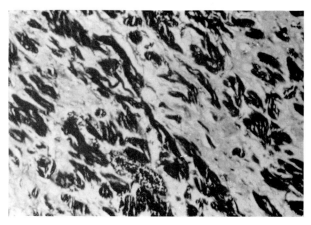

Figure 14.14. The myocardium showing interstitial fibrosis and loss of myofibrillar striations (Massons' trichrome stain × 120, reduced to 3/4). (Fleischer and Rubler, 1968)

exists between cor pulmonale (secondary to pulmonary artery thrombosis) and the presence of sickle-cell states, that is in persons where the erythrocytes contained large amounts of haemaglobin-S. Pulmonary thrombi were also likely to develop in conditions of low oxygen pressure such as would be present in these patients who have congestive heart failure.

The majority of these patients also have a history of acute or chronic alcoholism and this may be an associated cause of venous

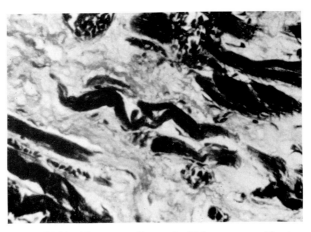

Figure 14.15. The myocardium under high-power magnification showing interstitial fibrosis and loss of myofibrillar striations (Masson's trichrone stain × 320, reduced to 3/4). (Fleischer and Rubler, 1968)

thrombosis, as alcohol is known to lower blood pH, and also to cause distinct haemodynamic alterations and disturbances of myocardial metabolism (Wendt *et al.*, 1966). It is also thought that alcohol may have an effect on the production of this congestive cardiomyopathy but the mechanism is not known at present.

References

Brugge, C. and Diggs, L. W. (1961). 'Unexpected death associated with the sickle cell trait.' A paper presented to the American Society of Clinical Pathology in Chicago, October 1951. Unpublished.

Diggs, L. W. (1965). 'Sickle cell crises.' *Am. J. clin. Path.* **44**, 1

Fleischer, R. A. and Rubler, S. (1968). 'Primary cardiopathy in non-anaemic patients. Association with sickle cell trait.' *Am. J. Cardiol.* **22**, 532

Lisker, S. A., Finkelstein, D., Schwartz, S., Marucyali, K. and Valdes-Dapena, A. (1965). 'The co-existence of acute rheumatic fever and sickle cell haemaglobin C disease.' *Circulation* **31**, 108

McCormick, W. F. (1961). 'Abnormal haemaglobins. II. Pathology of the sickle cell trait.' *Am. J. med. Sci.* **241**, 329

Moser, K. M. and Shea, J. G. (1957). 'The relationship between pulmonary infarction cor pulmonale and the sickle states.' *Am. J. Med.* **22**, 561

Oliviera, E. and Gomez-Patino, N. G. (1963). 'Falcemic cardiopathy. Report of a case.' *Am. J. Cardiol.* **11**, 686

Plachta, A. and Speer, F. D. (1952). 'The co-existence of rheumatic heart disease and sickle cell anemia.' *Am. J. clin. Path.* **22**, 970

Rubler, S. and Fleischer, R. A. (1967). 'Sickle cell states and cardiomyopathy—sudden death due to pulmonary thrombosis and infarction.' *Am. J. Cardiol.* **19**, 867

Smith, E. W. and Conley, C. L. (1955). 'Sickleimia and infarction of the spleen during aerial flight; electrophoresis of haemoglobin in 15 cases.' *Bull. Johns Hopkins Hosp.* **91**, 35

Uzsoy, N. K. (1964). 'Cardiovascular findings in patients with sickle cell anaemia.' *Am. J. Cardiol.* **13**, 320

Wendt, V. E., Ajluni, R., Bruce, T. A., Prasad, A. S. and Bing, R. J. (1966). 'The acute effects of alcohol on the human myocardium.' *Am. J. Cardiol.* **17**, 804

POLYCYTHAEMIA

In both primary and secondary polycythaemia, the incidence of thrombosis and consequent embolic episodes is greatly increased because of the increased viscosity and volume of blood in circulation. Although it has been thought that these changes impose a burden on the heart, leading to hypertension and cardiac failure, White (1951) stated that peripheral vasodilatation largely prevents such an additional cardiac burden. However, in the secondary polycythaemia associated with Fallot's tetralogy these thrombo-embolic episodes may lead to obstruction of small pulmonary blood vessels with consequential right-sided heart failure and hypertrophy.

A pericardial effusion may also be found in association with polycythaemia (Connolly *et al.*, 1959).

Although either or both of the above factors may clinically simulate a cardiomyopathy, no histological evidence of any specific myocardial changes have been found at autopsy in polycythaemia.

References

Connolly, D. C., Dry, T. J., Good, A. C., Clagett, O. T. and Burchell, H. B. (1959). 'Chronic idiopathic pericardial effusion without tamponade.' *Circulation* **20**, 1095

White, P. D. (1951). *Heart Diseases.* 4th Edition, p. 1015. New York: Macmillan

HAEMOLYTIC DISEASE OF THE NEWBORN

Pericardial effusion and an increase in heart weight are the two most frequent cardiac manifestations of haemolytic disease of the newborn. Recognizing that heart failure is a prominent clinical feature among infants with fatal haemolytic disease, Hogg (1962) studied the cardiac findings in 40 such infants, in about half of whom he found an increase in heart weight in relation to heel-to-crown length; in most instances dilatation of the chambers, frequently epicardial haemopoietic foci and intravascular nucleated red cells.

Manifestations of ischaemia and anoxia included enlargement of the myocardial nuclei and small foci of infarct-like necrosis. The latter was confined to the inner portion of the myocardium and the papillary muscles of either ventricle. Although no abnormalities of origin or course of the coronary arteries were detected, it has been suggested that arterial insufficiency may result from the dilatation of the heart with consequent overstretching of the intrinsic arteries and interference with blood flow. Varying degrees of microscopic endocardial fibro-elastosis may be present, in which anoxia and dilatation are the most obvious factors in its otherwise uncertain pathogenesis.

Reference

Hogg, G. R. (1962). 'Cardiac lesions in hemolytic disease of the newborn.' *J. Pediat.* **60**, 352

BERIBERI SYNDROME

Beriberi is intimately associated with a single essential vitamin, thiamine (vitamin B_1). It is widespread in the orient and was prevalent in Japanese prisoner-of-war camps. The important role of thiamine deficiency has been firmly established but the exact mechanism has not been elucidated (Bhuvaneswaran and Sreenivasan, 1962; Hicks *et al.*, 1962). Thiamine is essential for the metabolism of carbohydrates and the combination of a low thiamine intake with a high carbohydrate diet is the most common cause of thiamine deficiency syndromes, some of which are associated with cardiac failure. Other factors such as interference with absorption or utilization may be of some importance. The milled rice diets combined with the cooking habits and extreme poverty of large sections of the population in the orient are the principal factors. I agree with Follis (1958a) that undue emphasis has been placed on thiamine deficiency in the pathogenesis of this disease, which is actually a multi-factorial deficiency syndrome.

Clinical

The beriberi syndrome can be divided into three main types, all of which may present as an admixture: (1) the typical dry form; (2) the cardiac form; and (3) the wet or oedematous type.

(1) The classical or dry form is encountered as a primary disorder of the nervous system.

(2) The acute or cardiac form is characterized by sudden onset and often overwhelming heart failure which may be fatal within a few hours of onset or, relentlessly progressive, giving rise to the classic signs of congestive heart failure.

(3) Excessive anasarca characterizes the wet type of the beriberi heart syndrome and may be caused in part by cardiac failure and in part by hypoproteinaemia.

Heart failure is a cardinal manifestation of the beriberi syndrome. The cardiovascular manifestations are believed to result from peripheral vasodilatation with increased venous return and minute output; heart failure may be due to increased workload on a myocardium suffering from the biochemical lesions of thiamine deficiency (Hackel, Goodale and Kleinerman, 1953).

Evidence of beriberi heart disease includes palpitations, dyspnoea, dependent oedema and signs of increased enlargement of the heart. Failure of the right ventricle is accompanied by hepatomegaly, progressive ascites, hydrothorax and hydroperitoneum.

Blakenhorn (1945) has established the following diagnostic criteria for beriberi heart disease.

(1) An enlarged heart with sinoatrial rhythm.

(2) Dependent oedema.

(3) Elevated venous pressure.

(4) Peripheral neuritis.

(5) Non-specific changes in the electrocardiogram.

(6) Lack of other recognized causes of heart failure.

(7) Grossly-deficient diet for at least three months duration.

(8) Clinical improvement after treatment, i.e., administration of thiamine.

Occidental beriberi heart disease, popularized by Weiss (1940) is found almost exclusively amongst alcoholics. As this disorder responds very poorly to thiamine administration, it is probably in fact alcoholic cardiomyopathy (*see* Chapter 15).

Beriberi in infants often runs an acute course. The acute form of infantile beriberi is a striking condition (Ramalingaswami, 1958). The period from the first to the fourth month is the most dangerous one. The baby, apparently in good health and entirely nursed by the mother, is abruptly seized with a cry, the body shudders, the pulse becomes thready and the face cyanotic. The state may last from half an hour to one hour and may disappear spontaneously only to reappear with increasing frequency and severity: death usually occurs in one of these attacks.

The disease may affect infants or adults and in the former sudden death is a common occurrence. Disturbances of cardiac rhythm and congestive cardiac failure may occur in adults.

An injection of vitamin B_1 produces a dramatic response in a matter of a few hours as if a biochemical lesion has been reversed.

PATHOLOGICAL CHANGES

The changes described in the heart are non-specific and variable. There is a complete lack of any consistent 'pathognomonic' lesion in the heart in the beriberi syndrome. Early observers recorded inflammatory foci, scarring, hydropic degeneration and a host of additional non-specific histological changes. Grossly, the heart has been described as globose. Both ventricles are markedly dilated but paradoxically the right ventricle (the wall of which may measure as much as 7 mm in thickness) is most affected. In adults, the heart often weighs 500–600 g.

Microscopically, the myocardial fibres are usually markedly separated by oedema fluid. A central zone of basophilic hyaline degeneration is often seen in some myocardial fibres. There are often several areas of fibrous tissue proliferation in the myocardium. This fibrosis is usually found to be most marked around the small intra-myocardial blood vessels and also in many of the papillary muscles.

Besides oedema of the interstitial connective tissue and hydropic degeneration, slight scarring occurs, particularly in the subendo-cardial muscle fibres, and in the conduction tissue. Although there is an increase in the intercellular tissue, there is no alteration in the water content of the heart.

Clear-cut necrosis of muscle fibres, although reported in early descriptions, are not often seen and virtually no inflammatory re-actions are present (Follis, 1958b).

In infantile beriberi, the absence of morphological changes in the heart has been stressed (Fehily, 1944; Reid, 1961).

Since myocardial involvement in beriberi heart disease may reach a stage of advanced fibrosis, it is obvious that under these circumstances the condition has reached an irreversible stage and it is only possible to reverse the initial process of interstitial myocardial oedema.

Sometimes, advanced cases of beriberi may present as cases of ischaemic heart disease. Schlesinger and Benchimol (1951) described two patients who presented with congestive heart failure and a history of ischaemic chest pain. Both these patients also had electro-cardiograms typical of ischaemic heart disease and one had a conduction defect. These changes are almost certainly due to the severe degree of myocardial fibrosis found in advanced beriberi.

Similar cases of subendocardial fibrosis of indetermined origin have been reported as occurring in other vitamin-deficient patients (Dock, 1940). According to Smith and Furth (1943) these cases probably correspond to beriberi heart disease, since it is their belief that fibrosis may result not only from chronic myocardial ischaemia but also from a dietary deficiency.

In animals diffuse and focal necrosis of the myocardium has been produced in thiamine-deficient animals (Follis et al., 1943). It should also be mentioned that transient bundle branch block has also been seen in thiamine-deficient animals (Hundley, Ashburn and Sebrell, 1945).

References

Bhuvaneswaran, C. and Sreenivasan, A. (1962). 'Problems of thiamine deficiency states and their amelioration.' *Ann. N.Y. Acad. Sci.* **98**, 576

Blakenhorn, M. A. (1945). 'The diagnosis of beri-beri heart disease.' *Ann. intern. Med.* **23**, 398

Dock, W. (1940). 'Marked cardiac hypertrophy and mural thrombosis in the ventricles in beri-beri heart.' *Trans. Ass. Am. Physns* **55**, 61

Fehily, L. (1944). 'Human milk intoxication due to B, avitaminosis.' *Br. med. J.* **2**, 590

Follis, R. H., Jnr (1958a). *Deficiency Diseases.* Springfield, Ill: Thomas

— (1958b). 'The pathology of endemic beri-beri.' *Fedn. Proc.* **17**, Suppl. 2

— Miller, M. H., Wintrobe, M. M. and Stein, H. J. (1943). 'Development of myocardial necrosis and absence of nerve degeneration in thiamine deficiency in pigs.' *Am. J. Path.* **19**, 341

Hackel, D. B., Goodale, W. T. and Kleinerman, J. (1953). 'Effects of thiamin deficiency on myocardial metabolism in intact dogs.' *Am. Heart J.* **46**, 883

Hicks, C. S., Andrew, G. G., Willimot, S. G., Aitken, W. and Foley, D. P. (1962). 'Nutrition and beri-beri in a Japanese prisoner-of-war camp: a study of 500 daily food intakes in 35 months.' *Wld Rev. Nutr. Diet* **3**, 217

Hundley, J. H., Ashburn, L. L. and Sebrell, W. H. (1945). 'The electrocardiogram in chronic thiamine deficiency in rats.' *Am. J. Physiol.* **144**, 404

Ramalingaswami, V. (1958). 'Nutritional disease.' *Fedn Proc.* **17**, Suppl. 2, 43

Reid, D. H. S. (1961). 'Acute infantile beri-beri.' *J. Pediat.* **58**, 858

Schlesinger, P. and Benchimol, A. B. (1951). 'Cardiac beri-beri simulating arteriosclerotic heart disease.' *Am. Heart J.* **42**, 801

Smith, J. J. and Furth, J. (1943). 'Fibrosis of the endocardium and myocardium with mural thrombosis: notes on its relation to isolated

(Fiedler's) myocarditis and to beri-beri Heart.' *Archs intern. Med.* **71**, 602

Weiss, S. (1940). Occidental beri-beri with cardiovascular manifestations, its relation to thiamin deficiency.' *J. Am. med. Ass.* **115**, 832

CARCINOID HEART DISEASE

The association of endocardial fibrosis, valvular lesions and carcinoid tumours was first noticed by Rosenbaum, Santer and Claudon in 1953 and has since achieved considerable importance.

CARCINOID TUMOURS

MACROSCOPIC APPEARANCES

A carcinoid tumour arises from the enterochromaffin cells of Kulchitsky in the base of the crypts of Lieberkühn. These tumours are called carcinoids because of the fact that in their most common site in the appendix, they are usually benign, in spite of an appearance of infiltration. They are also sometimes found at routine necropsy or at surgery. Dische (1966) found that 19 (1·3 per cent) of 1426 appendices sliced longitudinally had an apical carcinoid, 10 of which were non-argentaffin. These tumours also occur occasionally in the stomach, frequently in the ileum and rarely in the rectum and other sites (Table 14.1). They are usually found in the appendix when

TABLE 14.1

Characteristics of Carcinoid Tumours derived from Different Embryonic Divisions of the Gut (Sandler, 1968)

	Foregut	*Midgut*	*Hindgut*
Argentaffin diazo reactions	Usually negative	Positive	Often negative
Associations with the carcinoid syndrome	Frequent	Frequent	None
Tumour 5-HT content	Low	High	Not detected
Urinary 5-HIAA	High	High	Normal
5-HTP secretion	Frequent	Rare	Not detected
Metastases to bone (usually osteoblastic and skin)	Common	Unusual	Common

present at the tip as a small yellowish brown nodule a few millimetres in diameter or even filling the distal lumen. In the small intestine, especially in the lower ileum, carcinoids are commonly multiple, forming small button-like swellings in the mucosa, one or more of which may show deep penetration of the muscular wall which may be greatly hypertrophied locally; lymphathic obstruction is often widespread in the affected segment.

Ileal carcinoids are never benign like the majority of those found in the appendix. In consequence, both intestinal obstruction and metastases to mesenteric lymph nodes and liver occur; characteristically these secondary deposits may grow exceedingly slowly.

MICROSCOPICAL APPEARANCES

A carcinoid tumour consists of small clear cells closely packed in alveolar formation throughout the whole thickness of the appendicular or ileal wall. The yellowish colour is due to the presence of lipids, some of which are doubly refractile.

The tumour cells contain granules which reduce silver salts— hence the name argentaffin cells. In the appendix carcinoid tumours are commonly related to old inflammatory lesions.

THE CARCINOID SYNDROME

Patients suffering from massive hepatic secondary growths of carcinoid tumours occasionally, but not invariably, exhibit a striking clinical syndrome of flushing, diarrhoea and sometimes pulmonary stenosis.

Massive secondary deposits are usually associated with the circulation of large amounts of 5-hydroxytryptamine (5-HT, serotonin) secreted by the tumour cells. It is not known why the syndrome is so inconsistent in its occurrence or if 5-HT is responsible for it.

Details of the various clinical signs associated with carcinoid tumour are given below.

CUTANEOUS FLUSHING

Cutaneous flushing may be spontaneous or may follow exercise, food, alcohol or manipulations of the tumour. This may possibly be due to the liberation of nor-adrenaline.

The colour ranges from bright red to violescent blue.

Rosacea may occur so that the margins of the eyelids show telangiectasia and the cornea small haemorrhages at the limbus (Starr and MacDonald, 1969). The precise mechanism of the flush is not known but it is not due solely to 5-HT. Oates, Pettinger and Doctor (1964) showed that the non-apeptide, bradykinin, is generated, the tumour containing a kinin-forming enzyme which acts on an α_2-globulin (kallidinogen) to produce lysyl bradykinin (kallidin) a decapeptide which is immediately degraded by a plasma esterase to form bradykinin (Oates, Pettinger and Doctor, 1960). Melmon, Lovenberg and Sjoerdsma (1965) demonstrated this reaction *in vitro*.

Cutaneous flushing may be absent in some cases of carcinoid heart disease.

CARDIAC LESIONS

Macroscopically the heart is usually of normal size or is only slightly enlarged. The *endocardium* on the right side often shows a diffuse grey-white thickening within both ventricle and atrium but more often thickening is patchy in distribution. This thickening may measure up to 2–3 cm in depth. The papillary muscles are markedly involved and the chordae are often almost obliterated, whilst pronounced shrinkage and perhaps fusion of some of them may also occur.

There may be complete loss of distinction between the cusps of the tricuspid valves and, sometimes, some degree of stenosis may be found. Both the base and free margins of the valves are often extensively thickened. The pulmonary valve is often severely stenotic with complete obliteration of the valve leaflets and with extensive fusion between them and a dense band of fibrous tissue may then form the pulmonary valve outlet. The pulmonary artery itself is not involved in this stenotic process.

The left atrium and ventricle sometimes show endocardial thickening the changes being similar to those described in the right side of the heart. Sometimes these changes are only seen on the left side of the heart as in the case reported by Goble *et al.* (1956).

The mitral valve may be involved, some thickening of the cusps along their borders and free margins being apparent but there is no fusing of the cusps or stenosis of the valves which are usually completely demarcated and the aortic valve is usually though not invariably normal.

Microscopic Examination

This endocardial thickening largely consists of collagenous and fibrotic tissue. It is relatively acellular but contains a few fibroblasts. Sometimes lymphocytes may be present in the endocardium and a few small dilated blood vessels may be present towards the junction of the endocardium and myocardium.

The junction between the thickened endocardium and myocardium is usually clearly differentiated. No strands of fibrous tissue pass down into the underlying myocardium but there is sometimes an increase in interstitial fibrosis (*Figure 14.16*).

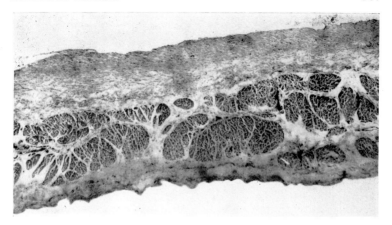

Figure 14.16. Left auricle in carcinoid heart disease showing considerable thickening of the endocardium by fibrous tissue while the underlying myocardium shows an increase in interstitial fibrosis (haematoxylin and eosin × 10, reduced to 2/3). (Reproduced by courtesy of Professor Hudson)

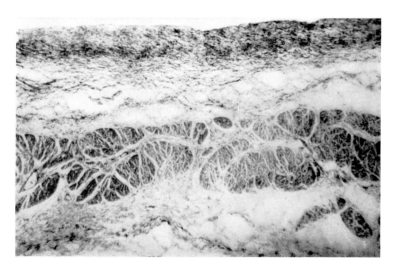

Figure 14.17. Carcinoid heart disease in the left auricle showing the thickened endocardium with an increase in elastic tissue fibres, the majority of which are situated towards the myocardium (van Gieson × 10, reduced to 2/3). (Reproduced by courtesy of Professor Hudson)

In some areas abundant myxoematous ground substance is present between the fibroblastic elements this particularly being seen in the pulmonary valve cusps. This material appears to be deposited on the atrial surface of the valves. Elastic tissue fibres are only few in number (*Figure 14.17*). Sometimes the surface of the endocardium is covered by small fibrin deposits which seem to be undergoing incorporation. They myxoematous substance is PAS, alcian blue positive for metachromasia. These reactions therefore imply the presence of a non-sulphated acid mucopolysaccharide. MacDonald and Robbins (1957) in their review state that most reports have not included details of vascular lesions in the carcinoid syndrome. They believe it is not possible to determine whether the valves on the left side of the heart may, in some instances, be markedly involved in the absence of a right to left shunt. They suggest that when both left- and right-sided heart valves are affected by carcinoid disease a careful histological study should be made to determine whether the left-sided involvement is due to previous rheumatic inflammation.

Mechanism for the Production of Endocardial Lesions

In Thorson and Nordenfelt's (1959) review, many hypotheses regarding the mechanism for the development of endocardial lesions in the carcinoid syndrome are discussed. Hedinger and Gloor (1954) first mentioned the possibility that the carcinoid tumour might liberate a substance stimulating connective tissue formation and Thorson et al. (1954) thought that 5-HT might in some way produce fibrosis; 5-HT might damage the endocardium and lead to reparative fibroblastic proliferation as was originally proposed by Waldenström and Ljungberg (1955). Goble, Hay and Sandler (1955) were impressed by the predominance of right-sided heart lesions and offered an explanation based on inactivation of a greater portion of circulating 5-HT during passage through the lungs, so that a lower concentration reached the left side of the heart.

Hedinger and Langemann (1955) postulated platelet deposition on the endocardial surface and Goble, Hay and Sandler (1955) expressed the opinion that the lesion was due to increased endocardial permeability and platelet deposition on the valve consequent to local 5-HT action. Thorsen and Nordenfelt (1959) have suggested that several mechanisms may participate in the production of the endocardial lesions, namely sudden dilatation of the endocardial structures in the right side of the heart, a local action of 5-HT to alter endothelial permeability or deposition of fibrin and platelets on the endothelial surface.

More recently, Bates and Clark (1963) have stated that the valvular lesions appear in several stages. Initially there is subendothelial oedema and damage to tissue from the direct action of circulating 5-HT on tissue mast cells; reactive fibrosis is a consequence with a subendocardial site of deposition. Fibrin is deposited upon the injured endocardium. These workers go on to postulate that the 'fibrin' is tanned, as a result of the interaction of 5-HT and ceruloplasmin in the process becoming resistant to fibrinolysis. The deposits of 'tanned fibrin' then enlarge by accretion and become organized and transformed to dense connective tissue.

Right-sided Carcinoid Heart Disease

The early reports of right-sided carcinoid heart disease seemed to indicate the great predominance of lesions involving the right side of the heart. More recently, however, reports would seem to indicate that perhaps mitral valvular involvement in the absence of a right to left shunt may not be as rare as originally supposed. Schrodt *et al.* (1960) and Jatlow and Rice (1964), for example, described left-sided lesions. Bates and Clark (1963) noted mitral valve involvement and suggested that the lesions of the mitral valve in their case represented the early phase of cardiac damage prior to fibrin accretion, and that the elastic tissue change in the endocardium of the right side of the heart was evidence of previous injury. These early changes were microscopic and consisted of two small metachromatic myxoematous areas in subendocardial locations. Roberts and Sjoerdsma (1964) found involvement of the left side of the heart in three of nine patients and in none of these was there an intracardiac communication. One patient who did have an intracardiac communication had no lesions on the left side. Fadell and Denham (1966) presented another case of carcinoid heart disease with lesions on both sides of the heart and no intracardiac communication. From these reports it seems that intracardiac communication is not important. Most observers believe that the direct action of 5-HT on the endocardium plays a leading role in the production of these valvular lesions. In all instances, however, the predominant involvement has been of the right side of the heart and this will be seen to indicate that factors other than local action of 5-HT are responsible.

Thorsen and Nordenfelt (1959) have observed striking haemodynamic changes during flushes with episodic increase of venous return and dilatation of the right side of the heart.

Oates *et al.* (1964) have suggested that the increased production of kinins associated with carcinoid disease may produce a high output state. These pharmacologically-active substances may also be active in altering endothelial permeability. Such an action could possibly play a role in the production of the heart lesions.

It has been stated that the cardiac lesions are due to the direct actions of 5-HT and so the reason that the right side of the heart is more commonly affected is due to the fact that 5-HT is broken down by enzymes while passing through the lungs.

The work of Vane (1957) in various experimental animals, particularly the dog, has shown that something over 95 per cent of free 5-HT is taken out of the circulation by the lungs.

Experimental Production of Cardiac Lesions

Animal experiments originally did not shed much light on the matter. Hamilton (1966) gave 0·2 ml of 1 per cent 5-HT creatinine sulphate intramuscularly twice daily to five 10 week old kittens for 28 days and produced no lesions. Spatz (1964) found it necessary to establish a triad of factors in experimental animals before it was possible to produce endocardial lesions resembling those seen in the carcinoid syndrome. The cardinal features of this triad are: (1) hyperserotoninaemia; (2) a relative tryptophan deficiency; and (3) a diminution of liver function produced by a hepatoxic agent.

It was concluded that tryptophan deficiency is an integral part of the total mechanism which results in endocardial fibroblastic proliferations. It also has an additional effect on the myocardium. The sensitivity of the myocardial lesions depend on the length of this deficiency state.

The 'protection effect' of 5-HT against myocardial injury in guinea-pigs on tryptophan deficient diets was striking (Spatz, 1969). The reason for tryptophan deficiency in patients with the carcinoid syndrome is due to the fact that a substantial percentage of dietary tryptophan is diverted into the serotonium pathway in patients with hyperserotoninaemia and then relative tryptophan or niacin deficiency may occur. The mechanism for the apparent increase in the incidence of pellagra which is sometimes seen in cases with the carcinoid syndrome is also easily explained by these results.

OTHER EVIDENCE OF CARDIOVASCULAR INVOLVEMENT

Hypotensive Crises

Hypotensive crises, which are very rare, may accompany attacks of flushing, diarrhoea, and/or bronchospasm; the fall of pressure may be gradual or rapid with fatal shock.

Congestive Heart Failure

Congestive heart failure occurs in patients with tricuspid regurgitation and/or pulmonary stenosis. Brauny oedema may occur early, producing stiff legs. The x-ray and electrocardiogram may give evidence of right heart enlargement; hypokalaemia may produce electrocardiogram changes. The cardiac output is probably unaltered.

The carcinoid syndrome has also been reported in association with widespread osteoblastic metastases of bronchial carcinoma. Flushing is severe, facial and periorbital oedema, with excessive lacrimation, anxiety, disorientation, explosive diarrhoea, and sudden death during an acute attack (Mengel, 1966).

Carcinoid heart disease with oat-cell bronchial carcinoma is rare: Monroe, Belter and Bates (1965) reported an example, and so did Bates (1967). A histological similarity between carcinoid tumours and oat-cell carcinoma was shown by Spencer and Corrin (1968) from an electron microscopic study. Kulchitsky-type cells with neurosecreting granules were found in both varieties of tumours. Similar granules were also found in normal bronchial epithelium. The authors, therefore, suggested that these tumours both arose from Kulchitsky cells.

Carcinoid Tumour of the Ovary

A case was reported by Bancroft, O'Brien and Tickner (1964) in a woman of 73 years of age who developed the carcinoid syndrome, starting with three years of abdominal pain and diarrhoea, then with flushing attacks, oedema, ascites and melaena (within final year). She died, and at necropsy the left ovary was found to contain 6 cm tumour, which was thought to be a carcinoid teratoma, containing a moderate amount of 5-HT (35 μg/g). The heart weighed 340 g and showed thickening of the endocardium of the right atrium and ventricle and of the tricuspid and pulmonary valves.

References

Bancroft, J. H. J., O'Brien, D. J. and Tickner, A. (1964). 'Carcinoid syndrome due to carcinoid tumour of the ovary.' *Br. med. J.* **2**, 1440

Bates, H. R., Jnr (1967). 'Oat cell carcinoma with quadrivalvular heart-disease.' *Lancet* **1**, 1111

— and Clark, R. F. (1963). 'Observations on the pathogenesis of carcinoid heart disease and the tanning of fluorescent fibrin by 5-hydroxytryptamine and ceruloplasmin.' *Am. J. clin. Path.* **39**, 46

Dische, F. E. (1966). 'Non-argentaffin carcinoid tumours of the appendix.' Communication to the 112th meeting (January 6–8) of the Pathological Society of Great Britain and Ireland. London: Pathological Society

Fadell, E. J. and Denham, R. M. (1966). 'Carcinoid heart disease with bilateral ventricular endocardial sclerosis.' *Am. J. Cardiol.* **17**, 259

Goble, A. J., Hay, D. R. and Sandler, M. (1955). 'Preliminary communication. 5-Hydroxytryptamine metabolism in acquired heart-disease associated with argentaffin carcinoma.' *Lancet* **2**, 1016

—— Hudson, R. and Sandler, M. (1956). 'Acquired heart disease with argentaffin carcinoma.' *Br. Heart J.* **18**, 544

Hamilton, J. M. (1966). 'The effect of serotonin on the pulmonary arteries of the cat.' *J. Path. Bact.* **91**, 249

Hedinger, C. and Gloor, R. (1954). 'Metastasiernende Dunndarmkarzinoide, Tricuspidalklappenveränderungen und pulmonal an Neues Syndrom.' *Schweiz. med. Wschr.* **84**, 942

— and Langemann, H. (1955). 'Ausgesprochene Thrombocytose bei Ratten unter Behandlung mit 5-Oxytryptamine experimenteller Beitrag zur Frage der endokrinen Aktivität der Karzinoide. *Schweiz med. Wschr.* **85**, 368

Jatlow, P. and Rice, J. (1964). 'Bronchial adenoma with hyperserotoninemia, biventricular valvular lesions and osteoblastic metastases.' *Am. J. clin. Path.* **42**, 285

MacDonald, R. A. and Robins, S. L. (1957). 'Pathology of the heart in the carcinoid syndrome, a comparative study.' *Archs Path.* **63**, 103

Melmon, K. L., Lovenberg, W. and Sjoerdsma, A. (1965). 'Characteristics of carcinoid tumour kallikrein: Identification of lysyl-bradykinin as a peptide it produces *in vitro*.' *Clinica chim. Acta* **12**, 292

Mengel, C. E. (1966). 'Carcinoid and the heart.' *Mod. Concepts. cardiovasc. Dis.* **35**, 75

Monroe, W. M., Belter, L. F. and Bates, H. R. (1965). 'Oat cell cancer of the lung—carcinoid heart disease.' *J. Am. med. Ass.* **192**, 1105

Oates, J. A., Pettinger, J. A. and Doctor, R. B. (1966). 'Evidence for the release of bradykinin in carcinoid syndrome.' *J. clin. Invest.* **45**, 173

— Melmon, K. L., Sjoerdsma, A., Gilespie, L. and Mason, D. T. (1964). 'Release of a kinin peptide in a carcinoid syndrome.' *Lancet* **1**, 514

Roberts, W. C. and Sjoerdsma, A. (1964). 'The cardiac disease associated with the carcinoid syndrome (carcinoid heart disease).' *Am. J. Med.* **36**, 5

Rosenbaum, F. F., Santer, D. G. and Claudon, D. B. (1953). 'Essential telongiectasia, pulmonic and tricuspid stenosis and neoplastic liver disease. A possible new clinical syndrome (Abstract).' *J. Lab. clin. Med.* **42**, 941

Sandler, M. (1968). 'The role of 5 hydroxyindoles in the carcinoid syndrome.' *Adv. Pharmacol.* **6**, 127

Schrodt, G. R., Dizon, F. Y., Peskoe, L. Y., Howell, R. S., Robie, C. H. and Stevenson, T. D. (1960). 'The effect of pyridoxine antagonists in the carcinoid syndrome.' *Am. Practnr. Dig. Treat.* **11**, 750

Spatz, M. (1964). 'Pathogenetic studies of experimentally induced heart lesions and their relation to the carcinoid syndrome.' *Lab. Invest.* **13**, 288

— (1969). 'Tryptophan metabolism and cardiac disease.' *Ann. N.Y. Acad. Sci.* **156**, 152

Spencer, H. and Corrin, B. (1968). 'Oat cell carcinoma of the lung; its origin and relationship to bronchial carcinoid tumours.' Communication to the 117th meeting (July 11–13) of the Pathological Society of Great Britain and Ireland. London: Pathological Society

Starr, P. A. J. and MacDonald, A. (1969). 'Oculocutaneous aspects of rosacea.' *Proc. R. Soc. Med.* **62**, 9

Thorsen, A. and Nordenfelt, O. (1959). 'Development of valvular lesions in metastatic carcinoid disease.' *Br. Heart J.* **21**, 243

— Bjorck, G., Bjorkman, G. and Waldenström, J. (1954). 'Malignant carcinoid of the small intestine with metastases to the liver, valvular disease of the right side of the heart (pulmonary stenosis and trycuspid regurgitation without septal defects), peripheral vasomotor symptoms, broncho-constriction and an unusual type of cyanosis.' *Am. Heart J.* **47**, 795

Vane, J. R. (1957). 'A sensitive method for the assay of 5-hydroxytryptamine.' *Br. J. Pharmacol.* **12**, 344

Waldenström, J. and Ljungberg, E. (1955). 'Studies on the functional circulatory influence from metastasizing carcinoid (argentaffine, enterochromaffine) tumours and their possible relation to enteramine production.' *Acta med. scand.* **152**, 293

CARDIAC CHANGES ASSOCIATED WITH INTRACRANIAL DISEASE

Over thirty years ago Aschenbrenner and Bodechtel (1938) reported electrocardiographic abnormalities in young patients with brain tumours. Despite electrocardiographic changes showing extensive myocardial infarction in association with cerebral disease, particularly cerebral haemorrhage, post-mortem examination commonly reveals normal coronary arteries. Sufficient myocardial necrosis to produce the electrical pattern of a transmural infarct is rare. Myocardial damage, however, occurs fairly frequently in humans with brain damage.

The extremely scattered distribution of small areas of focal necrosis of myocardial cells is more likely to produce the T wave changes of subendocardial ischaemia or infarction without the development of Q waves. Only Burch, De Pasquale and Malaret (1960); Eichbaum and Bissetti (1966); Hammermeister and Reichenbach (1969) and Connor (1969) have described any histological changes in the myocardium.

Eichbaum (1964) has also observed significant myocardial lesions in patients who incurred fatal injuries to the skull. The principal finding at autopsy was focal oedema of heart muscle with or without interstitial haemorrhage. Interfibrillar oedema is regarded by Eichbaum as the most serious form of focal myocardial oedema, because it is seen in patients who have died either immediately or very soon after injury. In instances of fatal injury, the interstitial oedema is accompanied by fragmentation of individual or large groups of muscle fibre structures (interfibrillar oedema). This oedematous interstitium was often said to contain numerous histiocytic cells, lymphocytes and isolated polymorphonuclear leucocytes. Apparently there was no site of predilection for the focal oedema.

Two pathological changes may be found in the myocardium, namely focal myocytolysis in some patients and fuchsinophilic degeneration in others.

MYOCYTOLYSIS

At autopsy about 8 per cent of patients dying from cerebral disease are found to have foci of myocytolysis in the myocardium (*Figure 14.18*). The most obvious abnormality is loss of sarcoplasm with retention of the sarcolemma, muscle nuclei and lipofuchsine. Polymorphs are rarely seen but histiocytes are present.

The sarcoplasm of the surrounding fibres may be vacuolated or shredded, but coagulative necrosis is not seen, the process is therefore basically different from infarction.

These lesions are usually small and affect only a few adjacent fibres. They may also not be found in every block of myocardium examined, and some blocks of myocardium only contain one small focus (*Figure 14.18*). These lesions are found most commonly in patients with spontaneous intracranial haemorrhage and in patients in their sixth or seventh decades. These lesions occur with equal frequency in men and women.

FUCHSINOPHILIC DEGENERATION

This term covers the lesser degrees of cardiac damage. Human cardiac tissue was first stained by Connor (1969), using the cresyl violet acid fuchsine technique of Bajusz (1963) to demonstrate myocardial damage in patients dying from intracerebral lesions, largely haemorrhages. Connor (1969) found that, of 92 patients dying with brain lesions, 20 showed significant degrees of fuchsinophilic damage.

The distribution of fuchsinophilia does not correspond to vascular territories; indeed it may sometimes end abruptly at an intercalated disc. This peculiar distribution of damage has also been found by others studying 'ischaemic' lesions in human hearts.

Intracranial haemorrhage is by far the most common cause of fuchsinophilic degeneration in the hearts of patients studied by Connor (1969).

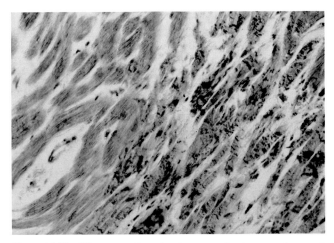

Figure 14.18. The myocardium showing severe focal myocytolysis with badly damaged fibres near the end of the foci (cresyl violet and fuchsine × 250, reduced to 8/10). (Reproduced by courtesy of Dr R. C. R. Connor)

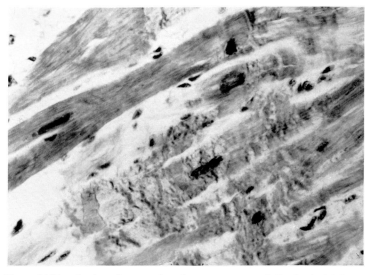

Figure 14.19. Section of myocardium from a woman aged 48 who died following the rupture of the cerebral aneurysm. Note the transverse bands of coagulated sarcoplasm and the denser appearance of the fuchsinophilia in part of the myocardium (cresyl violet and fuchsine × 400, reduced to 9/10). (Reproduced by courtesy of Dr R. C. R. Connor)

The age distribution is more even than in the cases of hearts found to show myocytolysis and there is no difference in sex distribution.

Microscopically, throughout the ventricle there are multiple foci of myocytolysis with loss of myocardial cells, collapse of the supporting stroma and a few surrounding mononuclear cells, frequently containing phagocytosed lipofuchsine pigment (*Figure 14.18*).

These extensive small foci of evolving cell necrosis do not follow a vascular distribution and are surrounded by myocardial cells of normal appearance, thus accounting for the inability of these lesions to be detected macroscopically.

It is likely that some of the myocardial damage seen in these patients is reversible, accounting in part for the previously reported normal pathological studies.

Lesser degrees of this type of change may be very subtle as fibrosis does not characteristically develop.

This diffuse myocardial necrosis, following no vascular pattern, is very similar to the focal myocardial necrosis of 'L-norepinephrine myocarditis' described by Szakăcs and associates (Szakăcs and Cannon, 1958; Szakăcs, Dimmette and Cowart, 1959; Szakăcs and Mehlman, 1960) (*Figure 14.19*).

It is postulated that acute intracranial disease stimulates sympathetic centres in the hypothalamus, which cause the release of catecholamines within the myocardium and/or systemically. These agents are presumably in sufficient concentration at the myocardial cellular level to cause damage to the contractile apparatus and to the cell membrane, thus accounting for the electrocardiographic changes.

Whether this represents focal ischaemia due to constriction of the myocardial microcirculation, or to a direct toxic effect of the catecholamines on the myocardial cells, is unknown.

Shkhvatsabaia and Men'shikov (1962) have shown that the catecholamine content is increased in the heart following cerebral stimulation and thus lends support to this being the aetiological mechanism.

In those cases of cerebral haemorrhage which do not exhibit hypertension or other findings of diffuse sympathetic discharge, the catecholamines' release may be localized to the myocardium.

A local increase of these substances may increase the metabolism of the sarcoplasm to a level at which the blood supply becomes insufficient.

The terminal effect may well be a failure of the mechanism by which a positive potassium-sodium balance is maintained in the cardiac muscle fibres (Bajusz, 1965).

References

Aschenbrenner, R. and Bodechtel, G. (1938). 'Über Ekg.-Veränderungen bei Hirntumorkranken.' *klin. Wschr.* **17**, 298

Bajusz, E. (1965). *Electrolytes and cardiovascular diseases: physiology, pathology, therapy.* Vol. 1 *Fundamental Aspects*, p. 274. Baltimore: Williams and Wilkins

Burch, G. E., De Pasquale, N. and Malaret, G. (1960). 'Selected problems in electrocardiography.' *Ann. intern. Med.* **52**, 587

Connor, R. C. R. (1969). 'Focal myocytolysis and fuchsinophilic degeneration of the myocardium of patients dying with various brain lesions.' *Ann. N.Y. Acad. Sci.* **156**, 261

Eichbaum, F. W. (1964). 'Myokardveränderungen nach Schädtraumen.' *Virchows Arch. path. Anat. Physiol.* **338**, 78

— and Bissetti, P. C. (1966). 'Cardiovascular disturbances following acute increase of intracranial pressure.' *Proceedings of the Fifth International Conference on Neuropathology*, pp. 1016–1020. Amsterdam: Excerptia Medica Foundation

Hammermeister, Karl E. and Reichenbach, D. D. (1969). 'QRS changes, pulmonary edema and myocardial necrosis associated with subarachnoid hemorrhage.' *Am. Heart J.* **78**, 94

Shkhvatsabaia, I. K. and Men'shikov, W. (1962). 'On the problem of the significance of catecholamines in the pathogenesis of neurogenic changes in the myocardium.' (Russian text.) *Kardiologia* **2**, 27

Szakăcs, J. E. and Cannon, A. (1958). 'L-Norepinephrine myocarditis' *Am. J. clin. Path.* **30**, 425

— and Mehlman, B. (1960). 'Pathologic changes induced by L-norepinephrine.' *Am. J. Cardiol.* **5**, 619

— Dimmette, R. M. and Cowart, E. C. (1959). 'Pathologic implication of the catecholamines, epinephrine and nor-epinephrine.' *U.S. arm. Forces med. J.* **10**, 908

Fifteen

Alcoholic cardiomyopathy

INTRODUCTION

Clinical experience indicates that alcoholism is often associated with heart disease. A relationship between chronic alcoholism and heart disease has been recognized since 1884 (Bollinger), but widespread interest in alcoholic heart disease did not develop until about 1930. In 1929 Aalsmeer and Wenckebach presented the first comprehensive description of beriberi heart disease, which was soon recognized in Europe and the USA where it was termed occidental beriberi (Weiss and Wilkins, 1936; Blankenhorn, 1945), and was found almost exclusively in chronic alcoholics. This explains why there was, and still is, a tendency for many doctors to have the impression that heart disease in many alcoholic cases is a form of beriberi.

The incidence of alcoholic heart disease is unknown, although it appears to be more common in adults with either thyrotoxic or congenital heart disease in the USA, although this does not appear to be so in England.

It appears that there are, however, three distinct mechanisms operative in the production of cardiomyopathies in alcoholic patients: (1) the toxic effect of alcohol on the myocardium; (2) general nutritional deficiencies and; (3) beriberi heart disease (thiamine deficiency). Many patients with heart disease and excessive intake of alcohol show predominant left-sided heart failure and high cardiac output. Toxic alcoholic cardiomyopathy may exist alone, but usually both nutritional factors and thiamine deficiency are associated with the toxic factor and, therefore, these cardiopathies have a multifactorial causation.

Within the last decade the opinion among many doctors, that alcoholic cardiomyopathy is a distinct entity, is shown by the fact that many people, who are heavy drinkers, develop congestive heart failure but do not respond to thiamine, whereas there are other heavy drinkers who show no sign of malnutrition and yet are similarly affected. Toxic cardiomyopathy is considered to be due to direct injury of the myocyte by alcohol. In addition it is now well established that metabolism of alcohol may lead to alterations in intermediary metabolism which in turn may result in pathological alterations (Lieber and Davidson, 1962). The administration of alcohol to patients (Wendt *et al.*, 1965) results in the loss of important Krebs cycle enzymes and electrolytes from the myocardium and, interferes with utilization of fatty acids for energy production and the accumulation of triglycerides (Regan *et al.*, 1964). The loss of these essential materials in the presence of a normal or increased cardiac output, and experimental evidence to suggest reduced coronary blood flow (Webb and Degerli, 1965), indicates that there is interference with the energy producing machinery of the heart.

These findings strongly suggest that oxidative phosphorylation via the Krebs cycle and fatty acid oxidation are seriously impaired in the patient with advanced alcoholic heart disease and explain the reduced myocardial contractility resulting in a heart which is massively enlarged. An intriguing concept is that beriberi is an early phase of alcoholic heart disease with high output failure and little or no cardiomegaly, ultimately progressing to massive cardiomegaly and low output failure, but it lacks the support of any experimental evidence. Excessive alcohol intake has been shown to produce a marked decrease in the myocardial uptake of free fatty acids, which is associated with an increase in the normally low uptake of triglycerides (Regan *et al.*, 1964).

Furthermore, excessive alcoholic intake may result in leakage of SGOT, phosphate, potassium and possibly magnesium from the myocardium. Myocardial hypertrophy with fibrosis has been recognized in chronic alcoholics, in whom no associated vitamin or nutritional deficiencies can be established (Eliaser and Giansiracusa, 1956). Excessive alcoholic intake has also been shown to produce myocardial degeneration in man (Alexander, 1966). Thus, there seems little doubt that alcohol may have a direct toxic effect on the myocardium.

It is often assumed that patients with alcoholic cardiomyopathy are malnourished, cachectic individuals with personalities of the 'skid-row' type. However, many patients with alcoholic cardiomyopathy are well-nourished, business and professional people who eat a perfectly normal balanced diet, but drink a considerable amount either for purely social reasons or in the course of their business when entertaining clients.

AETIOLOGY

It has been suggested by some workers (Burch and De Pasquale, 1969) that alcohol may have a direct toxic effect on the myocardium, but that poor nutrition and psychic factors may play a part in conditioning the myocardium to the toxic effects of alcohol. There are many patients suffering from alcoholic heart muscle disease for whom poor nutrition cannot be invoked as a cause of it. Recently, it has been suggested that some constituent of wine and beer, rather than the alcohol itself, may be responsible for this heart muscle disease.

Heavy alcoholic intake may be associated with skeletal as well as heart muscle disease. A syndrome consisting of muscle cramps, dark urine (myoglobinuria) and elevated serum creatine phosphokinase levels has been described in acute alcoholic intoxication (Perkoff et al., 1967). In addition blood lactic acid does not increase during ischaemic exercise. This fact that acute alcoholic intoxication may result in widespread injury to skeletal muscle suggests more strongly that alcohol itself is toxic and that other constituents of alcohol such as copper and iron play, at best, a secondary role in the production of this cardiomyopathy.

EXPERIMENTAL STUDIES

Burch et al. (1971a) have carried out a study to elucidate if alcohol directly damages the myocardium. These authors exposed 55 mice to long-term, unrestricted intake of alcohol in various forms, this being the only fluid the animals were allowed to drink. Ten additional mice, acting as controls, received water and no alcohol.

All mice were given access to a balanced diet of commercial laboratory food. The test animals were divided into four groups, each consuming various concentrations and volumes of alcoholic beverages. Group 1 was given beer (5 per cent alcohol); Group 2, 5 per cent ethyl alcohol; Group 3, 20 per cent ethyl alcohol and Group 4, a commercially available wine (20 per cent alcohol). The animals were killed after six months. The pathological changes were found in the hearts of all the animals drinking alcohol but not in any of the controls.

These changes were focal in distribution and consisted of focal areas of hydropic degeneration and loss of striations in some of the myocardial cells. Interstitial oedema with separation of myofibres, loss of cytoplasmic detail and shrunken, irregular nuclei indicated moderately advanced cellular damage. Occasionally areas of vacuolization within the muscle fibres, compatible with fatty degeneration, were observed.

More advanced stages of damage were indicated by areas of round-cell infiltration with fibroblast proliferation. These latter changes were usually confined to the myocardium, being most frequently seen in the subendocardial region.

In an earlier short-term study Burch *et al.* (1971b) maintained that mice drinking beer, wine and various concentrations of ethyl alcohol as their only liquid intake for 4–10 weeks had shown definite but only mild myocardial damage, both histologically and electron microscopically.

CLINICAL PRESENTATION

EARLY SIGNS

The patients may first present with atrial fibrillation or some other type of arrhythmia, such as a bundle branch block, but usually there will be no physical signs to be found.

SIGNS OF LATER STAGES

Alcoholic cardiomyopathy is more easily recognized in the later stages of the disease. The dominant complaints are palpitations, shortness of breath, orthophnoea and paroxysmal tachycardia. Although pain may not be present, it tends to be vague or not specific or pleuritic in type. Chest pain of anginal type does not occur. On physical examination the pulse pressure is small while the heart is diffusely enlarged. A booming apical systolic murmur is often present because of papillary muscle dysfunction secondary to left ventricular dilatations, or to electric and mechanical 'silence' of the papillary muscle due to extensive local disease. Peripheral oedema is present. Anasarca and scrotal oedema may also be found in patients with far advanced disease.

Chest radiogram demonstrates diffuse cardiac enlargement, pulmonary vein enlargement, prominent hilar blood vessels and blocking of both costophrenic angles due to pleural fluid accumulation. The heart is usually globular in configuration and often resembles the 'water-bottle' heart characteristic of pericardial effusions.

The electrocardiogram usually shows a low voltage pattern and various types of arrhythmias may be seen. Electrocardiographic changes, as evidenced by flattened or inverted T waves, may be produced in subjects with a known history of alcoholism by giving moderate quantities of alcohol (Wendt *et al.*, 1966). The administration of alcohol has also been shown to cause a rise in isocitric dehydrogenase and lactic dehydrogenase. These changes are non-specific when seen from a diagnostic viewpoint.

Although hepatomegaly may be present, clinical and laboratory evidence of hepatic failure is not usually seen. The mild liver failure, which is sometimes seen, is best explained on the basis of chronic congestive heart failure, since studies of liver function often show an improvement after the heart failure has responded to therapy. There is, at present, no explanation as to why patients with alcoholic heart disease rarely show liver failure. It is during the later stages of their disease that the patients appear malnourished and cachectic. In many patients the cachexia is due to chronic heart failure rather than to chronic alcoholism. This picture of a cachectic malnourished alcoholic patient, in congestive cardiac failure, represents a clinical stereotype for many doctors, who attribute all the findings to chronic alcoholism, malnutrition and vitamin deficiency.

In addition to chronic congestive heart failure, ventricular tachycardia, complete heart block and thrombo-embolism are often fatal complications of alcoholic cardiomyopathy.

MODE OF DEATH

Death usually occurs as a result of congestive heart failure although ventricular arrhythmias or complete heart block may play a part. During the later stages of the disease sensitivity to digitalis develops in many patients, possibly because of pulmonary hypertension which is secondary to the frequent occurrence of small pulmonary emboli or due to hypokalaemia secondary to prolonged diuretic therapy. Marked cardiac irritability, heart block, pulmonary and peripheral embolization may occur together with massive cardiac dilatation and sudden cardiac arrest which is characteristic of the later stages of the disease.

LABORATORY FINDINGS

The laboratory findings in alcoholic cardiomyopathy are non-specific. Liver function tests may show abnormal findings but improvement usually follows improvement to cardiac function. Hyponatraemia, hypokalaemia and hypomagnesaemia are often present in the later stages of the disease. The level of total body sodium is usually elevated, the hyponatraemia being dilatational in type. Hypokalaemia, when present, is usually due to diuretic therapy being used excessively.

PATHOLOGICAL FINDINGS

Gross examination of the heart with alcoholic cardiomyopathy usually demonstrates significant dilatation of all cardiac chambers. There is usually moderate hypertrophy of the left ventricle together with dilatation of the right ventricle and both atria. The principal structural alterations are small areas of fibrosis and cardiac enlargement, predominantly of the left ventricle. Two stages are recognized: (1) the stage where lesions are sparse; and (2) the stage when gross changes are present. The former, stage 1, may be associated with some enlargement owing to a compensatory hypertrophy of muscle fibres. Although the valves are normal, endocardial lesions consisting of patchy areas of fibro-elastic thickening, associated with overlying mural thrombi, usually in the septum and free left ventricular wall, may be present. The myocardium is pale and flabby and diffuse areas of fibrosis may often be seen on gross examination.

In stage 2 cardiac enlargement is marked and the fibrotic areas are large and often confluent.

In the mixed type of disease where there is also a degree of thiamine deficiency the added features of beriberi may make a precise diagnosis difficult. The coronary arteries are normal.

HISTOLOGICAL FINDINGS

Hypertrophied fibres are often present and may be seen adjacent to atrophic or degenerating muscle fibres. Various degrees of hyalinization and vacuolization of muscle fibres are present and cross striations may be lost in some areas. Some nuclei appear small and pyknotic, while others are large and blunt ended. Small areas of fibrosis are also present in the myocardium and are often accompanied by focal collections of inflammatory cells and interstitial oedema but this change is unusual. Elsewhere, there are areas of recent focal necrosis together with a mild cellular infiltrate. Often similar fibrotic lesions interrupt strands of conduction tissue. These small areas of muscle necrosis, with or without a slight cellular reaction, are present in all cases, even those of long standing, and therefore emphasizing that the toxic process is still continuing (Brigden and Robinson, 1964).

HISTOCHEMICAL STUDIES

Histochemical studies of the myocardium (Ferrans et al., 1965) demonstrate large amounts of neutral lipid material deposited within the myocardial fibres in the form of irregular droplets varying in diameter from 0·1 to 3·0 μm in size. Most of the lipid consists of triglycerides.

This neutral lipid is best demonstrated, at least in the early stages of the disease, by the use of fluorescent lipid stains such as phosphine-3R. Normal myocardium usually contains a few very small lipid

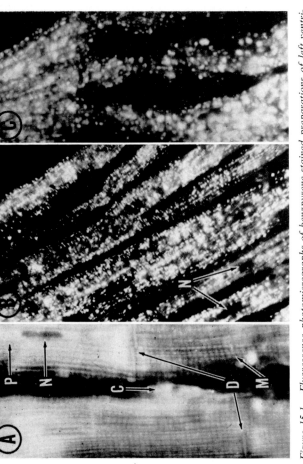

Figure 15.1. Fluorescence photomicrographs of benzpyrene-stained preparations of left ventricular myocardium. A. Normal human heart (× 1200). Showing a longitudinal section of myocardial fibres with the normal pattern of fluorescent lipid staining. Note the rows of mitochondria (M); the intercalated discs (D); the perinuclear area (P); and the unstained nucleus (N). An interstitial cell (C) is closely apposed to the adjacent myocardial fibre. B. Alcoholic cardiomyopathy (× 400) showing a moderately severe degree of neutral lipid deposition is illustrated. The outline of nuclei (N) is evident in several fibres. C. Alcoholic cardiomyopathy (× 800) showing an area similar to that of B. There is gross disorganization of the cytoplasm of the muscle fibres which are laden with numerous lipid droplets (reduced to 8/10 on reproduction) (Ferrans et al., 1965)

droplets (*Figure 15.1*) and also some small golden-brown lipofuchsine granules. In alcoholic cardiomyopathy these lipid deposits are much larger: in severe cases the lipid globules are so large that they completely obscure all other cytological detail (*Figure 15.1*). Sometimes the large hypertrophied fibres may only contain small lipid droplets while much larger ones are seen in normal-sized myocardial cells (*Figure 15.2*). It is important to remember that this lipid deposition is often very irregular, some cells being greatly involved while others are hardly affected.

Often these degenerative myocardial fibres, containing large quantities of lipid, are most commonly seen in the area of the myocardium immediately beneath the endocardium (*Figure 15.3*), especially in association with areas of endocardial thickening. It should also be noted that this excessive lipid deposition may only be found in parts of the conduction tissue, this involvement possibly accounting for the high incidence of arrhythmias and other conduction disturbances.

The concentration of lipofuchsine granules is increased. The lipofuchsine granules are acid-phosphatase positive and their relationship to myocardial lysosomes has been established by electron microscopy. The widespread and extensive mitochondrial degeneration in patients with alcoholic cardiomyopathy would be expected to be associated with defective myocardial oxidative activity and electron transport, and ultimately with defective energy production. Whereas the mitochondrial and enzymatic observations described are extensive it is unknown to what extent oxidative phosphorylation, high-energy phosphatase production and energy production are affected in alcoholic cardiomyopathy.

Studies of myocardial oxidative enzymes, show a decrease in cytochrome oxidase, succinic dehydrogenase, isocitric dehydrogenase, malic dehydrogenase, and DPN glycohydrolase activity (Ferrans *et al.*, 1965).

Methods used to demonstrate the presence of oxidative enzymes show that there is a marked reduction in the amount of succinic dehydrogenase present (*Figure 15.4*). That the alterations in the amount of oxidative enzyme found varies from case to case and in different parts of the myocardium is shown in *Figure 15.5*.

This diminution of enzyme activity is most markedly seen in degenerating or necrotic muscle fibres (*Figure 15.6*). In those parts of the connective tissue of the myocardium immediately below the endocardium, the enzymatic activity is often normal (*Figure 15.7*).

The plasmal reaction is usually decreased throughout all parts of the myocardium. The plasmal reaction is irregular in intensity in

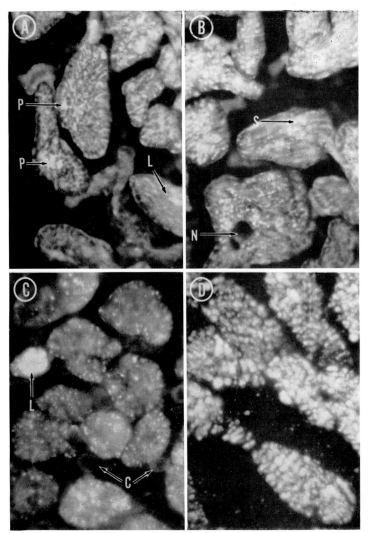

Figure 15.2. Fluorescence photomicrographs of left ventricular myocardium.
A. *Normal human myocardium showing a cross-section of fibres demonstrating the interfibrillary localization of lipid fluorescence. A few golden-brown lipofuchsine pigment granules (P) and very small lipid droplets (L) are visible.* B. *Alcoholic cardiomyopathy showing a moderate amount of lipid deposition is seen in the fibres at the top of the photograph. Streaks (S) of interfibrillary staining remain in the obliquely cut fibre in the centre. The large, hypertrophic fibre with the unstained nucleus (N) also contains many small lipid droplets.* C. *Alcoholic cardiomyopathy showing irregular lipid deposition. One fibre is heavily involved with lipid droplets (L). Capillaries (C) are seen in cross-section. There is loss of the normal interfibrillary fluorescence.* D. *Alcoholic cardiomyopathy showing the very severe degree of lipid deposition completely obscures all other cytological detail* (*benzpyrene × 1200, reduced to 9/10*) (*Ferrans* et al., *1965*)

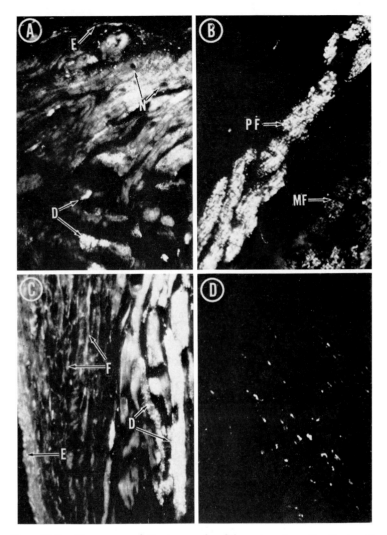

Figure 15.3. Fluorescence photomicrographs of the myocardium of patients with alcoholic cardiomyopathy. A. Alcoholic cardiomyopathy showing left atrial myocardium stained with benzpyrene (× 100). Degenerating myocardial fibres (D) with lipid droplets are scattered throughout an area immediately beneath the endocardium (E). Note the large, rounded nuclei (N). B. Alcoholic cardiomyopathy showing left ventricular subendocardium (benzpyrene × 600). Both Purkinje fibres (PF) and myocardial fibres (MF) are laden with lipid. C. Alcoholic cardiomyopathy showing an area of left ventricular endocardial thickening (benzpyrene × 200). Degenerating muscle fibres (D) with numerous lipid droplets are seen underlying the endocardium (E) and the layer of subendocardial collagenous and elastic fibres (F). D. Alcoholic cardiomyopathy showing unstained section of left ventricular myocardium (× 100) showing the autofluorescence of lipofuchsine in an area of fibrosis. Compare with C and D of Figure 15.5. (Ferrans et al., 1965)

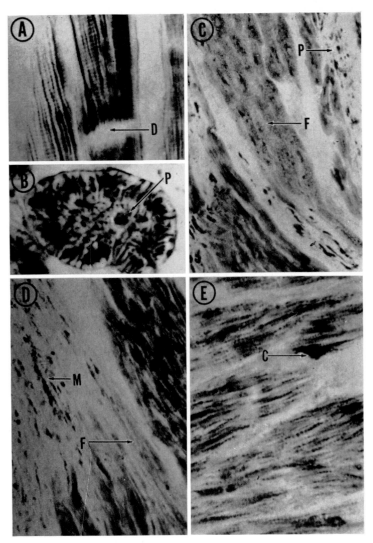

Figure 15.4. Histochemical reactions for oxidative enzymes in ventricular myo-cardium. A. Normal human heart (succinic dehydrogenase × 800) showing the reaction is localized to the mitochondria. Note the unstained intercalated disc (D). B. Same tissue as in A (lactic dehydrogenase × 1500). The interfibrillary staining is clearly demonstrated. A pigment granule (P) is seen near the centre of the fibre. C. Alcoholic cardiomyopathy (succinic dehydrogenase × 100) showing an area of necrosis and residual pigment (P), a zone of degenerating fibres (F), and relatively normal fibres (at the lower left corner) are illustrated. D. Alcoholic cardiomyopathy (succinic dehydrogenase × 100) showing fibres in various stages of degeneration (F) and pigment laden macrophages (M) are shown in an area similar to that of C. Compare with Figure 15.3, D, obtained from the same block of tissue. E. Alcoholic cardiomyopathy (succinic dehydrogenase × 800) showing marked reduction in the intensity of the reaction and areas of focal clumping of mitochondria (C) are present. Compare with the normal pattern seen in A (reduced to 9/10 on reproduction)
(Ferrans et al., 1965)

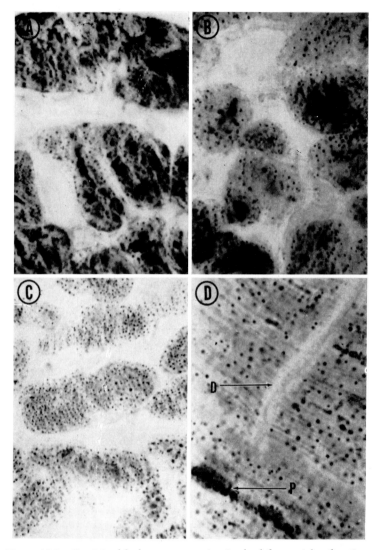

Figure 15.5. Succinic dehydrogenase reaction in the left ventricle of patients with alcoholic cardiomyopathy. A. Alcoholic cardiomyopathy (× 800) showing that there is moderate to marked reduction in the intensity of the staining reaction of the muscle fibres. C. Alcoholic cardiomyopathy (× 600) showing a pronounced decrease in the enzymatic reaction is evident. D. Alcoholic cardiomyopathy (× 1500) section showing the irregular arrangement of the formazan deposits. The intercalated disc (D) and the lipofuchsine granules (P) are unstained. Compare with the normal pattern of Figure 15.4, A (reduced to 9/10 on reproduction) (Ferrans et al., 1965)

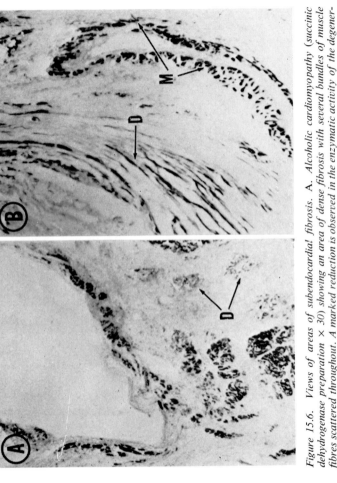

Figure 15.6. Views of areas of subendocardial fibrosis. A. Alcoholic cardiomyopathy (succinic dehydrogenase preparation × 30) showing an area of dense fibrosis with several bundles of muscle fibres scattered throughout. A marked reduction is observed in the enzymatic activity of the degenerating muscle fibres (D). B. Alcoholic cardiomyopathy (lactic dehydrogenase preparation × 30) showing a section through an area of subendocardial fibrosis with sparing (as in A) of the thin layer of muscle fibres (M) immediately beneath the endocardium. Note the degenerating muscle fibres (D) deeper to the zone of fibrosis (Ferrans et al., 1965)

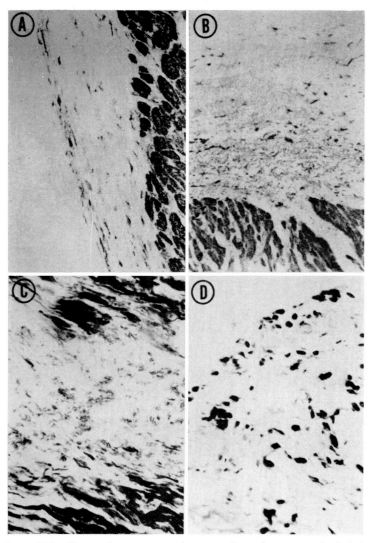

Figure 15.7. Enzymatic reactions in the myocardium of patients with alcoholic cardiomyopathy. A. Alcoholic cardiomyopathy, left ventricular myocardium (lactic dehydrogenase × 100), showing the positive reaction of the connective tissue cells in the subendocardium. B. Alcoholic cardiomyopathy, left atrial endocardium (malic dehydrogenase × 60) showing a positive reaction given by the myocardial fibres and the connective cells in the thickened endocardium. C. Alcoholic cardio-myopathy, left ventricular myocardium (lactic dehydrogenase × 100) showing a section through an area of necrosis shows disruption of the fibres and marked decrease in enzymatic activity. D. Alcoholic cardiomyopathy, left ventricular myocardium (× 300) stained for α-naphthyl acetate esterase activity. A strongly positive reaction is noted in the inflammatory cells present in a zone of fibrosis (reduced to 9/10 on reproduction) (Ferrans et al., 1965)

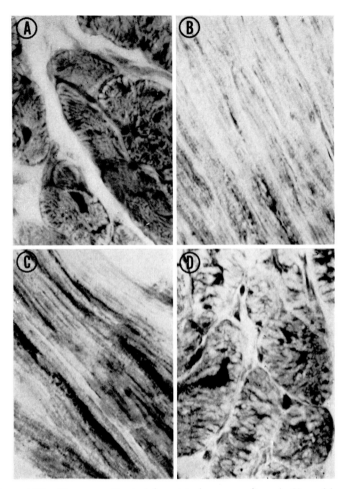

Figure 15.8.   Plasma reaction in left ventricular myocardium. A. Normal human heart (× 800) showing the interfibrillary distribution of the reaction. Compare with Figures 15.2A and 15.5B. B. Alcoholic cardiomyopathy (× 400) showing a marked decrease in the intensity of the staining reaction which is evident on comparison with the normal. C. Alcoholic cardiomyopathy (× 1200) showing the markedly increased reaction in the perinuclear areas and irregularly decreased elsewhere. D. Alcoholic cardiomyopathy (× 1200) showing an area similar to that of C, a decrease in the reaction at the top of the photograph, and an area of increased perinuclear reaction on the left (Ferrans et al., 1965)

various parts of the myocardium, although usually markedly diminished when compared with normal cardiac muscle. It is, however, markedly increased in perinuclear areas (*Figure 15.8*).

The widespread structural changes observed in histochemical studies of the myocardium are in marked contrast to the relatively minor structural alterations usually observed on ordinary light microscopy.

ELECTRON MICROSCOPIC EXAMINATION

It was originally said that the myocardium in alcoholic heart disease showed striking changes in subcellular elements (Hibbs *et al.*, 1965; Alexander, 1966).

The principal changes found in alcoholic cardiomyopathies are enumerated below, together with comments on their incidence in other disease states. These changes consist of the following.

(1) Roughening of the sarcoplasmic reticulum (*Figure 15.9*)—this change having been described in many pathological conditions including ischaemia (Miller, Rasmusen and Klionsky, 1964) and various forms of myocarditis (Hibbs *et al.*, 1965).

(2) Degenerative changes in the myofibrils (*Figure 15.10*), an alteration usually preceded by previous mitochondrial injury.

(3) Increased numbers of lipofuchsine granules and lysosomal body changes have been previously shown to occur in the aged and in various degenerative states (Streklar *et al.*, 1959).

(4) Large number of lipid droplet changes (*Figure 15.11*) is the most consistent finding in the alcoholic heart.

(5) Mitochondrial swelling (*Figure 15.12*) is a common finding in any cell which has been exposed for a long time to anoxia but is also commonly seen in other cases of congestive heart failure, as also seen in (6).

(6) Alterations of the mitochondrial cristae (*Figure 15.13*).

(7) The formation of dense intramitochondrial inclusions (*Figure 15.14*) which are thought by some (Hibbs *et al.*, 1965) to demonstrate evidence of mitochondrial degeneration.

It must, therefore, be emphasized that neither the histochemical nor the electron-microscopic findings are specific for alcoholic cardiomyopathy.

TREATMENT

There is little that can be done for these patients apart from treating the congestive heart failure. These patients should be very carefully watched as they very often become hypokalaemic and should,

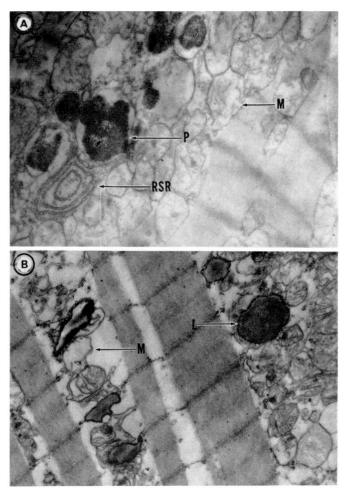

*Figure 15.9. Changes in pigment granules, lipid droplets, and sarco-
plasmic reticulum in the myocardium of two patients with alcoholic
cardiomyopathy. A. Area near the nuclear pole of a right ventricular
myocardial fibre in a case of alcoholic cardiomyopathy. Note the mitochondria (M) in various stages of degeneration: the membrane-enclosed
pigment granules (P), and the rough-surfaced sarcoplasmic reticulum
(RSR) (× 11 000). B. Section from an area of advanced myocardial
degeneration in the left ventricle of a case of alcoholic cardiomyopathy
showing disruption of mitochondria (M) and small dense particles forming
shells around the lipid droplets (L) (× 15 000) (Ferrans et al., 1965)*

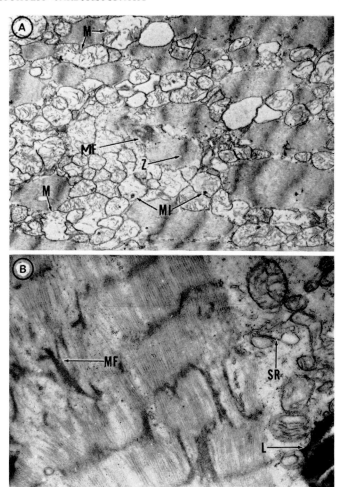

Figure 15.10. Changes in the contractile elements in the myocardium of two patients with alcoholic cardiomyopathy. A. Photograph of the right ventricular myocardium of a patient taken at low magnification showing swelling of the mitochondria (M); intramitochondrial inclusions (MI); and early degenerative changes in a myofibril (MF). The latter change begins at the level of the Z lines (Z). Compare with the more severe mitochondrial changes shown in Figure 15.2 obtained from the same patient (× 11 000). B. Photograph of the left ventricular myocardium of a patient taken at higher magnification, showing areas of disruption and granularity of myofibrils (MF); a few vesicles of the sarcoplasmic reticulum (SR), and the edge of a lipid droplet (L) (× 20 000) (Ferrans et al., 1965)

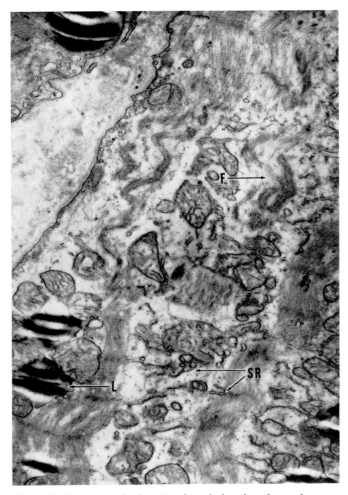

Figure 15.11. Longitudinal section through the edge of an oedematous muscle fibre from a case of alcoholic cardiomyopathy. Note the lipid droplets (L); the sarcoplasmic reticulum (SR); the localized loss of filament orientation (F); and the relative scarcity of mitochondria (× 20 000) (Ferrans et al., 1965)

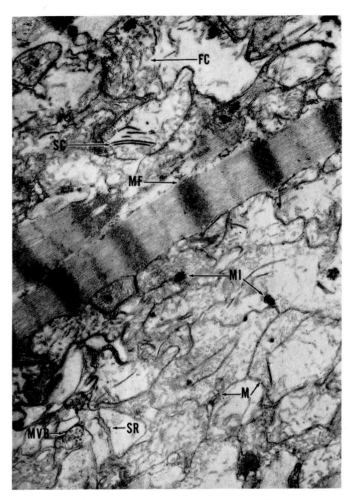

Figure 15.12. Longitudinal section through a muscle cell from a case of alcoholic cardiomyopathy showing pronounced degenerative changes in the densely packed and swollen mitochondria (M). Marked fragmentation of the cristae (FC) is seen in some of the mitochondria-dense intramitochondrial inclusions (MI) and stacks of parallel cristae (SC) are present in others. The myofibrils (MF) are in a state of contracture. A multivesicular body (MVB) is noted near some transverse elements of the sarcoplasmic reticulum (SR) (× 20 000) (Ferrans et al., 1965)

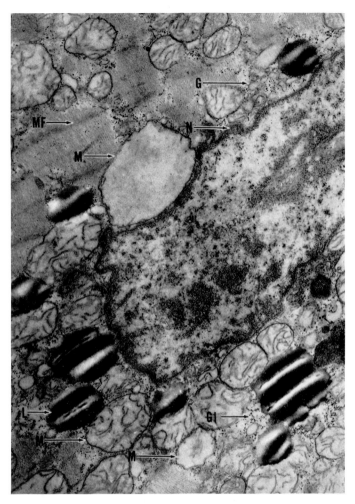

Figure 15.13. Central portion of a moderately damaged myocardial fibre from the right ventricle of a case of alcoholic cardiomyopathy, showing a nucleus (N) with margination of the chromatin. Various degrees of swelling and disruption of the cristae are seen in many mitochondria (M). Golgi membranes (G), numerous lipid droplets (L), glycogen granules (Gl), and normal myofibrils (MF) are indicated (× 18 750) (Ferrans et al., 1965)

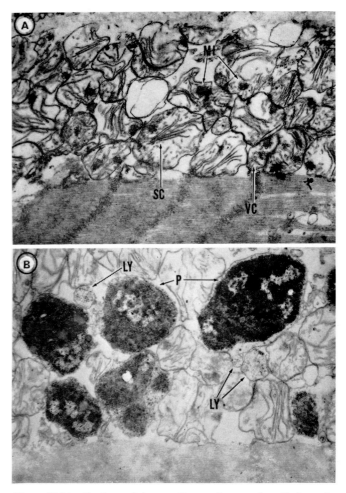

Figure 15.14. Sections of degenerating cardiac muscle cells from the left ventricle of a case of alcoholic cardiomyopathy. A. Longitudinal section through area of mitochondrial degeneration demonstrating numerous intramitochondrial inclusions (MI), vesiculation (VC), and stacking (SC) of the mitochondrial cristae (× 20 000). B. Perinuclear area of a myocardial fibre showing pigment granules (P), some of which are enclosed within membranes, and several lysosomes (LY) (× 16 000) (Ferrans et al., 1965)

therefore, receive potassium supplements. They should also be watched closely for electrolyte imbalance, particularly for hypo-kalaemic alkalosis. As the disease progresses, treatment becomes progressively more difficult and eventually fails completely.

It is unresponsive to administration of thiamine and may occur in well-nourished patients and, although the cause is unknown, it is most likely to be due to direct toxic action of alcohol on the myo-cardium; although viral infection, poor nutrition and non-alcoholic constituents of wine and beer may function as factors for the toxic effects of alcohol.

At present, however, it is most important to recognize that alco-holic cardiomyopathy, at least in its early stages, may occur in well-developed, well-nourished and productive people. The disease may be completely cured if recognized and treated at an early stage—the most important factor being complete abstention from alcohol, a close positive correlation having been shown between abstention from alcohol and waning of clinical severity, and between persistent drinking and increase in clinical severity (Tobin *et al.*, 1967).

It is, therefore, now recognized that the morphological findings in patients with alcoholic cardiomyopathies do not differ from those found in patients with other types of cardiomyopathies giving rise to congestive heart failure.

In a detailed study of the ultrastructure of the heart in primary myocardial disease and alcoholic cardiomyopathy, Ferrans *et al.* (1973) have said: 'Morphological findings in patients with alcoholic cardiomyopathy do not differ from those in patients with other types of congestive cardiomyopathy. The degree to which degenerative changes occur in individual biopsies generally correlates with the duration and severity of the patient's heart disease.'

References

Aalsmeer, W. C. and Wenckebach, K. F. (1929). 'Herz und Kreislauf bei der Beri-beri Krankheit.' *Wien Arch. inn. Med.* **16**, 193

Alexander, C. S. (1966). 'Idiopathic heart disease. I. Analysis of 100 cases with special reference to chronic alcoholism.' *Am. J. Med.* **41**, 213

Blankenhorn, M. A. (1945). 'Diagnosis of beri-beri heart disease.' *Ann. intern. Med.* **23**, 398

Bollinger, P. (1884). 'Ueber die Häufigkeit und Ursachen der idiopathis-chen Herzhypertrophie in München.' *Dt. med. Wschr.* **10**, 180

Brigden, W. and Robinson, J. (1964). 'Alcoholic heart disease.' *Br. med. J.* **2**, 1283

Burch, G. E. and De Pasquale, N. P. (1969). 'Alcoholic cardiomyopathy.' *Am. J. Cardiol.* **23**, 723

— Colcolough, H. L., Harb, J. M. and Tsui, C. Y. (1971a). 'The effects of ingestion of ethyl alcohol, wine and beer on the myocardium of mice.' *Am. J. Cardiol.* **27**, 522

— Harb, J. M., Colcolough, H. L. and Tsui, C. Y. (1971b). 'The effect of prolonged consumption of beer, wine and ethanol on the myocardium of the mouse.' *Johns Hopkins med. J.* **129**, 130

Eliaser, M. Jnr and Giansiracusa, F. J. (1956). 'The heart and alcohol.' *Calif. Med.* **84**, 234

Ferrans, V. J., Massumi, R. A., Shugoll, G. I., Nagab Ali and Roberts, W. C. (1973). 'Ultrastructural studies of myocardial biopsies in 45 patients with obstructive or congestive cardiomyopathy.' *Proceedings of a Conference on Cardiomyopathy Capetown*, South Africa, 1971 (In press)

— Hibbs, R. G., Weilbaecher, D. C., Black, W. C., Walsh, J. J., and Burch, G. E. (1965). 'Alcoholic cardiomyopathy. A histological study.' *Am. Heart J.* **69**, 748

Hibbs, R. G., Ferrans, V. J., Black, W. C., Weilbaecher, D. C., Walsh, J. J. and Burch, G. E. (1965). 'Alcoholic cardiomyopathy. (*An electron microscopic study.*) *Am. Heart J.* **69**, 766

Lieber, C. S. and Davidson, C. S. (1962). 'Some metabolic effects of ethyl alcohol.' *Am. J. Med.* **33**, 319

Miller, D. R., Rasmusen, P. and Klionsky, B. (1964). 'Cell damage after cardiac arrest.' *Am. Surg.* **159**, 208

Perkoff, G. T., Dioso, M. M., Bleisch, V. and Klinkerfuss, G. (1967). 'A spectrum of myopathy associated with alcoholism. I. *Clinical and laboratory features.*' *Ann. intern. Med.* **67**, 481

Regan, T. J., Moschos, C. B., Casanagra, P., Koroxenidis, G. and Hellems, H. K. (1964). 'Depression of cardiac function and altered myocardial metabolism after ethanol.' *Ann. intern. Med.* **60**, Abstracts 709

Streklar, B. L., Mark, D. O., Mildvan, A. S. and Malcolm, V. G. (1959). 'Rate and magnitude of age pigment: accumulation in the human myocardium.' *J. Gerontol.* **14**, 430

Tobin, J. R., Driscoll, J. F., Manuel, T. L., Sutton, G. C., Szanto, P. B. and Gunnar, R. M. (1967). 'Primary myocardial disease and alcoholism.' *Circulation* **35**, 754

Webb, W. R. and Degerli, I. U. (1965). 'Ethyl alcohol and the cardiovascular system: Effects on coronary blood flow.' *J. Am. med. Ass.* **191**, 1055

Weiss, S. and Wilkins, R. W. (1936). 'The nature of the cardiovascular disturbances in vitamin deficiency states.' *Trans. Ass. Am. Physns* **51**, 341

Wendt, V. E., Wu, C., Balcon, R., Doty, G. and Bing, R. J. (1965), 'Hemodynamic and metabolic effects of chronic alcoholism in man.' *Am. J. Cardiol.* **15**, 175

— Ajluni, R., Bruce, T. A., Prasad, A. S. and Bing, R. J. (1966). 'Acute effects of alcohol on the human myocardium.' *Am. J. Cardiol.* **17**, 804

Sixteen

Cardiac tumours

INCIDENCE AND HISTORY

Since a heart tumour was first described in 1835, about 500 tumours have been described up to 1957, over 100 being myxomas, which have been described since 1951 (Wharton, 1949; Prichard, 1951; Kaafman and Cohen, 1957).

Myxomas comprise 50 per cent and rhabdomyomas 20 per cent of the benign tumours while the remainder are comprised of fibromas, lipomas, angiomas, haemartomas, teratomas and epithelial inclusions, which occur at birth or in infants; the former usually being fatal and found at necropsy.

Myxomas are thrombus-like tumours which usually occur in the atria, arising from the interatrial septum, 80 per cent being polypoidal and about 75 per cent occurring on the left side of the heart. Sarcomas usually occur in the walls of both the atria and the ventricles, mainly on the right side, about 20 per cent being polypoidal in shape.

Primary heart tumours are stated to occur at all ages and to have an equal sex incidence, with the exception of the myxomas which are most frequently found between the ages of 30 and 60. Myxomas are also three times as common in women as in men (Harvey, 1957).

Malignant cardiac tumours are all sarcomatous.

CLASSIFICATION

All heart tumours should be considered together, as it may be difficult to differentiate between primary and secondary tumours and between benign and malignant primary heart tumours (Magna and Monahan, 1955). All types of heart tumour have to be differentiated from pericardial tumours and cysts, hydatid cysts and mediastinal growths (Wharton, 1949). Location, histology and whether or not they are polypoidal may also be used as a means of classification (Wall and Vickery, 1947; Goldberg and Steinberg, 1955).

Here it is proposed simply to list the different types of cardiac tumours. Little is, I think, to be gained from dividing them into polypoid and non-polypoid tumours, as has been done by some workers (Mahaim, 1945); because, while 80 per cent of the myxomas described have been found to be polypoid in nature, so have a quarter of the cardiac sarcomas. Few other cardiac tumours are polypoids; excepting rhabdomyomas, every tumour described so far has been within the myocardium.

Secondary tumours of the heart are at least sixteen times as common as primary heart tumours.

The complex of lesions characterized by endocardial thickening or fibro-elastosis and variously called foetal endocarditis, foetal endomyocarditis, endocardial sclerosis or foetal endocardial fibro-elastosis may, if involvement is sufficiently localized, simulate a cardiac tumour, numerous instances having been so reported. Although the cause is not known, and probably is not always the same, there is no reason to relate these findings to any of the cardiac neoplasms described in this section. Rarely other tumour-like lesions of unknown aetiology affect the heart, such as the involvement of the right coronary artery in Letterer–Siwe's disease, reported by Landing and Farber (1956) in their description of tumours of the cardio-vascular system. Epithelial cyst of the heart is a rare malformation, usually observed incidentally at *post mortem;* some reports of lymphangiomas of the heart appear to represent misinterpretations of this lesion.

Blood cysts are small (usually less than 2 mm in diameter). Red lesions most commonly present on the surface of atrioventricular valves of infants and their incidence becomes progressively less common with advancing age. Microscopically, they usually show a round thick vessel-like wall and a lumen filled with red cells. They are considered by many workers to be remnants of the foetal vascular system of the valves, but others believe that they are pinched-off or narrow-necked diverticula of the endocardium.

Usually these lesions have no clinical significance but are often of a sufficient size to produce a murmur.

References

Goldberg, H. P. and Steinberg, I. (1955). 'Primary tumours of the heart.' *Circulation* **11**, 963

Harvey, J. C. (1957). 'Myxoma of the left auricle.' *Am. intern. Med.* **47**, 1067

Kaafman, B. H. and Cohen, S. E. (1957). 'Primary tumour of the heart (Reticulum cell sarcoma).' *N.Y. St. J. Med.* **57**, 2, 652

Landing, B. H. and Farber, S. (1956). 'Tumours of the cardiovascular system.' In *Atlas of Tumor Pathology*. Section III, Fasicle 7, p. 138. Washington: Armed Forces Institute of Pathology

Magna, J. W. and Monahan, J. P. (1955). 'A case of primary sarcoma of the heart.' *J. Ir. Med. Ass.* **37**, 317

Mahaim, I. (1945). *Les Tumeurs et les Polypes du Coeur. Etude Anatomo-Clinique*. p. 568. Paris: Masson and Laussanne

Prichard, R. W. (1951). 'Tumour of the heart. Review of the subject and report of 150 cases.' *Archs Path.* **51**, 98

Wall, E. and Vickery, A. L. (1947). 'Primary fibrosarcoma of the heart with vertebral metastases.' *Archs Path.* **43**, 244

Wharton, C. M. (1949). 'Primary malignant tumour of the heart. Report of a case.' *Cancer, Philad.* **2**, 245

BENIGN PRIMARY CARDIAC TUMOURS

BENIGN MYXOMA

A benign myxoma is the most common primary tumour of the heart as several hundred cases have been described. About a third of all primary cardiac tumours are myxomas (Mahaim, 1945). Of the 125 reported cases reviewed by Prichard (1951) about 75 per cent were in the left atrium and most of the remaining cases in the right atrium, although there are cases of this tumour being found to arise in the ventricles or auricles. The age of cases has varied from 3 months to 68 years, but the sex incidence appears to be equal, although one gains the impression that women with this disease appear to be more severely affected than men in a similar age group.

Within the atria the most common site of attachment is to the fossa ovalis or to its rim (*Figure 16.1*). Macroscopically, the tumours vary in size from 1 to 7 cm in diameter. They are usually smooth, greyish-pink in colour but sometimes may be covered by a thin layer of blood clot or have a glistening surface, while the surface may be lobulated (*Figure 16.2*).

They are pedunculated tumours and are attached to the endocardium usually by a narrow stalk, although in some cases the attachment may be broader. Often the tumour is prolapsed through the valve ring so that the mitral or tricuspid valve cannot function efficiently, and the resultant back pressure may ensure that one or both atria are dilated.

Histology

The bulk of the tumour consists of myxomatous tissue composed largely of stellate cells or more rounded cells distributed sparsely or in

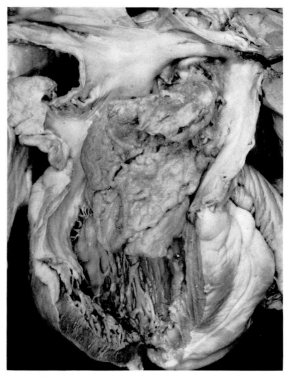

Figure 16.1. Myxoma of left atrium in a 51 year old male. A left atrium and left ventricle. A large myxoma arising from the atrial septum occupied a considerable portion of the left atrial cavity and protruded through the mitral valve (Sterns et al., 1966)

groups throughout the tumour (*Figure 16.3*). Haematoxylin and eosin-stained sections usually show a predominance of eosinophilic myxoid stroma containing many foci of haemorrhage. Sometimes individual cells or groups of cells are much enlarged and have an extensive eosinophilic cytoplasm (*Figure 16.4*) with irregular, slightly hyperchromatic nuclei. These cells may be multinucleate. Both types of cells may be enmeshed in the myxoid matrix. Adjacent cells are usually continuous with one another and assume a more cuboidal shape in papillary areas. The surface of the tumour is covered by a continuous layer of endothelium which covers myxoid, papillary formations which are sometimes partially hyalinized (*Figure 16.5*).

In some of these tumours small cystic endothelial-lined spaces are found (Orr, 1942; Boss and Bechar, 1959). In many areas these gland-

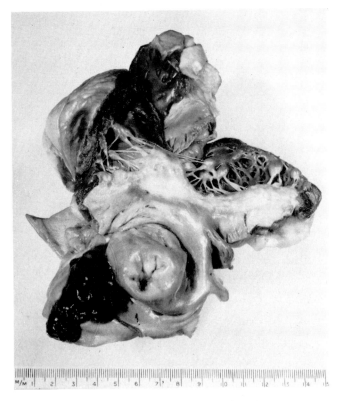

Figure 16.2. Photograph of atrial tumour before fixation showing gelatinous appearance. (Reproduced from Edwards and Johnson (1959) by courtesy of the authors and the Editor of the British Journal of Surgery)

like or cleft-like channels are found to lack a basement membrane and to contain eosinophilic material, while in other cases red blood cells may be present. These channels are usually lined by a single row of cells quite similar to those within the matrix (*Figure 16.6*). Syncitial groups of cells may be noted along the external borders of these channels. In these areas cells appear to stream from these clear-cut channels for a short distance into the matrix. Small groups of these myxoma cells are often circumscribed or are adjacent to true vascular channels. Focal areas of haemorrhage and deposition of haemosiderin are frequent and groups of lymphocytes may also be seen.

The stalk of the tumour is often fibrous and sometimes large vessels pass through the endocardium proper into the stalk. Delicate

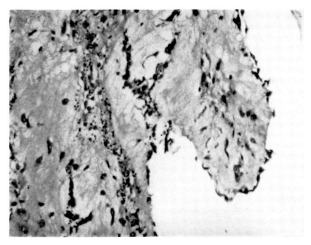

Figure 16.3. Section of cardiac myxoma (haematoxylin and eosin × 250, reduced to 3/4) (Skanse, Berg and Westfelt, 1959)

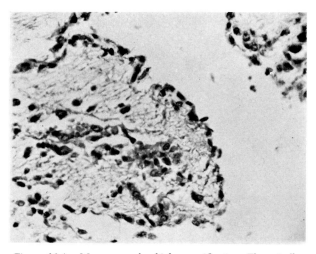

Figure 16.4. Myxoma under high magnification. The spindle-shaped cells are embedded in a thread-like myxomatous stroma. The cells are often arranged in sequestrial cords (Skanse, Berg and Westfelt, 1959)

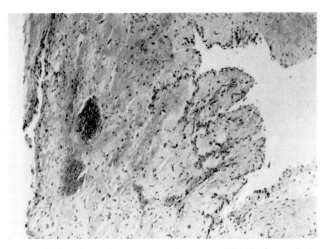

Figure 16.5.   General appearance of myxoma. This fairly accellular tumour shows a definitely papillary structure (haematoxylin and eosin × 50, reduced to 3/4). (Sterns et al., 1966)

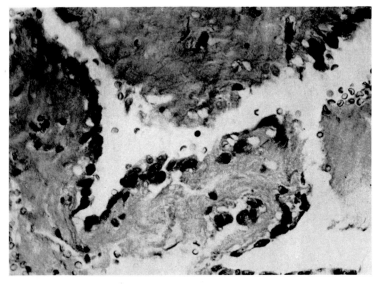

Figure 16.6.   Cells covering redundant myxomatous papillary stromal folds. The cells are arranged in a single row and assume cuboidal configuration (haematoxylin and eosin × 256, reduced to 2/3). (Skanse, Berg and Westfelt, 1959)

elastic tissue fibrils are often seen, particularly in association with blood vessels, and reticulin fibres may also be present. The surrounding endocardium shows no abnormality. The presence or absence of mucin has been a matter of dispute, largely because of the older histological methods of demonstrating mucin. In some cases, using mucicarmine, mucin can be demonstrated (Orr, 1942), but in other cases none can be found.

Acid mucopolysaccharides of various types are found in connective tissue and the staining reactions sometimes vary with the fixative. Mucicarmine and PAS stains are found to be positive in this tumour. Variations in intensity of staining and metachromasia are seen in different parts of this myxoid tumour. Fisher and Hellstrom (1960) found the matrix to be thionin positive, PAS positive and alcian blue positive. The metachromasia was removed by hyaluronidase and similar staining reactions were found in umbilical cord, and in a cutaneous myxoma.

Electron Microscopy

Often abundant fine intracytoplasmic parallel filaments (*Figure 16.7*), of a similar magnitude to those described for smooth muscle cells (Rhodin, 1962) can be seen in myxoma cells (Merkow *et al.*, 1969). These fibres, lacking periodicity, weave between organelles and fill the cytoplasm; these delicate filaments range from 85 to 125 Å in diameter.

This type of filament is believed to represent the contractile components of smooth muscle cells (Panner, 1967).

Pinocytotic vesicles have been observed beneath the plasmalemma of some neoplastic cells (Merkow *et al.* 1969). Chromatin may often be seen condensed along the inner nuclear membrane.

The surface of myxomatous cells displays many infoldings and redundant finger-like interdigitations between the surfaces of adjacent cells as well as in other cells in apposition with the myxomatous stroma (*Figure 16.8*).

Collagen fibrils and granular material are often noted within the myxoid matrix and in continuity with tumour cells.

Calcification in Myxoma

The surface of some myxomas shows small white flecks of calcium salts, but in a few cases these tumours may be very heavily calcified. Thus, Oliver and Missen (1966) found seven reports of major calcification of these tumours and it is interesting to note that six of these tumours had arisen in the right atrium.

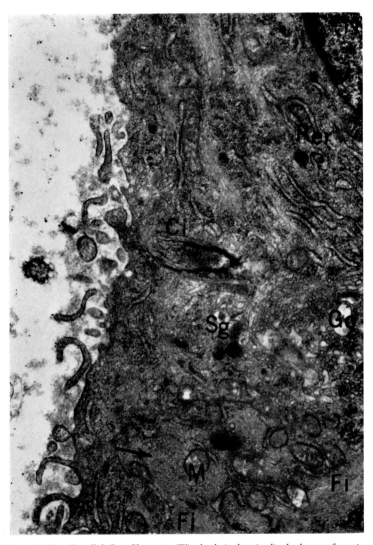

Figure 16.7. Parallel fine filaments (Fi), *both in longitudinal planes of section*
(arrow), interwoven with parallel arrayed rough endoplasmic reticulin (Rer), *small*
mitochondria (M), *prominent Golgi complex* (Go), *nucleus* (N) *is seen* (× *16 800).*
(Reproduced by courtesy of Dr Merkow)

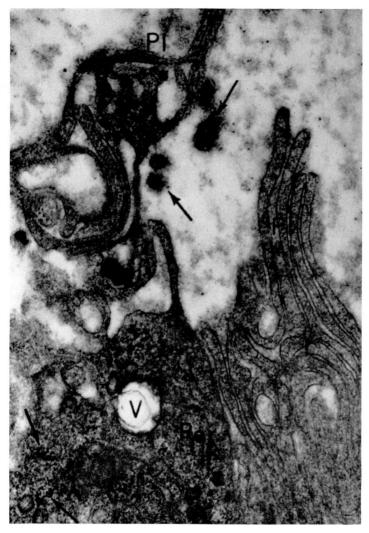

Figure 16.8. Plasmalemma (Pl) *displays complex finger-like processes and foldings. Ribosomes (bottom arrows), rough endoplasmic reticulum* (Rer), *vacuoles* (V) *and extra-cellular dense bodies (top arrows) are evident* (× 27 500). *(Reproduced by courtesy of Dr Merkow)*

Minor degrees of calcification are not uncommon and have been recognized in 3 left- and 3 right-sided myxomas, the first by Strause (1938).

Major calcification, recognized in life, has been noted in 7 reports, the tumour being in the right atrium in 6; the first was by Bayer *et al.* (1954), who did not confirm the nature of the tumour at operation. The first authentic example was that of a plum-sized spherical dense mass, moving with the heart's motion; on removal it measured 5·5 × 5·0 × 4·0 cm and was yellowish-white, smooth, glistening and slightly lobulated, and showed many foci of calcification on bisection. Wight, McCall and Weneer (1963) reported two cases, one in the left and one in the right atrium.

Mahaim (1945) in his monograph included 82 cases of atrial myxoma but none were described as calcified; in case 8 a man of 59 years, a heavily calcified sessile stony polyp (1·3 × 1 × 1 cm) attached to the left atrial septum was found incidentally at autopsy.

Oliver and Missen (1966) reported a 63 year old man whose symptoms started at 26 years, a calcified mass being discovered at 49, which was thought to be tuberculous constrictive pericarditis. Finally cardiac catheterization proved the presence of severe tricuspid regurgitation suggesting a calcified myxoma of the left atrium or calcified thrombus. This tumour, when removed, measured 6·1 × 6 × 3·0 cm in size and weighed 75 g; it was attached between the inferior vena cava and the coronary sinus and had a constricting ring made by the tricuspid valve (which was grossly dilated); it was brittle and portions of tumour had embolized to the pulmonary arteries.

Microscopy demonstrated extensive calcification (without bone formation) and typical mucoid myxoma tissue. The active surfaces showed buried remains of what could have been Lambl's excrescence. The heart weighed 825 g. Oliver and Missen postulated that the calcification was secondary to necrosis which is so common in myxomata and that, once started, haemodynamic trauma could aggravate the process by repeated fracture and healing of calcified areas. Although bone formation has been mentioned by several authors, no specific examples have been described.

Fleck and Lopez-Bescos (1968) described a man of 41 who had a calcified right atrial myxoma, similar to that in Oliver and Missen's (1966) case.

It was detected on routine x-ray screening as a calcified mass in the heart shadow, 5 cm in diameter, moving with respiration and associated with right bundle branch block. The ESR was only

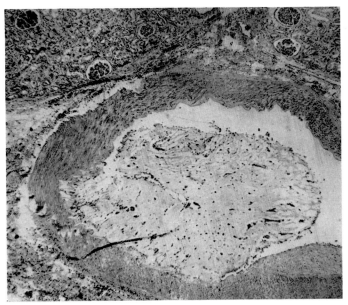

Figure 16.9. Myxoma of the left atrium in a 51 year old man. Photomicrograph of an intrarenal artery showing partial occlusion by an embolus of myxomatous tissue, which is believed to have originated in the tumour of the left atrium (haematoxylin and eosin × 57, reduced to 9/10).
(Sterns et al., 1966)

3 cm/hr. The tumour was excised at operation from a pedicle attached to the posterior rim of the fossa ovalis.

Embolic Phenomenon

Emboli occur fairly frequently and small emboli of myxomatous tissue may be found at post mortem in the absence of any clinical signs (*Figure 16.9*). On occasion the emboli may be the presenting feature (Silverman, Olwin and Graettinger, 1962).

The emboli occur most frequently in the systemic circulation, often involving the cerebral (*Figure 16.10*) or renal (*Figure 16.11*) circulation, but in the right atrial myxoma the pulmonary circulation is involved. Cumming and Finkel (1961) described a case in which a left atrial myxoma extended through the foramen ovale to the right atrium and emboli were then found in both circulations.

Although these tumours are regarded as benign and therefore will not metastasize, there have been a few reports of emboli from these tumours lodging in blood vessels and, apparently, infiltrating the vessel wall, although not very actively (Rimgertz, 1942).

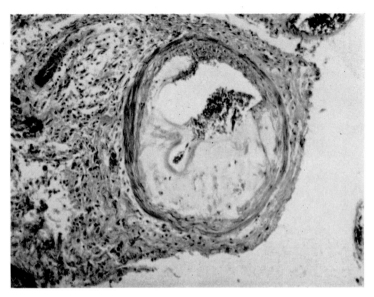

Figure 16.10.   Old tumour in an arachnoidal artery over right occipital lobe. The vessel is not completely obstructed with tumour masses. Note vigorous cellular reaction in surrounding arachnoid with round cells and histiocytes, some of which contain iron pigment (haematoxylin and eosin × 150, reduced to 9/10)

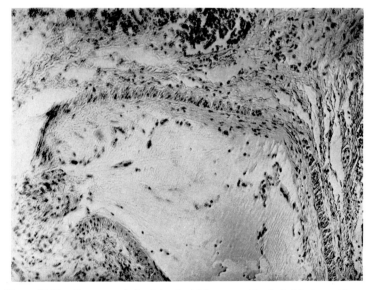

Figure 16.11.   Tumour embolus in an interlobar artery in the left kidney. Observe slight oedema of vessel walls and slight cellular infiltration of adventitia of vessel (haematoxylin and eosin × 150, reduced to 9/10)

Clinical Presentation

In the past stress has been laid on the haemodynamic and embolic features of this disease. Dyspnoea which is sometimes nocturnal and paroxysmal, pulmonary oedema, right ventricular failure, gangrene of the fingers, and sometimes the physical signs of mitral or tricuspid stenosis are often present.

During the past decade it has been noted that many patients with atrial myxomata show a generalized illness associated with fever, a raised serum globulin and a raised ESR, in addition to the other haemodynamic features (Goodwin *et al.*, 1962). Some other patients may present with Raynaud's phenomenon (Skanse, Berg and Westfelt, 1959) or a generalized arthralgia (Curry, Mathews and Robinson, 1967)—both of which may be cured after removal of the cardiac myxoma.

Disorder of Plasma Proteins

Increased serum gamma-globulin and altered albumin: globulin ratio are commonly seen—the serum albumin always being about 2 g per cent. The reason for this is unknown but may be related to the fever, anaemia, raised ESR and loss of weight. All these features could be explained by the generalized release from the myxoma of some abnormal substance with the generalized circulations or, less likely, repeated tiny emboli.

The myxoma itself may form excessive or unusual globulins but there is no abnormality in the serum gamma-globulin, and auto-antibodies to cardiac myxoma have not been discovered in the blood.

Anaemia

The haemoglobin level is usually about 10–12 g of haemoglobin per 100 ml of blood. The anaemia is non-specific with slight reduction in mean corpuscular haemoglobin concentration and anisocytosis and microcytosis suggesting iron deficiency or a toxic depression of bone marrow.

Nature of Myxoma

Two opposing theories as to the nature of these lesions are in vogue. One school of thought believes that they are true neoplasms, while the other is in favour of the view that they are organizing thrombi. The view that these are neoplastic and not true thrombi is based on the following reasons.

(1) Myxomata are, in the majority of cases, found in the atrium although ventricular thrombi are much more common.

(2)   In the atrium the most common site for a myxoma is attached to the atrial wall in the region of the fossa ovalis, but this is a most unusual site for thrombi, which are commonly seen in the auricular appendage where myxomata are only very infrequently found.

(3)   The absence of lamination in myxoma while they are commonly found in thrombi.

(4)   Myxomata are usually much less cellular than organizing thrombi.

(5)   In an organizing thrombus only the part of the thrombus adjacent to the endocardium is covered with endothelium, while the whole surface of a myxoma is covered with endothelium.

(6)   In myxoma there is not usually as much haemosiderin as one would expect in an organizing thrombus.

(7)   Sometimes embolic myxomatic tissue appears to invade the walls of blood vessels.

(8)   Simple thrombi do not give rise to generalized disease as myxomata sometimes do, or to changes in the levels of serum proteins or produce anaemia.

The presence of immunological-reacting, smooth muscle type filaments in endocardial cells and a similar morphological organelle in the myxoma cells (Merkow et al., 1969) lends support to the present concept of the latter's origin.

Since the cardiac myxoma most frequently takes origin in the left atrium one might surmise that endocardial cells, containing contractile elements, may also be abundant at this site, a finding supported by the work of Becker and Murphy (1969).

Ultrastructural studies add definitive morphological support to the belief that intracardiac myxomas are true neoplasms derived from certain morphological characteristics, observable only by electron microscopy. These observations seem to confirm the hypothesis that myxoma cells originate from endocardial type cells (Fine, Morales and Hones, 1968).

Abundant fine cytoplasmic filaments of a similar magnitude to that described in smooth muscle cells (Rhodin, 1962) have been described in myxoma cells (Merkow et al., 1969). Quite similar filaments have been noted in human fibromyxosarcoma cells (Leak et al., 1967). This type of filament is believed to represent the contractile components of smooth muscle cells (Leak et al., 1967; Panner, 1967).

The report by Becker and Murphy (1969) indicates that atrial endocardium contains smooth muscle cells which stain brilliantly, following the addition of fluorescein-labelled antiserum to human uterine actomyosin or myosin. The small amounts of cytoplasmic filaments observed by electron microscopy in human atrial endothelial cells

(Lannigan and Zaki, 1966; Sohal and Burch, 1969) originally only suggested that these cells possessed contractile elements, although smooth muscle cells have been reported within the subendocardial layer (Lannigan and Zaki, 1966).

With the later publication by Merkow *et al.* (1969) it will now be observed that these cells contain many intracytoplasmic filaments similar to those found in smooth muscle. The presence of immunological reacting smooth muscle type filaments in endocardial cells and a similar morphological organelle in the myxoma cells lends support to the concept that a myxoma originates from muscle cells in the endocardium. It thus appears that myxomas are true neoplasms which are derived from endocardial cells.

References

Bayer, D., Loogen, F., Vieten, H., Willman, K. H. and Wolter, H. H. (1954). 'Der Wert des Herzkatheterismas und die Angiokardiographie bei der Diagnostik intro und extrokardiolar tamorein.' *Dt. med. Wschr.* **79**, 619

Becker, C. G., and Murphy, G. E. (1969). 'Demonstration of contractile protein in endothelium and cells of the heart valves, endocardium, intima, arteriosclerotic plaques and Aschoff bodies of rheumatic heart disease.' *Am. J. Path.* **55**, 1

Boss, J. H. and Bechar, M. (1959). 'Myxoma of the heart. Report based on four cases.' *Am. J. Cardiol.* **3**, 823

Cumming, G. R. and Finkel, K. (1961). 'Intracardiac myxoma involving the right and left atria in a young patient.' *J. Pediat.* **58**, 559

Currey, H. L. F., Mathews, J. A. and Robinson, J. (1967). 'Right atrial myxoma involving rheumatic disorder.' *Br. med. J.* **1**, 547

Fine, G., Morales, A. and Hones, R. C., Jnr (1968). 'Cardiac myxoma: A morphologic and histologic appraisal.' *Cancer* **22**, 1156

Fisher, E. R. and Hellstrom, H. P. (1960). 'Evidence in support of the neoplastic nature of cardiac myxoma.' *Am. Heart J.* **60**, 630

Fleck, D. C. and Lopez-Bescos, L. (1968). 'Calcified right atrial myxoma producing tricuspid incompetence.' *Proc. R. Soc. Med.* **61**, 1115

Goodwin, J. F., Standfield, C. A., Steiner, R. E., Nemtall, N. H., Sayed, M. M., Bloom, V. R. and Bishop, M. S. (1962). 'Clinical features of left atrial myxoma.' *Thorax* **17**, 91

Lannigan, R. A. and Zaki, S. A. (1966). 'Ultrastructure of the normal endocardium.' *Br. Heart J.* **28**, 785

Leak, L. V., Caulfield, J. B., Burke, J. F. and McKann, C. F. (1967). 'Electromicroscopic studies on a human fibromyxosarcoma.' *Cancer Res.* **27**, 261

Mahaim, I. (1945). 'Les tumeurs et les polypes du coeur. Etude anatomoclinique.' Paris: Masson and Laussanne

Merkow, L. P., Kooros, M. A., Magovern, G., Hayslip, D. W., Weikers, N. J., Pardo, M. and Fisher, D. L. (1969). 'Ultrastructure of a cardiac myxoma.' *Archs Path.* **88**, 390

Oliver, G. S. and Missen, G. A. K. (1966). 'A heavily calcified right atrial myxoma.' *Guy's Hosp. Rep.* **115**, 37

Orr, J. W. (1942). 'Endothelioma (Pseudomyxoma) of the heart.' *J. Path. Bact.* **54**, 125

Panner, B. J. (1967). 'Filament ultrastructure and organisation in vertebrate smooth muscle: Contraction hypothesis based on localisation of actin and myosin.' *J. cell. Biol.* **35**, 303

Prichard, R. (1951). 'Tumours of the heart. Review of the subject and report of 150 cases.' *Archs Path.* **51**, 98

Rhodin, J. A. G. (1962). 'Fine structure of vascular walls with special reference to smooth muscle components.' *Physiol. Rev.* **42**, 48

Rimgertz, N. (1942). 'Über sogenannte endokardmyome.' *Acta path. microbiol. scand.* **19**, 262

Silverman, J. Olwin, J. S. and Graettinger, J. S. (1962). 'Cardiac myxoma with systemic embolisation. Review of the literature and report of a case.' *Circulation* **26**, 99

Skanse, B., Berg, N. G. and Westfelt, L. (1959). 'Atrial myxoma with Raynaud's phenomenon as the initial symptom.' *Acta. med. scand.* **164**, 321

Sohal, R. S. and Burch, G. E. (1969). 'Electron microscopic study of the endocardium in Coxsackie virus B4 infected mice.' *Am. J. Pathol.* **55**, 133

Strause, S. (1938). 'Primary benign tumour of the heart of 43 years duration.' *Acta intern. Med.* **62**, 401

Wight, R. P., McCall, M. M. and Weneer, Nanette K. L. (1963). 'Primary atrial tumour.' *Am. J. Cardiol.* **11**, 790

RHABDOMYOMA

The rhabdomyoma tumour, first described by von Recklinghausen in 1862, is a tumour-like formation which may occur in any part of the heart. It may occur as simple or multiple nodules and is most common in the newborn. Usually there may be several or many small tumours scattered throughout the myocardium, but only one tumour may be initially observed and the remainder are only seen after histological examination of the heart. These lesions may be widespread throughout the heart, as described in the case reported by Winstanley (1961) of a ten year old girl who died suddenly, but who had never previously complained of any cardiac symptoms. Some of the early cases reported as rhabdomyomata were, in actual fact, probably cases of Pompe's disease (type III glycogen storage disease).

The tumours are commonly associated with tuberose sclerosis as is shown in the paper by Batchelor and Maun (1945) who found associated tuberose sclerosis in 50 per cent of reported cases of rhabdomyoma. Taylor (1968) reported an Irish labourer of 23 years of age who had tuberose sclerosis, with mental deficiency, typical papillomatous rash with *cafe au lait* spots and arrhythmia, which electrocardiography showed to consist of multifocal extrasystoles in association with left bundle branch block. No cardiac tumour was demonstrated by cardiac catheterization and serum glucose was normal.

Age Incidence

The majority of cases which have been reported are in infants or in young children. Thus, Farber (1931) in his review of 41 cases of rhabdomyomata found that only 12 (29 per cent) were over the age of three years, a finding in keeping with a study of Batchelor and Maun (1945) who noted that approximately 85 per cent of cases were found in patients aged less than 15 years.

In children rhabdomyomas usually present as cardiac problems with congestive heart failure, cyanosis secondary to shunt reversal at atrial level, paroxysmal atrial tachycardia or significant sub-aortic stenosis as in the four cases of children with tuberose sclerosis reported by Shaher et al. (1972).

The reason for this type of age distribution is probably because many subjects with this disease, which is associated with tuberose sclerosis, are confined in mental hospitals, because of associated mental changes where post-mortems are only rarely carried out and the heart is even less frequently examined. Thus Steinbiss (1923) described finding 6 rhabdomyoma in 31 patients with tuberose sclerosis who died in mental institutions, one of which was in a 35 year old man.

Sex and Racial Incidence

The tumours are found with equal frequency in both sexes. Although the majority of cases have been reported in Caucasians there are two reports of the lesions in a Negro (Hueper, 1935; Pratt-Thomas, 1947). There are, at present, no reports of this disease in the Chinese or Japanese, but it almost certainly has not been carefully looked for.

Gross Appearance of Heart

The nodules are usually pale, isolated or numerous and usually lie in the cardiac septum. They have no capsule; large nodules simply compress the peripheral myocardium to give a fairly well-defined pseudocapsule. They are benign, never metastasize and are almost certainly not true tumours. They may extend into the heart, forming nodular projections which do not ulcerate.

Very commonly, especially in infants and young children, gross myocardial hypertrophy can be seen. The tumours are often yellow or gelatinous brown when sectioned. The parts most commonly affected, in those cases of diffuse cardiac involvement, are the papillary muscles, the main zones of both ventricles and the thickness of the septum. Firm elastic nodules of this yellowish-brown tissue may form low projections on both sides of the intraventricular septum.

Microscopical Appearance

A microscopic view shows a 'capsule' of compressed myocardium into which the nodule blends; most of the tumour shows an empty sponge-like appearance, probably due to the disappearance of glycogen which can be demonstrated only in very fresh tissue, say within an hour of death. It may be noted, however, that Mowry and Bangle (1951) demonstrated plentiful glycogen in normal infants' hearts, taking no special precautions to preserve it. Beaird, Mowry and Cunningham (1955) demonstrated abundant PAS-positive granules in a rhabdomyoma using alcoholic solutions; if the sections were floated on water only a few granules of glycogen remained.

They, therefore, suggested that the tumour contained water soluble polysaccharides. In places distinct striations may be seen, especially in those sections stained by phosphotungstic acid and haematoxylin. Many of these cells have a typical appearance and are called 'spider-cells'. It is usually a large cell, perhaps two or three times the diameter of a muscle fibre. It has a single nucleus attached to occasional myofibrils, and this gives it the 'spider hanging in a net' appearance described by Ziehfeldt (Steinbiss, 1921). Sometimes the histological appearance of these tumours may be different. Here it appears that muscle fibres from the affected parts of the myocardium are converted into tubes 30–60 μm in diameter. In some places cells are round or oval in transverse sections, but in most places they appear irregular and distended, though they have the staining properties of normal muscle. Striations in both longitudinal and transverse sections are seen in some areas. The centres of these tubes are empty except for some small granules which when stained with Best's stain are found to be glycogen. The endocardium overlying and adjacent to these tumorous nodules may show a considerable thickening and some elastic tissue proliferation. The other interesting feature of these hearts is that many of the medium-sized and small intramyocardial arteries show marked medial hypertrophy due to muscle fibre hypertrophy.

Origin of the Tumour

There are three main views concerning the nature of cardiac rhabdomyomata. The first considers them to be haemartomas, that is tumour-like masses of the cells from which the normal myocardium had evolved. The second view is that these tumour cells represent abnormal differentiation of embryonal myocardium at random and prematurely and result in a very large Purkinje-type of cell, especially as rhabdomyoma show a close resemblance to the normal Purkinje cell (Elliot and McGeachy, 1962).

The third view is that rhabdomyoma are congenital nodular glycogenic tumours (Batchelor and Maun, 1945). This is because they contain glycogen, but apart from this fact it is my opinion that they have nothing to do with glycogen storage disease. It is worth-while mentioning here the principal pathological features of tuberose sclerosis, as the reader may meet them while looking for a case of rhabdomyoma. In the brain, the characteristic features are hard nodules, better felt than seen and varying in size and number, and they lie scattered in the cerebrum, occasionally in the cerebellum, brain stem and cord, and they may calcify. Nissl staining shows deficient areas of staining in the cortex and glial method reveals areas of dense fibrosis in which the cortical lamination is lost, the nerve cells are fewer with shrunken, pyknotic or occasionally enlarged nuclei; glial cells, especially astrocytes, are increased and may have more than one nucleus; this being seen particularly in the nodules in the white matter. The bulk of the nodules is composed of a dense felt of glial fibres. Subependymal nodules in the lateral ventricles produce a well known 'candle guttering' appearance. Secondary changes of demyelination or softening may also be present.

In the skin, there is a characteristic facial rash, sebaceous adenoma, which is acneform, papular, colourless, reddish or brownish and distributed often as a 'butterfly' rash across the nose and cheeks; this may not appear until puberty. The superficial dermis shows a moderate increase and disordered arrangement of sebaceous glands, vessels and fibrous tissue and hyperkeratosis, thickening of the epidermis and irregularity in length of the rete pegs.

Several other skin changes may occur, *peau de chagrin* (areas of shagreen skin on the buttocks and thighs, close set, flattish or more elongated outgrowths of the superficial skin layer); other skin lesions include flat warts, haemangioma, fibroma, vertiligo, leucoderma and *cafe au lait* spots.

References

Batchelor, T. M. and Maun, V. M. E. (1945). 'Congenital glycogenic tumours of the heart.' *Archs Path.* **39**, 67
Beaird, J., Mowry, R. W. and Cunningham, J. A. (1955). 'Congenital

rhabdomyoma of the heart. Case report with histochemical study of tumour polysaccharides.' *Cancer* **8**, 916

Elliot, G. B. and McGeachy, W. G. (1962). 'The monster Purkinje-cell nature of so-called congenital rhabdomyoma of heart. A forme fruste of tuberose sclerosis.' *Am. Heart J.* **63**, 636

Farber, S. (1931). 'Congenital rhabdomyoma of the heart.' *Am. J. Path.* **7**, 105

Hueper, W. C. (1935). 'Rhabdomyoma of the heart in a negro.' *Archs Path.* **19**, 372

Mowry, R. W. and Bangle, R. (1951). 'Histochemically demonstrable glycogen in the human heart with special reference to glycogen storage diseases and diabetes mellitus.' *Am. J. Path.* **27**, 611

Pratt-Thomas, H. R. (1947). 'Tuberose sclerosis with congenital tumours of the heart and kidneys.' *Am. J. Path.* **23**, 189

Shaher, R. M., Mintzer, J., Farina, M., Alley, R. and Bishop, M. (1972). 'Clinical presentation of rhabdomyoma of the heart in infancy and childhood.' *Am. J. Cardiol.* **30**, 95

Steinbiss, W. (1923). 'Zur Kenntnis der Rhabdomyoma des Herzens und ihrer Beziehungen zur tuberohsen Gehirnsklerose.' *Virchows Arch. path. Anat. Physiol.* **243**, 22

Taylor, T. R. (1968). 'Tuberous sclerosis presenting as cardiac arrhythmia.' *Br. Heart J.* **30**, 132

Winstanley, D. P. (1961). 'Sudden death from multiple rhabdomyoma of the heart.' *J. Path. Bact.* **81**, 249

FIBROMA

These are tumours of fibrous tissue, usually arising in the interstitial tissue of the myocardium, and exclude those tumours arising from subendocardial tissue, which are often seen on heart valves (Mahaim, 1945). Perhaps the earliest report of a cardiac fibroma is that of Luschka (1855), who reported finding a 'tumor fibrosus' in the heart of a boy dying from diphtheria; he noted the resemblance of the tumour to a fibroma. This is a relatively rare tumour, so that Mahaim (1945) in his study of cardiac tumour could find only 37 (11.2 per cent) instances of fibromas in a total of 329 tumours reviewed.

Incidence

The sexes are equally affected and the majority of the cases are children under the age of 16, the majority being found in newborn and children of up to 2–3 years of age. In fact, endocardial fibroma is probably the cardiac tumour found most frequently in young children. Thus in 28 recorded cases of cardiac fibromata, 22 occurred in children (Freeman *et al.*, 1963). Sudden death has been reported commonly (Kalka, 1949; Freeman *et al.*, 1963).

Situation

The majority of these tumours are in the left ventricle or inter-ventricular septum but they have also, although rarely, been described in the wall of the right ventricle. All the tumours which have so far been described were solitary. Patients with intracardiac fibroma may present initially with paroxysmal tachycardia and multiple extra-systoles as in the case of James and Stansfield (1955).

Pathology

Gross appearance—These tumours are firm, without a capsule, and, when sectioned, have the appearance of a desmoid tumour (Geha *et al.*, 1967), and may, on occasions, be partially calcified, the calcifica-tion being visible radiologically (James and Stansfield, 1955).

Microscopic appearance—The tumours usually show interlacing bundles of spindle cells (fibroblasts) and about half the tumours contain strands of cardiac muscle. Some of these tumours only contain muscle fibres around their periphery because most of these reported tumours lack a capsule and it has been suggested as a suitable explanation that here the muscle fibres have been accidentally incorporated in the tumour (Kalka, 1949). In other cases the muscle fibres may be diffusely scattered throughout the whole tumour to give a histological picture which much more closely approximates to a leiomyoma and so should, more correctly, be regarded as a rhabdo-myoma (Clay and Shorter, 1957). In some tumours the occasional primitive cardiac muscle fibres are present in the centre of these tumours as well as at the periphery, and therefore an origin from primitive undifferentiated mesenchyme, either as a primitive fibroma or rhabdomyofibroma, has been suggested (Bigelow, Klinger and Wright, 1954).

Cardiac tumours made up entirely of fibrous tissue are extremely rare because, with few cases reported, several of these tumours contained interlacing strands of cardiac muscle and have, occasion-ally, been called 'fibrous haematomata' and this has caused some confusion in the histological diagnosis (Svejda and Tomasek, 1960; Parks, Adams and Longmire, 1962).

Van der Hauwaert, Corbell and MacDague (1965) in Louvain, Belgium, described a boy aged 16 months who had signs of severe tricuspid stenosis, with pulsatile liver, anaemia and a white cell count of 80,000 (87 per cent eosinophils). At operation a tumour was found embedded in the wall of the right ventricle, adhering to the tricuspid valve and impossible to remove; he died two days later. The heart weighed 130 g; the tumour was a firm non-capsulated pinkish-white mass like a uterine myoma embedded in the septum and free wall, stenosing the tricuspid orifice. Microscopy showed healthy myocardium interlaced with dense bundles of connective tissue like a myoma.

The author reviewed 29 previously reported cases. This tumour, according to a review by Geha *et al.* (1967) should be suspected in a child with unexplained heart failure or dysarrhythmia, intracardiac calcification, irregular shadow in angiocardiography and recurrent cardiac symptoms or murmurs. Four cases have been diagnosed in life or before operation. Ages of the 36 cases (21 males, 15 females) ranged from newborn to 65 years; 22 were under 2 years of age. Seventeen of 34 had cardiac symptoms and 30 per cent died suddenly; of 32 cases, the tumour was situated in the left ventricle in 22, and in the right ventricle or interventricular septum in 10; it resembled a non-capsulated desmoid.

Electrocardiography in 13 cases showed ventricular hypertrophy and strain, ectopic rhythms, bundle branch block or other conduction defects or 'healed infarction'.

Fibroma of the heart valves, a rare polypoid or papillary tumour, has many features in common with cardiac myxoma, described previously, and may represent the same process of development.

The symptomatology depends on the site of origin and the nature and severity of obstruction caused by the fibroma. Since most fibromas originate in the left ventricle from the interventricular septum, and very rarely from the right ventricle, the signs and symptoms of obstruction relate mostly to the left side of the heart (Nadas and Ellison, 1968).

References

Bigelow, W. H., Klinger, S. and Wright, A. W. (1954). 'Primary tumours of the heart in infancy and early childhood.' *Cancer* **7**, 549

Clay, R. D. and Shorter, R. G. (1957). 'Intra-mural fibroma of the heart.' *J. Path. Bact.* **74**, 163

Freeman, J. A., Greer, J. C., Randall, W. S., Jnr and Palfrey, W. G. (1963). 'Intra-mural fibroma of the heart'. *Am. J. clin. Path.* **39**, 374

Geha, A. S., Wiedman, W. H., Soole, E. H. and McGost, D. C. (1967). 'Intra-mural ventricular cardiac fibroma. Successful removal in two cases and a view of literature.' *Circulation* **36**, 427

James, V. and Stansfield, H. (1955). 'Fibroma of the left ventricle in a child.' *Archs Dis. Childh.* **30**, 187

Kalka, W. (1949). 'Intra-mural fibroma of the heart.' *Am. J. Path.* **25**, 549

Luschka, H. (1855). 'Ein Fibroid im Herzfleische.' *Virchows Arch. path. Anat. Physiol.* **8**, 343

Mahaim, L. (1945). *Les Tumeurs et les Polypes du Coeur. Etude Anatomo-Clinique*, p. 508. Paris: Masson

Nadas, A. S. and Ellison, C. R. (1968). 'Cardiac tumours in infancy.' *Am. J. Cardiol.* **21**, 363

Parks, F. R., Jnr, Adams, F. and Longmire, W. Q. (1962). 'Successful excision of a left ventricular hamartoma: report of a case.' *Circulation* **26**, 1316

Svejda, J. and Tomasek, V. (1960). 'Fibrous hamartoma or so-called fibroma of the myocardium.' *J. Path. Bact.* **80**, 430

Van der Hauwaert, L. G., Corbell, L. and MacDague, P. (1965). 'Fibroma of the right ventricle producing severe tricuspid stenosis.' *Circulation* **32**, 451

LIPOMA

Lipoma tumours are also very infrequent, and when present often show an odd mixture of lipomatous cells with other cell types, so that tumours such as fibrolipomata may be seen (Havier, Siska and Klein, 1956).

Hall, Kissane and Fidler (1955) could find only 33 examples of cardiac lipomata in the literature, to which they added a personal case of a patient who had a myolipoma arising in the right atrium.

Age Incidence

Due to the small number of cases described, one cannot state with any certainty what the age distribution is. Most of the cases described are in the middle and later years of life.

Sex Incidence

No preponderance of either sex in the distribution of this tumour has been noted.

Gross Appearance

These tumours are most frequently seen in the atrium and may achieve a very large size—thus Maurer (1952) described the successful surgical removal of a huge lipoma weighing $3\frac{1}{2}$ lb from the anterior surface of the left ventricle in the heart of a man aged 44 years.

Pearce (1968) successfully excised a lipoma from the right atrium of a woman aged 32; it had caused dyspnoea and heart failure and was diagnosed by angiocardiography. The tumour, which measured $6 \times 4 \times 1\cdot5$ cm in size was within the myocardium and extended into the right ventricle; its endocardial extent was covered by organizing haematoma; the tumour also lay beneath the tricuspid valve annulus which had to be detached temporally to allow excision of the tumour.

Histology

Histologically these tumours are made up of large lipoid filled cells but these may be admixed with cells showing a fibrous tissue origin or with myocytes. In a few tumours, cystic spaces have been seen, so that an endothelial origin may be suggested, as many of these cells resemble lymphangiomatous tissue.

The remaining myocardium in these hearts is normal and does not show an increased infiltration with lipophages nor does it show any signs of fatty infiltration.

References

Havier, V., Siska, K. and Klein, F. (1956). 'A successfully operated cardiac tumour of interesting biological structure.' *Cardiologia* **29**, 132

Hall, H., Kissane, R. W. and Fidler, R. S. (1955). 'Myolipoma of the heart—a case report.' *Expl Med. Surg.* **13**, 300

Maurer, E. R. (1952). 'Successful removal of a tumour of the heart.' *J. thorac. Surg.* **23**, 479

Pearce, C. W. (1968). 'Rare tumours removed from the heart muscle wall.' *Wld Med.* **3**, 53

TERATOMA

Teratoma is another exceedingly rare cardiac tumour. The first report of a cardiac terratoma was that of Joel in 1890, but Williams (1961), while finding some 21 reported cases in the literature, would only accept four as true cardiac teratomata, two of which were malignant. Nine of the reported cases consisted of cystic inclusions of respiratory ccll-type endothelium in the wall of the left ventricle and a further seven occurred in the region of the atrioventricular node causing heart block.

The case reported by Williams (1961) was a male infant who died at 20 days and at autopsy was found to have a tumour filling the right atrium and projecting through the pulmonary valve. The cut surface of the tumour showed numerous thin-walled cysts up to 4 mm in diameter, containing clear mucinous fluid. The capsule was 1 mm thick. All three germ-cell layers could be seen microscopically; the cysts were lined by pseudostratified, ciliated, simple columns of non-keratinized squamous epithelium. Between the cysts there were cartilage, pancreas, embryonic liver tissue and primitive renal tissue. There were no hairs, sebaceous glands or keratinizing squamous epithelium.

Fibrous ventricular tumours, which are apparently fibro-elastic haematomas, are comparatively common, 40 cases having been described (Folger and Peters, 1968). The majority of these tumours are found in children aged 6 years or less, but have been found in patients of all ages.

At autopsy the heart is usually found to be significantly enlarged. These tumours are usually in the myocardium or may increase in size

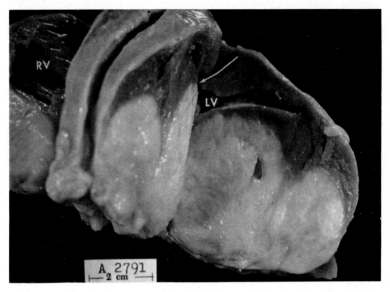

Figure 16.12. Gross appearance of a fibro-elastic tumour (nodular fibroelastosis). The heart is opened from the apex. The tumour is apparent in the interventricular septum, and the entire apex is obliterated. The left ventricle (LV) is compressed to a narrow slit, and distortion of the right ventricle (RV) is also seen. Arrow indicates the left ventricular outflow area. (Reproduced from Folger and Peters (1968) by courtesy of the authors and Editor of the American Journal of Cardiology)

to such an extent that the ventricular cavities may be markedly diminished in size or almost obliterated (*Figure 16.12*).

Microscopically the tumour usually consists of slender cells having pale staining nuclei and often containing eosinophilic granules.

These 'tumours' are not sharply demarcated from the surrounding myocardium, although this is often assumed from an examination of the gross specimen. No capsule separates the 'tumour' from the adjacent myocardium, but the adjacent myocardial fibres often appear atrophied. Death is most commonly sudden.

Detailed histological examination of these tumours often shows multiple areas within the tumour in which the tissue closely resembles that seen lining the endocardial surface in fibro-elastosis, thus suggesting an aetiological relationship between these two conditions (*Figure 16.13*).

Nodular fibro-elastosis is probably a better word to use to describe this condition than fibrous haematoma. The condition probably has

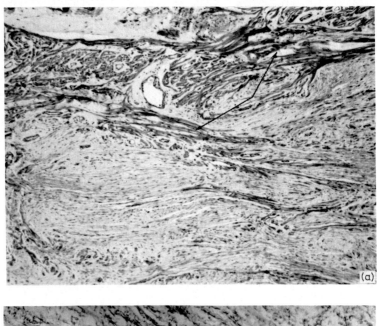

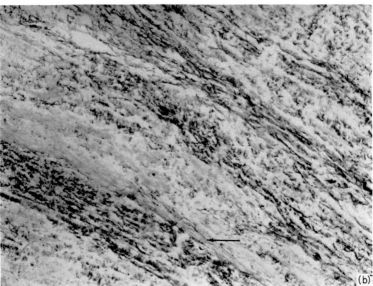

Figure 16.13. Low-power photomicrographs of the tumour. (a) *A fibro-elastic stroma comprises the bulk of the tumour. Arrows indicate myocardial fibres included within the stroma (haematoxylin and eosin × 10, reduced to 4/10).* (b) *The elastic component of the tumour is represented as darkly staining material. Myocardial fibres are seen with the stroma (arrow) (Resorcin and fuchsine stain × 10, reduced to 4/10)*

its origin in the supporting tissue found within the myocardium and is the result of an abnormal proliferation during cardiogenesis.

It is assumed that such hyperplastic connective tissue within the myocardium proliferates with the developing myocardial fibres in the embryonic heart and ceases with cessation of myocardial fibre growth. Examples of this process may be found in the cardiac 'fibromas' which are occasionally seen in the myocardium in the elderly (Naeve, 1955).

References

Folger, G. M. and Peters, H. J. (1968). 'Nodular fibro-elastosis (fibro-elastic hamatoma). A tumorous malformation of the heart.' *Am. J. Cardiol.* **21**, 420

Joel, J. (1890). 'Ein Teratom aus der arteriea Palmonalie annerhalb der Acarzbeutek.' *Virchows. Arch. path. Anat. Physiol.* **122**, 38

Naeve, W. (1955). 'Ploetzlicher Tod eines saenglings bei fibro-elastose Harmartie des Myokards (Sogor Herzfibrom).' *Kinderärztl. Prax.* **23**, 304

Williams, G. E. G. (1961). 'Teratoma of the heart.' *J. Path. Bact.* **82**, 281

MESOTHELIOMA

Mesothelioma is a rarely encountered tumour, involving a part or parts of the conduction system, particularly the atrioventricular node. This tumour is referred to by a variety of different names; lymphangioma (Lloyd, 1929; Perry and Rogers, 1934), mesothelioma (Mahaim, 1942), lymphangitis, epithelial inclusions or developmental heterologia (Rabson and Thill, 1948; Morris and Johnson, 1964; Willis, 1968).

Other writers have included it with cysts of the interatrial septum which are of entodermal origin and, thus, its incidence and histogenesis have been obscured (Marshall, 1957).

Macroscopic Findings

This tumour is commonly found as a small grey, firm, poorly-defined nodule in the myocardium in some areas associated with part of the conduction system, such as the atrioventricular node or bundle of His. This tumour is distinctly different from the surrounding red muscle and yellow adipose tissue.

Microscopic Findings

Microscopically, this tumour seems usually to be confined to a particular part of the conduction system such as the atrioventricular node. If, however, the entire conduction system is examined in any heart where a mesothelioma has been found, additional involvement of other parts of the conduction system is also seen in about a third of the cases.

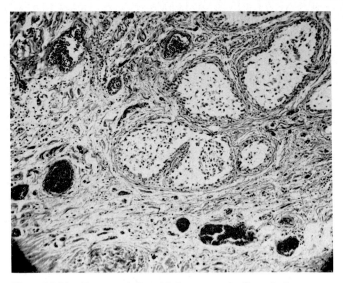

*Figure 16.14.   Tumour tubules with desquamated cells in the lumen, i.e.,
in a fibrovascular stoma containing lymphocytes (haematoxylin and eosin
× 150, reduced to 6/10) (Fine and Morales, 1971)*

These tumours are commonly composed of varying layers of tubules, lined by a single layer or multiple layers of cuboidal cells, some of which are desquamated into the lumen (*Figure 16.14*). Homogeneous eosinophilic material frequently occupies part of the lumen of some tubules and, occasionally, small irregular foci of calcification are also present. Squamous cell transformation in the lining cells of the tubules varies from simple squamous to stratified squamous type with intercellular bridges and keratinization (*Figures 16.15* and *16.16*)

Fibrous tissue and lymphocytes are distributed irregularly throughout the area involved by the tumour. The inner aspect of the tubule is often sharply outlined by a distinct radially arranged layer of cells having a moderate amount of slightly eosinophilic cytoplasm. In a number of tubules the cells peripheral to the inner cell layer lose their alignment and often appear as piled up nuclei with little visible cytoplasm (*Figures 16.17* and *16.18*). No cilia may be seen. Elastic tissue fibres are scattered haphazardly throughout the tumour although they often appear as discrete bands around many of the tubules. Reticulin fibres are also commonly seen scattered throughout the tumours as are mast cells.

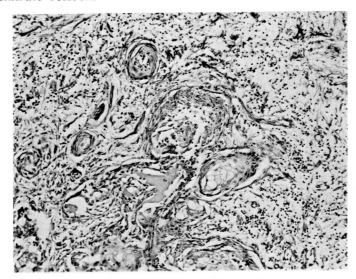

Figure 16.15. Squamous metaplasia of tubular epithelium has reached the stage of keratinization with pearl formation in this area (haematoxylin and eosin × 150) (Fine and Morales, 1971)

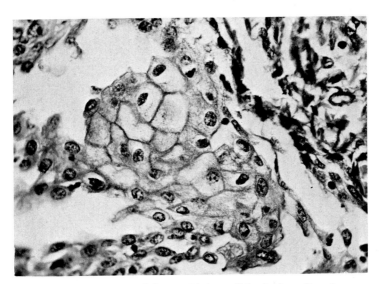

Figure 16.16. Squamous epithelioma with intercellular bridges. Cytoplasm contains diastase-digestible polysaccharides but no vacuoles to suggest lipoid can be seen (haematoxylin and eosin × 600) (Fine and Morales, 1971)

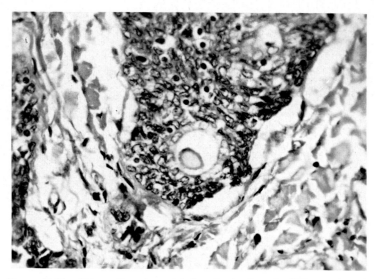

Figure 16.17.   This section shows tubules, the lamina of which contain poly-saccharides (haematoxylin and eosin × 600) (Fine and Morales, 1971)

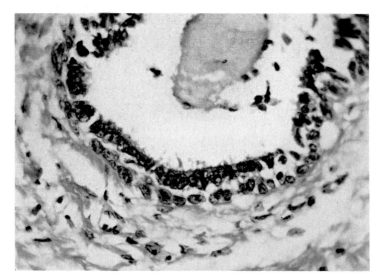

Figure 16.18.   A higher magnification of part of Figure 16.17, *showing that the tubules consist of two layers (haematoxylin and eosin × 600) (Fine and Morales, 1971)*

Clinical Presentation

Clinical presentation is varied and these tumours are often asymptomatic. Sometimes syncope or heart failure both occur or, infrequently, it produces partial or complete heart block.

Histogenesis of the Tumour

The mesothelial-cell derivation, suggested by Mahaim (1942) has an embryological, as well as a histochemical and histological basis. The intimate association of the epicardial cells (cells of the myo-epicardial mantle) to the atrioventricular node begins in the embryo and the similarity in morphology and staining reactions, using the PAS stain, between these tumours and mesotheliomas of other serosal surfaces supports this concept (Fisher and Hellstrom, 1960).

Additional support for a mesothelial cell origin of these tumours is the study of Fine, James and Morales (1971) of a large tumour, limited to the area of the tricuspid valve which was found to be identical to the mixed tubular and fibrous mesotheliomas of the pleura and peritoneum (Fine and Morales, 1971).

References

Fine, G. and Morales, A. R. (1971). 'Mesothelioma of the atrioventricular node.' *Archs Path.* **92**, 402
— James, T. and Morales, A. R. (1971). 'Mesothelioma of the atrioventricular node.' *Archs Path.* **92**, 402
Fisher, E. R. and Hellstrom, H. R. (1960). 'The periodic acid Schiff reaction as an acid in the classification of mesothelioma.' *Cancer* **13**, 837
Lloyd, P. C. (1929). 'Heart block due to primary lymphangio-endothelioma of the atrio-ventricular node.' *Bull. Johns Hopkins Hosp.* **44**, 149
Mahaim, I. (1942). 'Le coelothéliome tawarien bênin: Un tumeur sui generis du noeud du tawara avec bloc du coeur.' *Cardiologia* **6**, 57
Marshall, F. C. (1957). 'Epithelial cyst of the heart.' *Archs Path.* **64**, 107
Morris, A. W. and Johnson, I. M. (1964). 'Epithelial inclusion cysts of the heart. A case report and review of the literature.' *Archs Path.* **77**, 36
Perry, C. B. and Rogers, H. (1934). 'Lymphangioendothelioma of the heart causing complete heart block.' *J. Path. Bact.* **39**, 281
Rabson, S. M. and Thill, L. J. (1948). 'Epithelium-like inclusions in the heart.' *Am. J. Path.* **24**, 655
Willis, R. A. (1968). 'Some unusual heterotopias.' *Br. med. J.* **3**, 267

MALIGNANT PRIMARY CARDIAC TUMOURS

MALIGNANT PRIMARY SARCOMA

In the past, sarcomas primarily involving the endocardium and myocardium have been variously classified as giant-cell, round-cell, spindle-cell, polymorphous cell and fibromyxosarcoma.

A more precise classification of prognostic and therapeutic import has virtually eliminated the old descriptive terms from the more recent literature. However, in view of different histological criteria employed by various authors, it is impossible to determine the number of tumours in each category; what might indicate rhabdomyosarcoma to one author may indicate a fibrosarcoma of indetermined type to other workers.

Incidence and Location

Approximately 200 primary sarcomas of the myocardium have been reported: 178 prior to 1960 (Somers and Lothe, 1960). Although found in patients of all ages, they occurred in men more frequently than women (97 to 67 cases) and most often during the third and fifth decades. The right side of the heart is more frequently involved than the left (95 to 48 cases). The right atrium, left atrium, right ventricle and left ventricle are affected in that order of frequency.

Clinical Presentation

The signs and symptoms have been varied, and in rare instances totally absent, even in patients with large tumours. The most frequent manifestations are intractable heart failure, superior vena cava syndrome, dry cough, precardial pain, haemopericardium (in 25 per cent of the cases) and cardiomegaly. Ball valve obstruction of the mitral and tricuspid valves and chylous hydrothorax were less often seen. Some primary sarcomas have caused sudden death both in patients with and in those without previous symptoms.

Pathology

Almost invariably the myocardium of one or more chambers is infiltrated; a number of these tumours are polypoid, projecting into a cardiac chamber (*Figure 16.19*) and malignant vascular tumours are especially prone to infiltrate the epicardium. Metastases occur in the majority of cases for which descriptive details are available. The lungs, thoracic lymph nodes, and mediastinum are most frequently involved, the liver, kidneys, adrenals, pancreas, bone, spleen, and bowel less often. Round-cell, spindle-cell and polymorphous-cell sarcomas were the diagnoses rendered in 58 of 178 myocardial sarcomas reviewed in the period from 1865 to 1960. While a definite classification of a sarcoma is not always possible, it seems highly probable that many of the tumours so labelled would be classified today as rhabdomyosarcoma, malignant haemangio-endothelioma or malignant lymphoma.

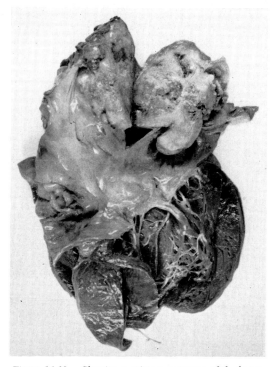

Figure 16.19. Showing a primary sarcoma of the heart. The tumour is seen bulging into the left atrium. (Reproduced from Gudsonsdottir and Hagerstrand (1971) by courtesy of the authors and Editor of Acta pathologica et microbiologica scandinavica)

Course and Prognosis

The interval between the onset of symptoms and death, although varying from a few weeks to several years, is usually very short. The infiltrative growth and ability of the sarcoma to metastasize render its prognosis grave; early diagnoses of the polypoid intraluminal sarcomas offer the only real hope of successful treatment.

FIBROSARCOMA

Incidence and Location

Sixteen of the 178 myocardial sarcomas collected prior to 1960 were recorded as fibrosarcomas and, since then, sporadic cases have been reported (Becker *et al.*, 1961; Cayley and Bisapur, 1963;

Johnson and Stokes, 1964). Among 19 patients, the ages varied from 9 months to 75 years, and the incidence was approximately the same for both sexes. The sites of origin for these tumours were the right atrium (9) and the left atrium (6), and the left and right ventricles, and the intraventricular septum in one instance each. Also in one instance both the right atrium and the right ventricle were involved and therefore a definite origin could not be demonstrated.

Pathological Changes

The growths usually were infiltrative but three were polypoid. Haemopericardium was present in five cases and hydropericardium in two. One tumour was diagnosed clinically but was inoperable (Johnson and Stokes, 1964). Eight tumours metastasized, five to the lungs and three each to the lymph nodes and bone. Other metastatic sites included the liver, mediastinum and soft tissues of the buttocks.

Evaluation

Although the occurrence of fibrosarcoma of the heart is undisputed, its true incidence is difficult to determine since a number of the reported cases appear to be fibromas as judged from the published gross and microscopic photographs (Fidler, Kissane and Koons, 1937; and Jackson and Jacobson, 1939).

RHABDOMYOSARCOMA

Incidence and Location

To the 24 rhabdomyosarcomas among the 178 cardiac sarcomas reported previous to 1960, at least 7 new cases have been added. The age of the 30 patients ranged from 3 months to 80 years (Porter, Berroth and Bristow, 1961). Twenty of the 30 patients for whom data were available were in the 4th to 8th decades, 17 were males and 19 were females.

The right side of the heart was involved more often than the left (14–8); in 5 instances both sides were involved. The right atrium, left atrium, right ventricle and left ventricle were affected in that order of frequency.

Signs and Symptoms

The signs and symptoms of rhabdomyomas were similar to those for sarcoma in general. Among 22 rhabdomyomas patients with available pertinent information, pericardial effusions were present in 11, and, of these cases, was grossly bloody in 8.

Pathology

As a rule the myocardium is infiltrated but occasionally a polypoid tumour projects into the cardiac chamber and produces valvular obstruction. The consistency of the tumour varies with the degree of cellularity and the type of stroma. A polypoid tumour that is abundant and mucoid may resemble the botryoid rhabdomyosarcoma and thus closely resemble a cardiac myxoma (Fine, 1970).

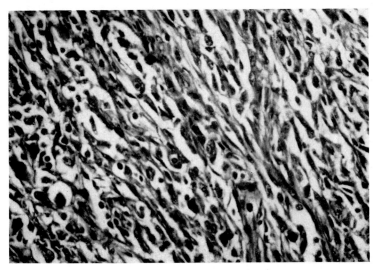

Figure 16.20.   Rhabdomyosarcoma showing the tumour consisting of polymorphic spindle cells (haematoxylin and eosin × 300, reduced to 2/3). (Reproduced from Gudsonsdottir and Hagerstrand (1971) by courtesy of the authors and Editor of Acta pathologica et microbiologica scandinavica)

Microscopically, these tumours manifest various patterns of growth of extra-cardiac rhabdomyosarcoma—pleomorphic, embryomal or alveolar. In addition to cross striations which constitute unequivocal evidence of tumour origin, hallmarks for the diagnoses of rhabdomyosarcoma are the presence of cells with abundant unipolar or bipolar eosinophilic cytoplasm and 'spider cells' containing a fine reticulated web-like clear cytoplasm (*Figure 16.20*). The eosinophilic cells may be arranged in tandem, in patterns reminiscent of muscle, either singly or in small groups, and are characterized by unipolar, streaming cytoplasm, so called 'strap' or 'tennis racket' cells. The 'spider cells' may be associated with areas of round cell or polygonal cells having varying amounts of eosinophilic clear or vacuolated cytoplasm. Special stains may be helpful in the diagnosis of rhabdomyosarcoma. A variable amount of glycogen can be demonstrated especially in the 'spider cells' by using the PAS stain with and without previous diastase digestion. Trichrome and PTAH stains may be useful in demonstrating cross striations or longitudinal cytoplasmic fibrils. In contrast with fibrosarcoma collagen and reticulin are scarce.

Metastases

Data regarding 27 cases indicate dissemination of the tumour in 24 of these. Sites of metastases are lungs in 12, lymph nodes in 6, liver in 8, bone, kidney, small intestine, pleura in 4 cases, adrenal gland, pancreas, brain, lungs, myocardium in 3 cases each, thyroid in 2, omentum, breast, uterus, ovary, stomach, thymus, diaphragm, carotid gland, pulmonary vein and pulmonary artery in 1 case each.

Evaluation

The variable histological appearance and the failure to detect cross striations have undoubtedly resulted in the erroneous classification of some rhabdomyoma as other types of sarcoma. Whether the demonstration of striations is essential for the diagnosis of rhabdomyosarcoma is controversial. Since we know that cross striations may be associated with certain patterns of neoplastic growth, it seems that identical patterns should permit recognition of rhabdomyosarcoma in the absence of striations. The need for other means of identification of rhabdomyosarcoma was acknowledged years ago by McCallum when he so aptly said: 'Since the criteria demanded before an origin from muscular tissue will be admitted is the demonstration of characteristic cross striations, it is not at all improbable, indeed it is almost certain, that many tumours truly of such origin are not recognised as such, and are relegated to the tumour scrapheap of sarcoma'.

NEUROSARCOMA

Primary neurosarcoma of the heart is very rare. Yanguas (1955) reviewed the literature of primary heart tumours and reported an example of a neurosarcoma appearing as a mass in the left chest. Although the intraventricular septum and both atria were invaded, there were no cardiovascular symptoms or signs.

RETICULOSARCOMA

Reticulosarcoma of an infant heart was reported by Gillet and Parmentier (1953).

References

Becker, K. L., Gross, J. B., Dearing, W. H., Parkin, T. W. and Sayre, G. P. (1961). 'Fibrosarcoma of the heart masquerading clinically as a malignant tumour of the stomach or pancreas. Report of a case.' *Gastroenterology* **41**, 585

Cayley, F. E. and Bisapur, H. I. (1963). 'Fibrosarcoma of the left atrium.' *Br. med. J.* **3**, 1134

Fidler, R. S., Kissane, R. W. and Koons, R. A. (1937). 'Primary fibrosarcoma of the heart.' *Am. Heart J.* **13**, 736

Fine, G. (1970). 'Neoplasms of the pericardium and heart.' In *Pathology of the Heart and Blood Vessels*. Ed. by S. E. Gould, Chapter XIX, p. 870. Springfield, Ill: Thomas

Gillet, P. and Parmentier, R. (1953). 'Reticulosarcoma a depart cardiaque chez un enfant de seize mois.' *Acta paediat. belg.* **7**, 27

Gudsonsdottir, A. and Hagerstrand, I. (1971). 'Primary sarcoma of the heart.' *Acta path. microbiol. scand.* **79**, 604

Jackson, M. N. and Jacobson, J. G. (1939). 'Primary fibrosarcoma of the heart—report of a case.' *Lancet* **2**, 740

Johnson, A. G. and Stokes, J. F. (1964). 'Fibrosarcoma of the heart diagnosed during life.' *Br. med. J.* **1**, 480

Porter, G. A., Berroth, M. and Bristow, J. D. (1961). 'Primary rhabdomyosarcoma of the heart and complete atrio-ventricular block. A case report and review of the literature.' *Am. J. Med.* **31**, 820

Somers, K. and Lothe, F. (1960). 'Primary lymphosarcoma of the heart— Review of the literature and report of three cases.' *Cancer* **13**, 449

Yanguas, M. G. (1955). 'Primary neurosarcoma of the heart.' *Am. J. Roentg.* **73**, 590

RETICULUM CELL SARCOMA AND LYMPHOSARCOMA

Primary reticulum cell sarcoma of the heart is one of the most frequently found varieties of this rare disease.

The term 'reticulum-cell sarcoma' is applied to these tumours because many of the cells morphologically resemble reticulum cells and are associated with fine reticulum fibres. However, because reticulum fibres are not uniformly present in close association with these cells, it may be called, by some, a lymphoblastic cell lymphosarcoma.

Deposits of lymphosarcoma may similarly be found in the heart, being either primary or due to direct extension of the tumour from adjacent lymph glands—as, for instance, the para-aortic glands.

The tumour may be found at any age, reported cases having occurred in patients aged between 3 days (Schink, 1941) and 84 years (Brucker and Glassy, 1955).

About 35 per cent of cases are found at autopsy to have a haemorrhagic pericardial effusion.

Microscopically, nodules of tumour may be found only in the heart, where the primary growth is commonly situated at its base. The deposits of lymphosarcomatous tissue are often haemorrhagic and may be found within the myocardium but are often found projecting through the endocardium or pericardium. In other cases deposits of reticulum cell sarcoma are seen in other organs such as

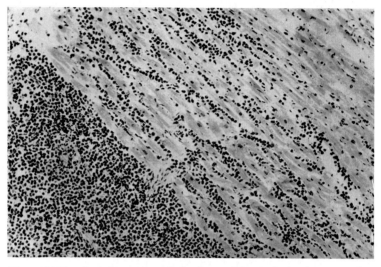

Figure 16.21. Lymphosarcoma of the heart. Metastasis in the myocardium showing that there is no clear line of demarcation between the lymphomatous deposit and the surrounding myocardium (haematoxylin and eosin × 240, reduced to 2/3)

lung, liver or intestine. It is not, in these cases, possible to say if the tumour originated primarily in the myocardium or is only a metastatic deposit.

The deposits of lymphosarcoma in the heart are found not commonly in the ventricles and usually appear, macroscopically, to be clearly separated from the surrounding myocardium. However, microscopically, it can be seen that this is not so. Although in most places the lymphoma cells are quite distinct from the surrounding tissue, there are some places where they seem to spill over into the myocardium and interstitial tissue (*Figure 16.21*).

Other types of lymphosarcoma may also involve the heart, as, for example, the three cases of Burkitt's tumour (malignant lymphoma) described by Somers and Lothe (1960). In all these cases, however, the authors were uncertain whether these tumours first originated in the heart.

References

Brucker, E. A., Jnr and Glassy, F. J. (1955). 'Primary reticulum-cell sarcoma of the heart with review of the literature.' *Cancer* **8**, 921

Schink, W. (1941). 'Über primare Herztumoren. Ein Beitrag zur Pathologie derselben.' *Virchows Arch. path. Anat. Physiol.* **307**, 20

Somers, K. and Lothe, F. (1960). 'Primary lymphosarcoma of the heart— Review of the literature and report of three cases.' *Cancer* **13**, 449

ANGIOSARCOMA

Angiosarcoma is a particularly uncommon tumour, the first detailed report being that of Hewer and Kemp, who in 1936 reported a patient with malignant haemangio-endothelioma of the heart. This tumour has also been described as malignant angio-endothelioma and angioreticulo-endothelioma. Mahaim's (1945) series of 87 sarcomata (from 329 primary heart tumours) included three examples of angiosarcoma—the first being that of Mennig in 1888. It is thought that these tumours arise from angioblasts, normally dormant in the myocardium. McClane (1921) said that primitive mesenchymal tissue in any part of the body could produce angioblasts and Tacket, Jones and Kyle (1950) considered that the origin of primary cardiac tumours from the septal areas of the heart was related to these being the situations where structures were finally completed.

Stout (1943) said that the criteria of angiosarcoma were the occurrence of atypical endothelial cells in excess, thus forming anastomotic channels, the cells being polygonal to spindle-shaped, in a single layer, heaped in the lumen or in sheets outside the vascular channels.

Harris (1960) added one case to the 16 she found in the literature and from these reports the following conclusions may be drawn. The ages of these patients varied from 18 to 32 years, and the majority (13) arose in the right atrium, while the remaining 3 arose from the left atrium, the tricuspid valve and the right ventricle respectively.

At autopsy the heart is found to be enlarged (*Figure 16.22*) and may weigh 600–700 g or more. The cut surface of the tumour is purplish and haemorrhagic, often with white specks (*Figure 16.23*). Histology shows variously sized blood-filled spaces forming ill-defined vascular channels; the larger sinuses show marked proliferation of the endothelial lining cells and they are surrounded by small, thick-walled capillaries. The endothelial cells vary in size and shape, have pale eosinophilic cytoplasm, hyperchromatic nuclei with a fine network of chromatin and a few small indistinct nucleoli, while

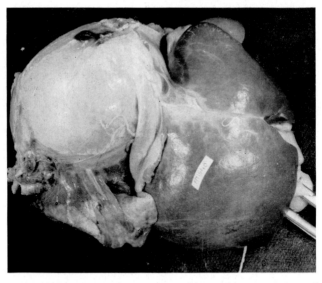

Figure 16.22. External appearance of heart showing gross atrial distension caused by cardiac angiosarcoma

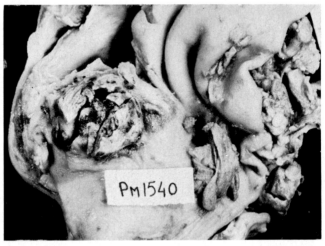

Figure 16.23. The right atrium opened. The necrotic haemorrhagic tumour occupies the whole of the right appendage and protrudes into the atrial cavity (Aikat and Nirodi, 1971)

mitoses are usually frequent. Areas of necrosis and haemorrhage were also seen. In other areas the capillaries had thick walls composed of concentric layers of plump rounded pericytes. The angiomatous nature of the tumour is usually clearly demonstrated by its being largely composed of plump spindle cells, which have proliferated to a marked degree (*Figure 16.24*). Reticulin stains will often clearly demonstrate that the tumour is formed of endothelium containing many vascular spaces (*Figure 16.25*). These tumours often metastasize to the lungs and liver.

McNalley *et al.* (1963) reviewed 14 cases, only 4 of which were diagnosed in life; the tumour occurred in the right atrium in 13 and in the left atrium in 1; in 4 no metastasis occurred.

Svejda *et al.* (1966) of Brno, Czechoslovakia, described an example of this rare tumour, variously known as malignant endothelioma, angiosarcoma or haemangio-endothelioblastoma. The patient was a 46 year old man who had had recurrent heart failure, first degree heart block, ESR 31 mm/hr and blood stained pericardial effusion. Later, despite antibiotic therapy, thrombophlebitis and oedema of both legs with gangrene of the right foot occurred and he died in six weeks. The heart weighed 720 g and the right atrium contained a tumour 6 × 5 × 4 cm in size, which was nodular, red, white and yellow and attached to the anterior septum which it had penetrated. Nodules were also present in a mediastinal node in both lungs and in the liver.

Microscopy showed small elongated, or spindle cells with dark nodes in fascicular or elongated pattern; tortuous blood channels lined with endothelial cells were present and there were dense fibrous bundles between the capillaries. The tumour cells infiltrated the myocardium.

The authors remarked that this was the first to be seen in Brno among 30,202 necropsies in 12 years. The usual presentation is an obstruction of the superior vena cava, as cardiomegaly or as pleural effusion.

Dissemination of this tumour is usually restricted to the pericardium and lungs, the latter being involved by embolism from the right atrium. In the case reported by Svejda *et al.* (1966) there were pulmonary secondaries that resembled haemorrhagic infarcts and also lymph node and hepatic metastases. Of the 14 cases of McNalley *et al.* (1963) only 4 had not metastasized. In a further report of angiosarcoma of the heart, Aikat and Nirodi (1971) described a case with secondary deposits in the lungs (*Figure 16.26*) which were haemorrhagic and partially or completely necrotic. Many tumour emboli, both viable and necrotic, were also found in branches of the pulmonary artery (*Figure 16.27*).

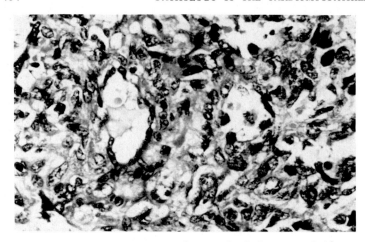

Figure 16.24.   Angiomatous nature of tumour clearly demonstrated with pro-liferation of plump spindle cells (haematoxylin and eosin × 120, reduced to 8/10) (Aikat and Nirodi, 1971)

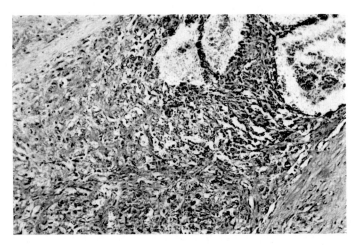

Figure 16.25.   Reticulum preparation and sharp outlining of the vascular channels (× 120, reduced to 8/10)

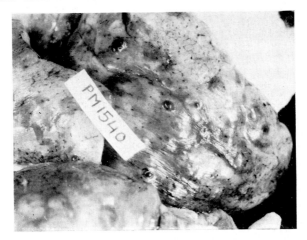

*Figure 16.23. Multiple haemorrhagic subpleural nodules in
the lung (× 2, reduced to 2/3) (Aikat and Nirodi, 1971)*

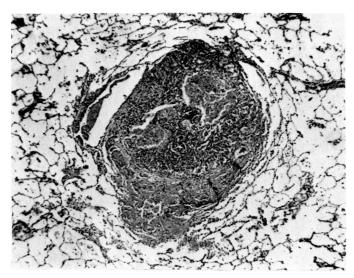

*Figure 16.27. Intravascular metastasis in the lung (haematoxylin and
eosin × 60) (Aikat and Nirodi, 1971)*

In their report of 14 cases, McNalley *et al.* (1963) noted that the tumour was located in the right atrium in 13 cases and in the left atrium in only one case. In the case reports of both Svejda *et al.* (1966) and Aikat and Nirodi (1971) a right atrial origin was similarly noted, but no reason is known for this location.

The tumour is largely haemorrhagic and necrotic. It is usually found to be invading the atrial myocardium and is partially covered by thrombus where it projects into the right atrial cavity, where usually it is characterized by the formation of vascular channels associated with a proliferation of plump spindle cells, which are hyperchromatic and display a moderate degree of mitotic activity.

The angioblastic features of the tumour are well shown with anastomotic channels lined by one or more layers of atypical endothelium. A reticulin stain demonstrates the highly vascular structure of the tumour. In other areas the cells are arranged in solid masses but still with vasoformative tendencies.

A chest x-ray usually reveals cardiomegaly and a pleural effusion but lack of other findings makes diagnosis during life extremely difficult.

References

Aikat, B. K. and Nirodi, N. S. (1971). 'Angio-sarcoma of the heart.' *J. Path. Bact.* **104**, 73

Harris, Hilda R. (1960). 'Angiosarcoma of the heart.' *J. clin. Path.* **13**, 205

Hewer, T. F. and Kemp, R. P. (1936). 'Malignant haemangio-endothelioma of the heart; report of a case.' *J. Path. Bact.* **43**, 511

McClane, C. F. W. (1921). 'The endothelial problem.' *Anat. Rec.* **22**, 219

McNalley, M. C., Kelble, D., Pryor, R. and Blount, S. G., Jnr (1963). 'Angiosarcoma of the heart. Report of a case and review of the literature.' *Am. Heart J.* **65**, 244

Mahaim, I. (1945). *Les Tumeurs et les Polypes de Coeur.* Paris: Masson

Mennig (1888). 'Primarem sarkom des Herzens.' *Dt. med. Wschr.* **14**, 1073

Stout, A. P. (1943). 'Haemangio-endothelioma: a tumour of blood vessels featuring vascular endothelial cells.' *Ann. Surg.* **118**, 445

Svejda, J., Dvorak, R., Melichar, F. and Jedlicka, V. (1966). 'Primary malignant haemangioma of the heart.' *J. Path. Bact.* **92**, 564

Tacket, H. S., Jones, R. S. and Kyle, J. W. (1950). 'Primary angiosarcoma of the heart.' *Am. Heart J.* **39**, 912

KAPOSI'S IDIOPATHIC HAEMORRHAGIC SARCOMA

Kaposi's idiopathic haemorrhagic sarcoma, sometimes known as a haemangiosarcoma, usually presents itself as skin nodules, most commonly seen in lower limbs and later spreading to the trunk, upper limbs and viscera. The disease was said originally to be most commonly found among Jews but more than half the cases of this disease in the world literature come from Africa and are in Negroes. It is also frequently associated with cases of malignant reticuloses or lymphosarcoma (Allen, 1957).

The heart has been found to be involved in 19 reported cases and involvement occurs in a similar proportion in all racial groups. The lesion, however, has been restricted to primary involvement of the myocardium in only six cases (Epstein, 1957; Tedeschi, 1958; Templeton, 1972). In all other cases with cardiac involvement the pericardium has been involved first, and only later is the myocardium involved by direct extension of the tumour into the myocardium. The patient reported by Tedeschi (1958) died as a result of myocardial involvement but in all other cases no clinically detectable disease was produced by these deposits. The findings in the heart in cases with pericardial involvement are illustrated by the following three case reports.

Choisser and Ramsey (1939 and 1940) described 2 cases in which the lesions were located in the heart but not in the skin; death occurred from tamponade and proliferative lesions were found in the right atrium, spreading to the myocardium and pericardium. Gelfand (1957) described a 38 year old African (Negro) who died from congestive heart failure and, at autopsy, the whole heart was found to be covered with raspberry like tumours of varying sizes and shapes, from 6 to 18 mm in diameter (*Figure 16.28*). These tumours invaded the outer quarter of the myocardium but the endocardium was left intact.

It is possible that other heart tumours which have been previously diagnosed as angiosarcomas are, in fact, Kaposi's sarcoma. Histologically Kaposi's sarcoma shows small newly-formed blood vessels with walls consisting of a layer of spindle cells on a reticular base; but, in other places, these blood sinuses may be filled with blood. Small foci of lymphocytes and polymorphs are usually present and there are more solid parts of the tumour with proliferative spindle cells, differing in size and arrangement, some large and some small and all with hyperchromatic nuclei and a few undergoing mitosis (*Figure 16.29*). Although Kaposi's sarcoma as a cause of heart failure is very uncommon, it should be remembered as a possibility in a male African when the aetiology is not immediately obvious.

Kaposi's sarcoma is a lesion, generally considered a form of angiosarcoma, which occurs most commonly in the fifth to seventh decades. It occurs less commonly in children. It is also rare in females (6 per cent of the 434 collected cases in the study of Choisser and Ramsey (1967)) but since it seems to show a predilection for

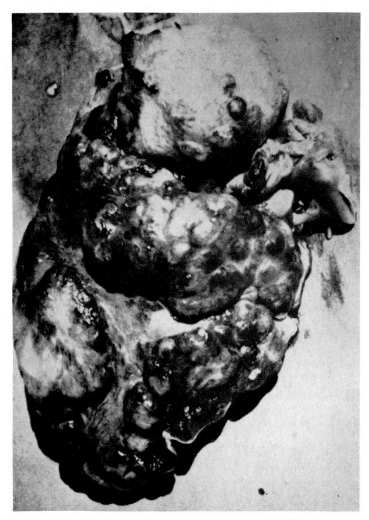

Figure 16.28.   Heart of a 38 year old African male who died of congestive heart failure. Deposit of Kaposi's sarcoma present over the whole of the epicardial surface of the myocardium which was invaded to about a quarter of its depth. (Reproduced from Gelfand (1957) by courtesy of the author and Editor of the British Heart Journal)

labourers and outside workers this sex difference may be an occupational one. This disease most commonly arises on the skin of the lower extremities as red marks or papules of no characteristic shape. The lesions slowly spread proximally; eventually, in many cases, visceral metastasis leads to death. The gastro-intestinal tract, liver, lungs, spleen and lymph nodes are the most common sites of

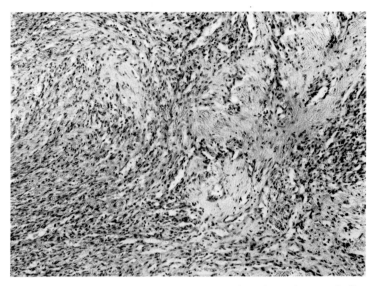

Figure 16.29. Showing a section of myocardium where the cardiac muscle fibres have been largely replaced by the spindle cells of Kaposi's sarcomas. This section also contains a few remaining muscle fibres surrounded by areas of fibrosis (haematoxylin and eosin × 80, reduced to 2/3). (Reproduced by courtesy of Dr A. Templeton)

metastasis and gastro-intestinal bleeding is perhaps the most common cause of death. The majority of patients showing massive visceral involvement were found to have large tumours of the cardiac atria and, in many of these cases, involvement of other organs was minimal.

Visceral primary lesions with late or with no skin involvement have been reported. Since, as will be discussed, the tumour can simulate sarcomas of other types, the actual nature of many of these reported tumours is doubtful.

On other occasions the Kaposi sarcoma may have a long-standing history and appear to have reached a chronic stage. Thus in one of the patients described by Ager, Paul and Capps (1962), a 59 year old white female who had had cutaneous manifestations of the disease for 11 years showed at autopsy widespread nodules in the gastro-intestinal tract. In addition a massive tumour was found in the left atrium which appeared similar in all respects to those reported by other workers.

With time the skin lesions tend to progress from red or mottled red-grey to yellow, white or brown. Microscopically early lesions most commonly suggest capillary or cavernous haemangioma, with intervascular proliferation of spindle-shaped tumour cells, varying degrees of inflammatory reaction (lymphocytes, macrophages, eosinophils and rather rarely neutrophils), and varying amounts of collagenous or myxoid stroma. Infiltration of adjoining tissue is usual but is not of diagnostic value since many benign haemangiomata are also interspersed throughout the involved tissue. Older lesions show progression to greater degrees of cellular proliferation and fibrosis with progressive obliteration of the vascular channels, the end stage of this process resembling fibrosarcoma or neurosarcoma. Sponta-neous haemorrhage with accumulation of haemosiderin in macro-phages is common in the earlier stages and is partly responsible for the colour of the lesions described. Different stages of this process often occur in the same lesion as well as in different lesions in the same patient.

This variation in microscopic appearance, with resultant difference of opinion as to the basic nature of the lesion and the basic cell type, is responsible for the extensive synonomy; thus one paper (Choisser and Ramsey, 1939) lists 28 synonyms for Kaposi's sarcoma. Some of these cardiac tumours may represent a particularly aggressive form of Kaposi's sarcoma, although in some cases these have probably been confused with other entities which are histologically similar.

Whether Kaposi's sarcoma is truly a malignant tumour and, if so, whether it is a well-vascularized fibrosarcoma or a sclerosing angio-sarcoma remain to be established.

It used to be thought that Kaposi's sarcoma was not common in children, but the paper by Slavin and Cameron (1967) gave a comprehensive account of this disease, including 2 necropsies, as seen in 51 Negro children in Uganda and Tanzania; the manifestations differed from those in adults in that skin lesions were few and atypical, the dominant features being polyadenopathy and ocular lesions.

Lee (1968) in Uganda compared the biopsy skin lesions in 91 patients with Kaposi's sarcoma with those of 47 with granuloma pyogenicum. Both conditions were common. Kaposi's sarcoma affected adult males and contained a sarcomatous element; it progressed slowly without regression. The tissue was vascoformative, comprising intertwining bundles or sheaves of spindle cells and vascular spaces. There was a lobulated appearance, cells radiating from a central 'arteriole' as 'rays of a sunburst', and intracytoplasmic inclusions (resembling erythrocytes) were also seen. Granuloma pyogenicum affected immature males or females; it developed quickly but was self-limiting. Lee postulated that both diseases were due to the response of vascoformative elements of the skin to a similar stimulus and that hormonal or sex-linked genetic factors determined which lesions developed.

Other workers (McKinney, 1967) have postulated that a virus infection may be the aetiological cause for Kaposi's sarcoma, especially taking into account the fact that it is commonly associated, in the same patient, with tumours of the reticulo-endothelial system, many of which are also thought to have a viral aetiology and that, in places like East Africa, with a high incidence of lymphoma in children, adults appear to be protected from this disease and to develop Kaposi's sarcoma.

This theory, however, needs much more work before it can be thought of as anything but speculation.

References

Ager, J. P., Paul, O. and Capps, R. B. (1962). 'Clinico-pathologic conference.' *Am. Heart J.* **63**, 566

Allen, A. C. (1957). 'The skin (tumours of vessels).' In *Pathology* Ed. by W. A. D. Anderson, 3rd Edition, p. 1172. St. Louis: Mosby

Choisser, R. M. and Ramsay, Elizabeth M. (1939). 'Angioreticuloendothelioma (Kaposi's disease) of the heart.' *Am. J. Path.* **15**, 155

— — (1940). 'Etiology of Kaposi's disease. Preliminary report of investigations.' *Sth. med. J.* **33**, 392

Epstein, E. (1957). 'Extracutaneous manifestations of Kaposi's sarcoma. A systemic lymphoblastoma.' *Calif. Med.* **87**, 98

Gelfand, M. (1957). 'Kaposi's haemangiosarcoma of the heart.' *Br. Heart J.* **19**, 290

Lee, F. D. (1968). 'A comparative study of Kaposi's sarcoma and granuloma pyogenicum.' *J. clin. Path.* **21**, 119

McKinney, B. (1967). 'Kaposi's sarcoma and Burkitt's lymphoma. Report of a case where the two tumours occurred simultaneously.' *E. Afr. med. J.* **44**, 417

Slavin, G. and Cameron, H. McD. (1967). 'Kaposi's sarcoma in African children.' Communication to the Pathological Society of Great Britain and Ireland. January 4–7 London: Pathological Society

Tedeschi, C. G. (1958). 'Some considerations concerning the nature of the so-called sarcoma of Kaposi.' *Archs Path.* **66**, 656

Templeton, A. (1972). 'Kaposi's sarcoma in Uganda—a post mortem study.' *Cancer* **30**, 854

SECONDARY CARDIAC TUMOURS

METASTASES FROM SOLID TUMOURS

Data regarding metastases of tumours to the heart are difficult to assess because of the variability of criteria followed by various authors. Some workers include only gross involvement by the tumours and many do not notice the precise site of the metastases.

The kneeding action and metabolic peculiarities of the myocardium, rapid blood flow and limited lymphatic connections are explanations offered for the low incidence of metastases. The incidence of metastasis of carcinoma and sarcoma to the heart varies, depending upon the type of neoplasm, sampling, as in certain hospitals, admitting a high proportion of referred patients with cancer accounting for a higher reported incidence of sarcoma or carcinoma, as for example, leukaemia, lymphoma, melanoma, or carcinoma of the lung or breast, all of which metastasize frequently to the heart. By the same token inclusion in the reports of sarcoma of a large number of cases of plasma cell myeloma, mycoses fungoides or thymoma tends to lower the apparent incidence of sarcoma.

SITE OF PRIMARY TUMOUR

Almost every variety of malignant neoplasm of various organs and tissue has been reported to metastasize to the heart with the notable exceptions of tumours of intracranial and intraspinous nervous system and parathyroid carcinoma.

The neoplasms that tend to metastasize most frequently to the heart are: (1) carcinoma of the lung and breast (19–35 per cent); (2) melanoma (33–50 per cent); (3) malignant lymphoma (15–37 per cent).

AREA OF THE HEART INVOLVED

Certain tumours such as lymphomas seem to select the myocardium preferentially. The mural endocardium and valvular endocardium are rarely involved, especially when other parts of the heart are free of tumour (Herbert and Maisel, 1942). Metastasis to the region of the AV node has been reported (Mahaim, 1945). As a rule (Herbert and Maisel, 1942) tumour metastasis to the heart is associated with metastasis to other organs. The frequency of involvement of other organs by secondary tumours is greater if the heart is also involved. In the presence of metastases to the heart, organs other than the heart rarely escape involvement.

PATHOLOGY

Metastatic growths usually develop as isolated multiple nodules, rather than as a solitary nodule. Their growth, however, may be diffuse and simulate a diffuse mesothelioma, myocarditis, pericarditis or endocarditis. Endocarditis, as well as interstitial granulomas, may be associated with disseminated carcinoma not necessarily involving the heart (Eger, 1941).

MODE OF SPREAD TO THE HEART

Metastatic growths may reach the heart by way of the blood stream or lymphatic system, by direct extension or by a combination of these routes. Haematogenous and retrograde lymphatic embolization are probably the most frequent methods of spread, but venous invasion and endocardial implantation by way of the venae cavae or pulmonary veins have also been reported (Coller, Inkley and Maragues, 1950; Lam, Webb and Green, 1966).

Signs and symptoms are usually absent even in the presence of extensive involvement.

References

Coller, F. C., Inkley, J. T. and Maragues, V. (1950). 'Neoplastic endocardial implants. Report of a case.' *Am. J. clin. Path.* **20**, 159

Eger, W. (1941). 'Verondeanger, des Myocards und Endocards bei Karzinoum.' *Beitr. path. Anat.* **105**, 219

Herbert, P. A. and Maisel, A. L. (1942). 'Secondary tumours of the heart.' *Archs Path.* **34**, 358

Lam, C. R., Webb, D. and Green, E. (1966). 'Primary liver tumour presenting as a right atrial tumour. A case report.' *Surgery, St. Louis* **59**, 872

Mahaim I. (1945). 'Les Tumeurs et les Polypes du Coeur.' *Etude Anatomo-Clinique Paris* (Masson & Laussanne Rotha, p. 568)

METASTASES CAUSING CONDUCTION DEFECTS

Space-occupying lesions, including both primary and secondary tumours are infrequently the cause of AV conduction defects (Perry and Rogers, 1934; Pieoff and Petenyi, 1970).

It is infrequent, however, for them to cause chronic heart block although this has been recorded (Manion *et al.*, 1971)—the case referred to being a lymphangio-endothelioma which caused AV block lasting for fifteen years, until the patient finally died.

References

Manion, W. G., Nelson, W. P., Hall, R. J. and Brierty, R. E. (1972). 'Benign tumour of the heart causing complete heart block.' *Am. Heart J.* **83**, 535

Perry, C. B. and Rogers, H. (1934). 'Lymphangioendothelioma of the heart causing complete heart block.' *J. Path. Bact.* **39**, 281

Pieoff, R. C. and Petenyi, C. (1970). 'Primary mesothelioma of the atrioventricular node.' *Archs Path.* **89**, 84

LEUKAEMIA

The heart is frequently involved in leukaemias of all types but the incidence given in various series seems very low. This can probably be explained by the care with which the heart has been examined histologically.

Cardiac hypertrophy may accompany leukaemia, the enlargement being attributed, in part, to associated anaemia and, in part, to the increased metabolic rate. Gross and microscopic involvement of the heart in the lymphomas and leukaemias is fairly common. This has been given as 34 per cent of 123 cases in the series reported by Kirshbaum and Preuss (1943) and as 30 per cent in the series of 66 cases reported by Javier *et al.* (1967); while Saphir (1960) found involvement in 36 per cent of cases.

Roberts, Bodey and Wertlake (1967) studied 420 patients at necropsy at the National Heart Institute, Bethesda. The heart wall showed haemorrhages in 132, infiltration in 60 and both in 96. In life, however, clinical involvement was rare; 13 had chest pain (9 had pericarditis) or dyspnoea. Pleural, pericardial or peritoneal effusions occurred, as did oedema and tachycardia.

Sometimes the infiltrate is detectable macroscopically but frequently only histologically. The incidence of cardiac involvement is higher in acute rather than in chronic leukaemia (Kirschbaum and Preuss, 1943).

The pericardium, myocardium and subendocardium are involved in that order of frequency. There is a direct relationship between myocardial infiltrate with leukaemic cells and their numbers in the peripheral blood, a fact also found in other organs. There is, however, no causal relationship between the leucocyte cell count and myocardial involvement. Saphir (1958) has stated that infiltration of the myocardium occurs more frequently with myelocytic than with lymphoblastic leukaemia. Leukaemic infiltrates tend to exhibit a perivascular deposition. Haemorrhages, due to the associated thrombocytopenia are often found, especially beneath or within the endocardium and around small blood vessels.

Although clinical evidence of cardiac involvement may be present in addition to the infiltration by leukaemic cells, the heart frequently shows fatty changes and petechial haemorrhages associated with the accompanying anaemia and thrombocytopenia, and it is possible that some of the cardiac symptoms are the result of degenerative changes.

The extent of the infiltration varies from gross diffuse infiltration to small microscopic collections of leukaemic cells. With the use of cytotoxic drugs leukaemic infiltrations are often not conspicuous at autopsy.

Childhood Leukaemia

The response to therapy for malignancy in adults varies from the response observed in children suffering from the same neoplastic disease (Burchenal et al., 1962). Consequently the course of leukaemia in children will differ from that observed in adults.

Cardiac infiltration by tumour cells in children with leukaemia may be marked by the many manifestations of this disease and is usually an incidental autopsy finding.

In addition to these differences, recent therapeutic advances have markedly altered the natural history of the disease and extended the survival time in children with leukaemia (Saunders, Kauder and Mauer, 1967).

In only one study have the myocardial changes in children with leukaemia been studied specifically (Sumners, Johnson and Ainger, 1969). Other studies such as those of Javier et al. (1967) and Roberts, Bodey and Wertlake (1968) have included children, but no distinction has been made as to myocardial changes in different age groups.

In children post-mortem examinations of the heart reveal that the principal macroscopic changes are cardiomegaly, pericardial effusion and myocardial haemorrhages.

The principal histological findings consist of myocardial leukaemic infiltrate, myofibre damage of varying severity and intramyocardial haemorrhage.

Sumners, Johnson and Ainger (1969) have found a leukaemic cell infiltrate of the myocardium in forty-four per cent of their cases. A significantly higher incidence of cardiac infiltration is found in cases of acute myeloid leukaemia than in acute lymphoblastic leukaemia. The damage to the myofibres includes shrinkage, pyknosis and loss of myofibre nuclei in addition to shrinkage and vacuolation of myofibres.

Apart from *cell type* and the *level of circulating leucocytes*, the third factor which is responsible for myocardial cell involvement is the *survival* time, because the duration of anaemia and consequently the degree of cardiac cell infiltration is roughly equivalent to *survival time*.

The clinical and pathological changes found in *eosinophilic leukaemia* are similar to those described under the title Loeffler's syndrome (Chapter 12).

Bousser (1957) summarized the clinical and pathological findings in 13 patients with eosinophilic leukaemia reported between 1944 and 1956; and Odeberg (1965) summarized the observations in 12 additional necropsy patients with eosinophilic leukaemia reported between 1957 and 1963.

These 25 patients ranged from 7 to 49 years of age (average 32) 18 males and 7 females; all had blood eosinophilia (up to 98 per cent); only 5 patients survived longer than 2 years following the onset of cardiac failure. At necropsy over half the subjects had extensive endomyocardial fibrosis with mural thrombosis; nearly all also had infiltration by mature eosinophils into one or more other organs (usually the liver, kidney or lung).

It seems probable that the eosinophils or some associated breakdown products derived from this cell are able to stimulate the formation of fibrous tissue by the endocardium and underlying myocardium.

References

Bousser, J. (1957). 'Eosinophillie et Leucemie.' *Sang* **28**, 553

Burchenal, J. H., Murphy, M. L., Tan, C. T. and Dargeon, H. D. (1962). 'Chemotherapy of neoplastic disease in children.' *Adv. Pediat.* **12**, 189

Javier, B. V., Young, W. J., Crosby, D. J. and Hall, T. C. (1967). 'Cardiac metastasis in lymphoma and leukemia.' *Dis. Chest.* **52**, 481

Kirschbaum, J. D. and Preuss, F. S. (1943). 'Leukemia. A clinical and pathologic study of one hundred and twenty three cases in a series of 14,400 necropsies.' *Archs intern. Med.* **71**, 777

Odeberg, B. (1965). 'Eosinophilic leukaemia and disseminated eosinophilic collagen disease—a disease entity?' *Acta med. scand.* **177**, 129

Roberts, W. C., Bodey, G. P. and Wertlake, P. T. (1967). 'Heart in acute leukaemia; study of 420 autopsy cases.' *Am. J. Cardiol.* **21**, 388

Saphir, O. (1958). *Systemic Pathology.* Vol. 1, p. 116. New York: Grune and Stratton

— (1960). 'Neoplasms of the pericardium and heart.' In *Pathology of the Heart*, Ed. by S. E. Gould 2nd Edition. Springfield, Ill: Thomas

Saunders, E. F., Kauder, E. and Mauer, A. M. (1967). 'Sequential therapy of acute leukemia in childhood.' *J. Pediat.* **70**, 632

Sumners, J. E., Johnson, W. W. and Ainger, L. E. (1969). 'Childhood leukaemic heart disease. A study of 116 hearts of children dying of leukaemia.' *Circulation* **40**, 575

Seventeen

Cardiomyopathies caused by drugs and poisons and physical trauma

DRUGS

IMMUNOSUPPRESSIVE THERAPY

Myocardial changes have been found in the hearts of a considerable number of patients who have had renal transplantations and who then have been treated with immunosuppressive drugs. It is also, at present, well recognized that a considerable number of people who are on long-term immunosuppressive drugs eventually develop congestive heart failure, which seems, in some cases, to be the final cause of death.

Chatty and Deodhar (1969), in a survey of 85 patients who had received immunosuppressive therapy following renal transplantation, found interstitial myocardial fibrosis in 24 (28 per cent) (*Figure 17.1*) and in 14 of these 24, the fibrosis was associated with an active myocarditis manifested by interstitial and perivascular infiltrates of inflammatory cells consisting of lymphocytes and a few plasma cells, monocytes and macrophages, together with a focal necrosis of some myocardial fibres (*Figure 17.2*). The fibrosis was usually more prominent in the left ventricular wall and interventricular septum than in the right ventricular wall. This fibrous tissue was relatively poor in cellular elements and did not contain any elastic tissue fibres (*Figure 17.3*).

As previously stated, 14 of the hearts which showed fibrosis also showed an active myocarditis in some areas of the myocardium.

All stages of myocarditis ranging from the active cellular phase to the dormant, acellular, fibrotic phase, with intermediate healing stages were seen in some of these hearts (*Figure 17.4*).

Five hearts in the transplant group showed myocardial lesions of an infectious type, three of which were fungal in origin, while two were caused by parasites, one of which was *Toxoplasma gondii*, while the other was indeterminate in origin. It seemed likely that many of the

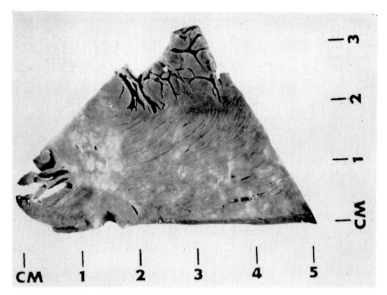

Figure 17.1.   Section of the left ventricle showing increased thickness and patchy fibrosis of the myocardium after methotrexate therapy (Chatty and Deodhar, 1969)

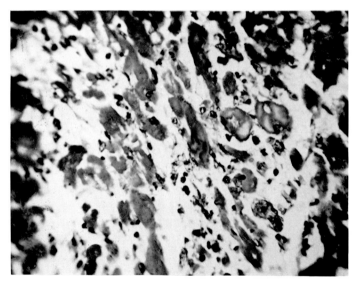

Figure 17.2.   Focus of necrosis in myocardium, showing myoclasis, loss of striations of myofibrils, macrophage activity, and round-cell infiltration (× 350, reduced to 7/10) (Deodhar and Chatty, 1969)

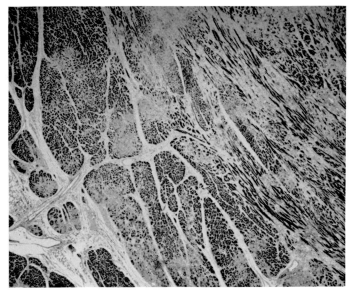

Figure 17.3. Extensive patchy fibrosis of myocardium with few cellular elements (Masson's trichrome × 25, reduced to 7/10) (Deodhar and Chatty, 1969)

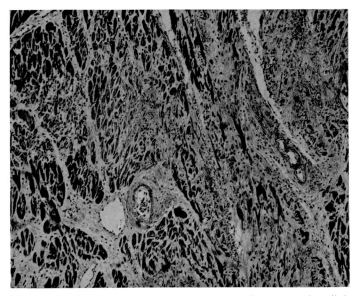

Figure 17.4. Varying stages of myocarditis, ranging from active phase (left middle portion of the microphotograph) to fibrotic-healed stage—here present simultaneously (haematoxylin and eosin counterstained with methylene blue × 60, reduced to 7/10) (Deodhar and Chatty, 1969)

other cases of myocarditis were due to viral infection, especially as many of these hearts showed the association of necrosis of individual muscle fibres and an adjacent inflammatory exudate; a finding said by some workers to be characteristic of viral myocarditis (Saphir and Cohen, 1957).

It has also been suggested that antilymphocytic globulin, one of the immunosuppressives used by Chatty and Deodhar, is associated with an increased susceptibility to viral infections (Hirsch and Murphy, 1968).

It was found that this myocarditis in the transplant group could not be related to any particular immunosuppressive drug.

References

Chatty, A., Eyad and Deodhar, S. D. (1969). 'Myocardial changes and kidney transplantation.' *Archs Path.* **88**, 602

Hirsch, M. S. and Murphy, F. A. (1968). 'Antilymphocyte serum and viral infections.' *Lancet* **2**, 37

Saphir, O. and Cohen, N. A. (1957). 'Myocarditis in infancy.' *Archs Path.* **64**, 446

DAUNORUBICIN

Daunorubicin was introduced by French workers to treat leukaemia, and may cause electrocardiogram changes and heart failure which may be fatal (Tan *et al.*, 1967; Macrez *et al.*, 1967; Malpas and Scott, 1968).

Bonnadonna and Monfardini (1969) reported sudden acute heart failure in 16 patients receiving the drug; 5 died within 1–5 days having received total dosages of 2·2–8·0 mg/kg. Clinically there was dyspnoea, hypertension and tachycardia with ST depression and flattened T waves.

The cause of cardiac arrest appears to be a selective deposition of the drug in the cardiac nerve ganglia—as has been demonstrated by the studies of Macrez *et al.* (1967)—and which prevents these cells from functioning correctly.

Marmont, Damasio and Rossi (1969) of Genoa also reported death from heart failure in 3 out of 4 patients over 45 years; and one death from the same cause in a group of 8 patients under 45 years.

References

Bonnadonna, G. and Monfardini, S. (1969). 'Cardiac toxicity of dauno-rubicin.' *Lancet* **1**, 837

Macrez, C. L., Marneffe-Lebrequier, H., Ripault, J., Claudez, J. P., Jacquillat, C. and Wetl, M. (1967). '*Accidents* cardiaques observés au cours des traitements par la rubidomycine.' *Path. Biol., Paris* **15**, 949

Malpas, J. S. and Scott, R. B. (1968). 'Rubidomycin in acute leukaemia in adults.' *Br. med. J.* **3**, 227

Marmont, A. M., Damasio, E. and Rossi, E. (1969). 'Cardiac toxicity of daunorubicin.' *Lancet* **1**, 837

Tan, C., Tasaila, H., Yu K-P., Murphy, M. L. and Karnoesky, D. A. (1967). 'Daunomycin, an autotumour antibiotic, in the treatment of neoplastic disease.' *Cancer, N.Y.* **20**, 333

EMETINE

There are many reports of the cardiotoxic effects of emetine. By far the largest number describe the changes in the heart rate, blood pressure and electrocardiogram. Klatskin and Friedman (1948) in a study of 93 healthy young soldiers under treatment for intestinal amoebiasis with emetine found that 83 per cent displayed some cardiovascular effect. Dack and Moloshok (1947) have observed that the cardiac abnormalities may occur even after a course of emetine has been completed, and that, in some instances, the electrocardiographic abnormalities persist for weeks.

Reports of human deaths due to emetine are exceedingly rare, so that Brown in 1935 was able to find only ten cases in the world literature. Two of the reports (Levy and Rowntree, 1916; Leibly, 1930) are convincing, but although post-mortem examinations were carried out, descriptions of the hearts were often absent or inadequate. The only cases in which electrocardiogram abnormalities have been reported in life—presumably due to emetine therapy—and a detailed description of the heart after death has been obtained are those of Kattwinkel (1949) and those of Brem and Konwater (1955).

Other descriptions of the myocardial lesions are those limited to studies in experimental animals given varying amounts of emetine (Anderson and Leake, 1930; Rinehart and Anderson, 1931).

PATHOLOGY

Macroscopically, the heart appears normal and, on section, the myocardium shows the normal reddish-brown colour. Microscopically the heart may show, in all areas, evidence of an interstitial myocarditis. In the more seriously involved areas, there may be separation of muscle fibres and infiltration of the interstitium by atypical cells, most of which resemble histiocytes, and only rarely are polymorphs seen. Many of the myocardial cells have 'caterpillar' nuclei and resemble the Anitschkow myocyte or cardiac histiocytes. Definite evidence of destruction of myocardial fibres may also be seen. Where this is present the nuclei are pyknotic and sometimes take up bizarre appearances.

The striking finding is the relative absence of inflammatory cells. Neither the epicardium nor the endocardium appears to be involved in this process.

References

Anderson, H. H. and Leake, C. D. (1930). 'The oral toxicity of emetine hydrochloride and certain related compounds in rabbits and cats.' *Am. J. trop. Med. Hyg.* **10**, 249

Brem and Konwater (1955). 'Fatal myocarditis due to emetine hydrochloride.' *Am. Heart J.* **50**, 476

Brown, P. W. (1935). 'Results and dangers in the treatment of amoebiasis. Summary of 15 years clinical experience at the Mayo Clinic.' *J. Am. med. Ass.* **105**, 1319

Dack, S. and Moloshok, R. E. (1947). 'Cardiac manifestation of toxic action of emetine hydrochloride in amoebic dysentery.' *Ann. intern. Med.* **79**, 228

Kattwinkel, E. E. (1949). 'Death due to cardiac disease following the use of emetine hydrochloride in the conditioned reflex treatment of chronic alcoholism.' *New Engl. J. Med.* **240**, 995

Klatskin, G. and Friedman, H. (1948). 'Emetine therapy in man.' *Ann. intern. Med.* **28**, 892

Leibly, F. J. (1930). 'Fatal emetine poisoning due to cumulative action in amoebic dysentery.' *Am. J. med. Sci.* **179**, 834

Levy, R. L. and Rowntree, L. G. (1916). 'Toxicity of commercial preparations of emetine.' *Archs intern. Med.* **17**, 420

Rinehart, J. F. and Anderson, H. H. (1931). 'The oral toxicity of emetine hydrochloride and artaus related.' *Am. J. trop. Med.* **10**, 249

PHENYLBUTAZONE

Phenylbutazone is given for osteoarthritis, rheumatoid arthritis and related disabilities to relieve aches, pains, stiffness and swelling of joints.

In 1957 Hodge and Lawrence reported two fatal cases. The first was a woman of 38 suffering from rheumatoid arthritis who developed arrhythmia, oedema of the face and limbs and then jaundice; the drug was stopped but ten weeks later she developed fatal hypotension and tachycardia; at necropsy pericardial effusions and myocarditis were found.

The other was a woman aged 70 with osteoarthritis. After three weeks therapy she developed fever, erythema, bronchitis and fatal status epilepticus. Necropsy revealed perivascular granulomata in the heart.

Reference

Hodge, P. R. and Lawrence, J. R. (1957). 'Two cases of myocarditis associated with phenylbutazone therapy.' *Med. J. Aust.* **1**, 640

SULPHONAMIDES

Various reports have appeared suggesting that myocarditis can result from sulphonamide therapy in the absence of an arteritis.

French and Weller (1942) reported 126 cases of interstitial cellular lesions in patients receiving sulphonamide drugs. The cellular components were mainly mononuclear but many of these had eosinophilic cytoplasm. A few eosinophils were also present. They claimed similar changes after experimental administration of sulphonamides to mice and rats.

Fawcett (1948), using a control series and a cell counting technique, cast doubt on these findings, but could not exclude sulphonamides in a few cases.

Blanchard and Mertens (1958) reported three cases with distinctive lesions, some with fibrinous exudate and some distinctly granulomatous. All were associated with many eosinophilia.

More recently MacSerraigh and Patel (1968) in Kampala, Uganda, reported on an African boy of 12 years who developed fulminating, generalized skin lesions in two days and cardiomyopathy with heart failure in 28 days following 6 g of sulphadimidine for otitis media. He survived after prednisone and digitalis therapy.

Sulphonamide therapy is also associated with periarteritis nodosa; Simon (1943) reported this condition, together with eosinophilic myocarditis, occurring 30 days after sulphonamide therapy.

References

Blanchard, A. J. and Mertens, G. A. (1958). 'Hypersensitivity myocarditis occurring with sulphamethoxypyridazine therapy.' *Can. med. Ass. J.* **79**, 627

Fawcett, R. M. (1948). 'Myocarditis after sulphonamide therapy.' *Archs Path.* **48**, 25

French, A. J. and Weller, C. V. (1942). 'Interstitial myocarditis following the clinical and experimental use of sulphonamide drugs.' *Am. J. Path.* **18**, 109

MacSerraigh, E. T. M. and Patel, K. M. (1968). 'Cardiomyopathy as a complication of sulphonamide therapy.' *Br. med. J.* **3**, 33

Simon, M. A. (1943). 'Pathologic lesions following the administration of sulphonamide drugs.' *Am. J. med. Sci.* **205**, 439

ANTIBIOTICS

There are few reports of myocardial lesions produced by antibiotics.

Waugh (1952) reported the case of a patient who died of congestive heart failure. At necropsy areas of necrosis were found in the cardiac muscle together with giant cells and eosinophils. These changes were believed to be due to penicillin sensitivity.

Streptomycin sensitivity was believed to be the basis for a myocarditis with widespread necrosis and large numbers of eosinophils occurring eight days after an injection (Chatterjee and Thakre, 1958).

It is difficult to be certain of the nature of some of the cases described. These antibiotics are very widely used and the association may be fortuitous.

References

Chatterjee, S. S. and Thakre, M. W. (1958). 'Fiedler's myocarditis: Report of a fatal case following intramuscular injection of streptomycin.' *Tubercle, Lond.* **39**, 240

Waugh, D. (1952). 'Myocarditis, arteritis and focal hepatic, splenic and renal granulomes apparently due to penicillin sensitivity.' *Am. J. Path.* **28**, 437

PARACETAMOL

Paracetamol has been suggested as a safe alternative to phenacetin, but it is a metabolite of both phenacetin and of acetanalide and open to suspicion.

MacLean *et al.* (1968) reviewed 6 reported cases and described 5 of their own suffering from paracetamol poisoning (20 g and upwards). They had electrocardiogram changes of myocardial damage, hypoalbuminaemia, a tendency to bleeding and liver cell damage. One patient died and necropsy showed massive liver necrosis, renal distal tubular necrosis and cerebral oedema; the heart was not studied, but severe myocardial damage was reported in a fatal case by Pimstone and Vys (1968).

References

MacLean, D., Peters, T. J., Brown, R. A. G., McCathie, M., Baines, G. T. and Robertson, P. G. C. (1968). 'Treatment of acute paracetamol poisoning.' *Lancet* **2**, 849

Pimstone, B. S. and Vys, C. J. (1968). 'Liver necrosis and myocardiopathy following paracetamol overdosage.' *S. Afr. med. J.* **42**, 259

OTHER ANAESTHETIC AGENTS

Practically all drugs administered as anaesthetic agents may affect the heart either by acting directly on the cardiac muscle itself or by altering the sympathetic or vagal tone. The effects on the autonomic nervous system may include: (1) direct action on autonomic nervous centres; (2) inhibition or stimulation of autonomic ganglia; and (3) secondary autonomic reflexes initiated by peripheral effects, for instance, changes in arterial pressure.

FUNCTIONAL CHANGES

Gravenstein (1965) has briefly summarized the functional effects of various anaesthetics. Atropine sulphate and scopolamine hydrobromide (0·1–0·2 mg/70 kg of body weight) cause bradycardia, but additional doses of either will accelerate the pulse to a state of tachycardia. This phenomenon is related to increased peripheral blockade, which masks the central vagal stimulation produced by these two alkaloids. In the isolated heart neither ether nor cyclopropane alters the rate significantly.

Cyclopropane, when administered alone, produces little change in the heart rate in man, while ether causes only a mild bradycardia. These changes in rate, in the intact individual, are most likely alterations in the autonomic tone. Both agents increase sympathetic activity differences in the peripheral effects of cyclopropane and ether and probably account for the different effects on heart rate.

Halothane depresses the autonomic centres, decreases the body's ability to respond to surgical stress with increased sympathetic tone and has a direct negative chronotropic effect on the pacemaker, which leads to bradycardia. This depression does not indicate an antagonistic effect of halothane to the catecholamines but, rather, a direct effect of halothane on the pacemaker.

Barbiturate poisoning is often associated with hypothermia and asystole. Linton and Ledingham (1966) reviewed this aspect and reported a man of 27 years whose temperature fell to 23°C and who had ventricular fibrillation which responded only to defibrillation through a thoracotomy, with direct warming of the mediastinum. On re-warming, the antidiuretic action of the barbiturate necessitated forced diuresis. Recovery was complete, although only one such recovery had been reported previously; his serum barbiturate was 5·7 mg/100 ml. Fell *et al.* (1968) reported the case of a woman, aged 42, who took excessive barbiturates and then tried to drown herself in a canal; when found, her temperature was 22°C (71·6°F). She recovered after external cardiac massage for $3\frac{1}{2}$ hours, intermittent positive pressure ventilation, internal defibrillation and re-warming on a by-pass machine.

ARRHYTHMIAS

Cyclopropane is capable of rendering a heart susceptible to arrhythmias induced by epinephrine; clinical experience cautions against the use of cyclopropane and epinephrine together. Although halothane is also capable of sensitizing the heart, its use in combination with epinephrine during anaesthesia is permissible if dosage and rate of injection are carefully regulated.

SUMMARY

All anaesthetics, local barbiturates, vapours and gases depress the contractile force of the heart, especially the heart devoid of its autonomic innervation. Barbiturates may also induce hypothermia.

References

Fell, R. H., Gunning, S. J., Bardhan, K. D. and Triger, D. H. (1968). 'Severe hypothermia as a result of barbiturate overdosage complicated by cardiac arrest.' *Lancet* **1**, 397

Gravenstein, J. S. (1965). 'Effects of anaesthetics on the heart.' *Am. Surg.* **31**, 159

Linton, A. L. and Ledingham, I. McA. (1966). 'Severe hypothermia with barbiturate overdosage.' *Lancet* **1**, 24

PHAEOCHROMOCYTOMA

The well-known clinical picture of paroxysmal hypertension occurring in cases of phaeochromocytoma is mainly due to the vasoconstrictional effect of catecholamines on peripheral blood vessels. The central effects of catecholamines on the heart itself are less well recognized, but it seems possible that these are of much greater importance than the peripheral effects in determining prognosis.

Kline (1961) described focal necrosis of cardiac muscle, cellular infiltrates of lymphocytes and histiocytes and focal fibrosis in 4 of 7 cases of phaeochromocytoma.

Similar lesions have been described in patients treated with adrenaline and related substances and in experimental animals injected with adrenaline and noradrenaline (Szakacs and Cannon, 1958; Szakacs, Dimmette and Cowart, 1959; Namas, Manion, and Bronson, 1959).

Northfield (1967) described the cardiac complications in those patients dying with phaeochromocytoma. These included paroxysmal supraventricular tachycardia, ventricular fibrillation and diffuse myocardial damage. Northfield suggested that ventricular fibrillation is the cause of the sudden death in many cases of this disease. In two of his cases there were diffuse myocardial changes which may have been caused by the effect of catecholamines on the myocardium. The changes were a diffuse infiltration of lymphocytes, eosinophils and monocytes throughout the myocardium, together with a few small foci of fibrosis.

Gruber, Olca and Blades (1933) had earlier shown that high levels of circulating adrenaline may be used experimentally to produce a haemorrhagic myocarditis.

These lesions are similar to the severe haemorrhagic myocarditis and severe myocardial oedema which has been found, at necropsy, in patients following the use of noradrenaline or adrenaline, even in therapeutic doses.

Similar lesions have been produced experimentally in animals following the infusion of noradrenaline and in a heart-lung preparation following the infusion of both adrenaline and noradrenaline. The workers also observed similar lesions in a phaeochromocytoma.

References

Gruber, C. M., Olca, I. Y. and Blades, B. (1933). 'Myocarditis produced experimentally in rabbits by drugs.' *J. Pharmaco. exp. Ther.* **49**, 300

Kline, I. K. (1961). 'Myocardial alterations associated with phaeochromocytoma.' *Am. J. Path.* **38**, 539

Namas, G. G., Manion, W. C. and Bronson, D. (1959). 'Lésions cardiaques par excès de norepinephrine.' *Presse méd.* **67**, 1079

Northfield, J. C. (1967). 'Cardiac complications of phaeochromocytoma.' *Br. Heart J.* **32**, 588

Szakacs, J. E. and Cannon, A. (1958). 'L-Norepinephrine myocarditis.' *Am. J. clin. Path.* **30**, 425

— Dimmette, R. M. and Cowart, E. C., Jnr (1959). 'Pathologic implication of the catecholamines, epinephrine and norepinephrine.' *U.S. armed Forces med. J.* **10**, 908

LITHIUM CARBONATE

Lithium carbonate has been used in treating manic depression in mental patients since 1949 (Cade, 1949) and Schou, Andisen and Trap-Jensen (1968) reported 8 cases of lithium carbonate poisoning with 3 deaths; among these patients 3 showed electrocardiogram abnormalities, one among the 3 deaths and another 2 among the 5 cases which recovered. Horowitz and Fisher (1969) also reported electrocardiogram changes in one case who had injected large amounts of lithium carbonate in a suicidal attempt, while Wilbanks, Bresler and Peete (1970) reported a case with cyanosis, flaccid muscular tone and a loud systolic murmur in an infant born to a mother receiving lithium carbonate. The lithium level in the infant's blood in the first two days was 2·4 and 2·2 mol/l but had dropped to 0·6 mol/l on the third day, when all the signs and symptoms had disappeared, including the cardiac murmur. There is, however, only one report on their pathological findings in the heart of a patient who had died from lithium carbonate poisoning (Tseng, 1971). At autopsy the heart was enlarged, 510 g, and the left ventricle was both dilated and hypertrophied, the myocardium being 2 cm thick. The entire myocardium of the left ventricle, including the septum, showed many greyish-pink and gelatinous areas 0·3–0·8 cm in diameter, in contrast to the dark red appearance seen in other areas. A yellow-grey iridescent area was also seen in the anterior septum near the apex. All the coronary vessels were normal.

Microscopically, the myocardium of the left ventricle showed marked and diffuse myocarditis—at differing stages of development and healing. Some of these areas were recent, showing lymphocytes, plasma cells and macrophages with lipochrome pigments and also Anitschkow myocyte in between the degenerated myocardial fibres (*Figure 17.5*). The older areas showed more fibrosis and less inflammatory cells (*Figure 17.6*). Here, occasional muscle giant cells were also recognized. The lithium content of the heart muscle was 214 m Eq/l. These histological findings demonstrate that these pathological findings had been present for many months. It seems very unlikely that the aetiology of these pathological findings is due to a direct toxic action of lithium on the myocardium and not allergic in nature as no eosinophils were seen. Their patient also had complete right bundle branch block, auricular-ventricular dissociation with idioventriculous rhythm and multiple premature ventricular contractions. The conducting system was not, however, examined in this case.

References

Cade, J. F. J. (1949). 'Lithium salts in the treatment of psychotic excitement.' *Med. J. Aust.* **36**, 349

Horowitz, L. C. and Fisher, G. V. (1969). 'Acute lithium toxicity.' *New Engl. J. Med.* **289**, 1369

Schou, M., Andisen, A. and Trap-Jensen, J. (1968). 'Lithium poisoning.' *Am. J. Psychiat.* **125**, 1443

Tseng, H. Len. (1971). 'Interstitial myocarditis, probably related to lithium carbonate intoxication.' *Archs Path.* **92**, 444

Wilbanks, G. D., Bresler, B. and Peete, C. H., Jnr (1970). 'Toxic effects of lithium carbonate in a mother and newborn infant.' *J. Am. med. Ass.* **213**, 865

PHENOTHIAZINES AND DERIVATIVES

Tranquillizing drugs such as phenothiazines are prescribed widely. Richardson, Graupner and Richardson (1966) studied the records of 2,156 patients dying in a mental hospital in the period 1944–65 and

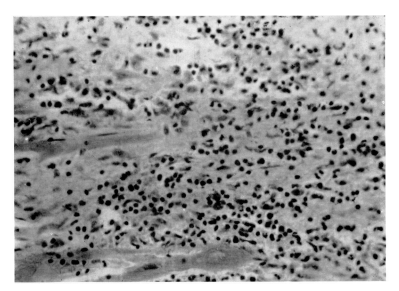

Figure 17.5. Section of the myocardium showing scattered inflammatory cells and necrosis of muscle fibres (haematoxylin and eosin × 100). (Reproduced from Tseng (1971) by courtesy of the author and Editor of the Archives of Pathology)

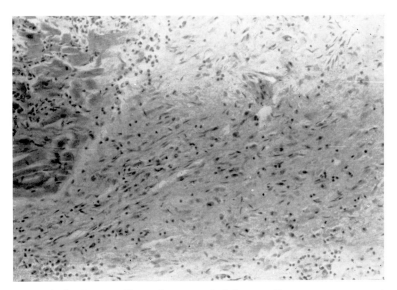

Figure 17.6. Section of heart showing marked chronic inflammatory reaction and mild fibrosis (haematoxylin and eosin × 430). (Reproduced from Tseng (1971) by courtesy of the author and Editor of the Archives of Pathology)

noted the sudden increase of unexpected deaths since the introduction of phenothiazine in 1957; 21 of 87 such patients died, 12 from obscure causes. Two-thirds of these had abnormal electrocardiograms before death; 3 had heart block and the remainder had ST depression or low T waves.

The heart sections from 8 pre-1962 cases were re-examined and compared to 150 control hearts. These hearts showed an increase in acid mucopolysaccharides between muscle bundles and around arterioles. A detailed study of the hearts of four patients receiving tranquillizers, who died suddenly in 1964–68, was then made. The hearts of 49 non-tranquillized patients were used as controls.

The cardiac changes in these four cases were similar. There was some irregularity of nuclear size and shape. Interstitial spaces between the myocardial fibres and around some blood vessels contained a loose fibrillary network. In the inner one-third of the heart, adjacent to the endocardium, there were triangular and wedge-shaped areas of myofibrillary degeneration.

The lumina of some arterioles were patent but the endothelium was prominent. The vessel walls were composed of multi-layered hyperplastic smooth muscle cells with prominent nuclei and abundant cytoplasm. Cell boundaries appeared to be interlaced together by a diamond-shaped fibrillary membrane. Between the vessel and the myocardial muscle fibres was a fine fibrillary network, which stained positively for acid mucopolysaccharides, but was PAS negative. Smaller vessels of the arteriocapillary bed (14–40 μm) were especially prominent in these areas of myofibrillary degenerative change and often showed proliferation of the lining endothelial cells.

A dense, celloidal-iron negative, PAS positive, bright circular protein band was deposited in the middle of the vessel's wall. This clearly separated the endothelial cells from the underlying muscle cells of the small arterioles.

Focal or diffuse myocardial degenerative changes were spotty and appeared to be dependent on the extent of the small arteriocapillary bed involvement.

In many instances there was basophilic degeneration of nearby muscle fibres and formation of hydrocolloid bodies of various shapes and sizes. These bodies contain a PAS positive diastase resistant material.

The myocardial nuclei were frequently box-like with peripheral condensation of nuclear chromatin.

There were only rare vascular myofibrillary changes in the outer two-thirds of the ventricular myocardium.

The walls of some arterioles were extremely hyperplastic; degeneration and fragmentation of the hyperplastic smooth muscle common; and acid mucopolysaccharides were sometimes found in huge pools within the intima, media, adventitia and surrounding interstitial tissues.

Excessive AMPS deposition was also seen in areas where conducting tissue is present and just under the endocardium of both ventricles. The lesions were also seen in 70 per cent of those receiving the drug but dying of other causes. Leesma and Koenig (1968) also discussed the relationship of sudden death to phenothiazine therapy, and Alexander (1968) reviewed the whole question of the permanent cardiotoxic damage which could follow the administration of the phenothiazines and imipramine type drugs. Some workers reported arrhythmias, widened QRS and marked ST changes in two females aged 17 and 46 who took overdoses of amitriptyline (Tryptizol). The elder woman died and the younger woman had electrocardiogram changes simulating cardiac infarction.

References

Alexander, C. S. and Nino, A. (1969). 'Cardiovascular complications in young patients taking psychotropic drugs—a preliminary report.' *Am. Heart J.* **78**, 757

Leesma, J. E. and Koenig, K. L. (1968). 'Sudden death and phenothiazide. A current controversy.' *Archs gen. Psychiat.* **18**, 137

Richardson, H. L., Graupner, K. E. and Richardson, M. E. (1966). 'Intramyocardial lesions in patients dying suddenly and unexpectedly.' *J. Am. med. Ass.* **195**, 254

POISONS

CARBON MONOXIDE

Inhalation of coal gas or exhaust gases are the most common causes of carbon monoxide poisoning.

Carbon monoxide has 300 times the affinity of oxygen for haemoglobin.

The toxicity of carbon monoxide is directly related to its great affinity for haemoglobin and to the low disassociation rate of carbon methaemoglobin. The carbon monoxide forms carboxyhaemoglobin, exactly replacing the oxygen, volume for volume, so that the blood is unable to carry oxygen. Petrol exhaust also contains benzol which increases the toxicity (Winslow, 1927). Its effect on the heart depends on the intensity and duration of the anoxaemia produced and on the state of the heart. The signs and symptoms of cardiac injury from carbon monoxide poisoning may be delayed or masked by its more prominent effects on the nervous system. Objective evidence of myocardial injury may not be manifested until several days after exposure, sometimes even in those who appear to be recovering from the toxic effects of carbon monoxide. Haggard (1921) showed that acute oxygen deficiency causes impaired atrioventricular conduction and Steinman (1937) found that electrocardiographic changes were common in coal gas poisoning.

Lewis, White and Meakins (1913–14) demonstrated, in cats, the sensitivity of conducting tissue to asphyxia, and Green and Gilbert (1921) considered that any disturbance below the bundle of His was permanent; Colvin (1928), however, demonstrated that such changes might only be temporary, in a healthy young man poisoned by carbon monoxide. A variety of electrocardiographic changes have been observed, the most common of which are abnormalities of the T waves and ST segments. In the earlier stages there is shortening of the PR interval, but later there is a tendency for the atrioventricular node to take over as pacemaker with slowing of the heart. Other changes encountered include ventricular extrasystole, atrial fibrillation, AV nodal rhythm and bundle branch block. Relapse is common and can occur up to several weeks later, but is rarely fatal. It is less likely to occur if bed rest is enforced as long as needed (British Medical Journal, 1968). Death occurs in up to 40 per cent of cases, but 60 per cent of those who survive recover completely.

PATHOLOGY

In acute deaths all the organs are pink and show congestion and haemorrhage. In fatal carbon monoxide poisoning, the heart invariably exhibits focal areas of necrosis, most marked in the sub-endocardial region of the left ventricle and its papillary muscles. Gurich (1925) described haemorrhagic necrotic foci with surrounding leucocyte infiltration of the septum and papillary muscles in four previously healthy victims of carbon monoxide poisoning. Small foci of intramyocardial haemorrhage and perivascular infiltrates have also been observed. The histological features resemble those produced by prolonged coronary insufficiency, even though the coronary arteries are not occluded. Heart muscle damage was also reported by Hadley (1952), who reviewed the 272 cases of coal gas poisoning admitted to the Edinburgh Royal Infirmary; 0·7 per cent suffered major cardiac sequelae. He further described the case of a fit man aged 53 who, being overcome by petrol exhaust, remained unconscious for 36 hours; 14 days later he developed angina pectoris and electrocardiogram evidence of a myocardial infarction and died within 24 hours. He further considered it to have been directly precipitated by the toxic action of carbon monoxide on the cardiac muscle. Various authors disagree as to whether carbon monoxide produces direct injury to the coronary vessels. Beck, Schulze and Suter (1940) contend that there is damage to endothelial cells which promotes intravascular thrombosis and culminates in small myocardial infarcts. It is more probable, however, that coronary artery injury or thrombosis is a consequence of pre-existing atherosclerosis.

References

Beck, H. G., Schulze, W. H. and Suter, G. M. (1940). 'Carbon monoxide, a domestic hazard.' *J. Am. med. Ass.* **115**, 1

British Medical Journal (1968). 'Coal gas and the brain.' **1**, 398

Colvin, L. T. (1928). 'Electro cardiographic changes in a case of severe carbon monoxide poisoning.' *Am. Heart J.* **3**, 484

Green, C. W. and Gilbert, N. C. (1921). 'Studies on the response of the circulation to low oxygen tension. III. Changes in the pacemaker and in conduction in extreme oxygen want as shown in the human electrocardiogram.' *Archs intern. Med.* **27**, 517

Gurich, I. (1925). 'Herzmuskelveränderungen bei Leucht-gasvergiftung.' *Munchen med. Wschr.* **72**, 2194

Hadley, M. (1952). 'Coal gas poisoning and cardiac sequelae.' *Br. Heart J.* **14**, 534

Haggard, H. W. (1921). 'Studies in carbon monoxide asphyxia. I. The behaviour of the heart.' *Am. J. Physiol.* **56**, 390

Lewis, T., White, P. D. and Meakins, D. (1913–14). 'The susceptible region in AV conduction.' *Heart* **5**, 289

Steinman, B. (1937). 'Über das Elektrokardiogram bei Khlenoxyct vergiftung.' *Z. Kreislaufforsch* **29**, 281

Winslow, C. E. A. (1927). 'Summary of the Natural Safety Council study of benzol poisoning.' *J. ind. Hyg. Toxicol.* **9**, 61

SCORPION VENOM CARDIOMYOPATHY

Cardiomyopathy produced by scorpion sting remains a constant problem in different parts of the world; case reports of stings from these animals have come from places as far apart as Israel (Gueron and Yarom, 1969), Malaya (Poon-King, 1963), Arizona (Stahnke, 1950), and the West Indies. The venom is believed to be mainly neurotoxic but potent cardiovascular responses have been observed both in man (Gueron, Stern and Cohen, 1967) and in experimental animals (Paterson, 1960).

In Egypt and Israel—like elsewhere in the East—the most dangerous scorpion is the *Buthus Quinquestriatus*.

The sting is characterized by local pain, anxiety and profuse perspiration. Hypertension usually ranging from 100 to 130 mmHg, diastolic, is found in about half the patients seen. This hypertension is also usually accompanied by excessive tachycardia and restlessness, and persists for a few hours before returning to normal levels.

In a smaller proportion of patients, usually about 15–20 per cent, the blood pressure, on admission to hospital, is seen to be very low— usually about 80 mmHg systolic and accompanied by the clinical signs of peripheral vascular collapse. Later, about a further 30 per cent of these patients develop signs of peripheral circulatory collapse without preceding hypertension. The patient is often seen in peripheral circulating failure and may subsequently die. This clinical presentation is much more serious in young children, the majority of whom are brought into hospital in a collapsed state, and subsequently die—usually without regaining consciousness.

LABORATORY INVESTIGATIONS

The urinary catecholamines have been estimated in some cases. Epinephrine and norepinephrine levels are elevated in about a third of these cases but the levels of urinary vanillylmandelic acid, the breakdown product of these catecholamines, which may be slightly elevated initially, are later found to be normal.

As almost all these patients complain of abdominal pain, serum amylase levels have been estimated and are found to vary from normal, often being elevated, while the blood sugar is found to be above the normal levels of 95 mg per cent in about a third of the cases.

SGOT levels have similarly been estimated and have similarly been found to be elevated in about 70 per cent of cases examined.

PATHOLOGY

Of the patients who die from scorpion sting cardiomyopathy, the cause of death in the majority of them is pulmonary oedema, but a certain number (about 30 per cent) die suddenly and unexpectedly.

All heart specimens examined with this disease are grossly normal but many changes may be seen microscopically, and usually show similar changes, although of varying intensity. These changes are usually most prominent in the papillary muscles and in the subendocardial region but are found in all locations in some cases. The following changes may be met: (1) interstitial oedema accompanied by an increased cellularity (*Figure 17.7*), the cells being mostly lymphocytes and monocytes while a few polymorphs and Anitsch-kow-type myocytes may sometimes be seen. (2) In several cases more marked focal interstitial accumulations of cells may be seen and consist mainly of lymphocytes, but some polymorphs are also present—these areas have all the appearance of focal myocarditis. (3) Degeneration or necrosis of small groups of myocardial fibres may be recognized by eosinophilic swelling of the fibres, loss of cross

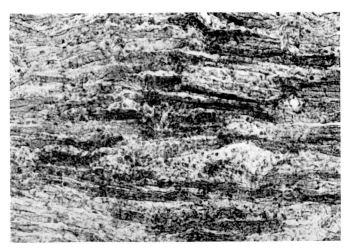

Figure 17.7. Myocardium diffusely infiltrated with lymphocytes and some polymorphs. Most of the myocardial cells have lost their usual striations and their cytoplasm has a hyaline appearance (haematoxylin and eosin × 50, reduced to 6/10). (Reproduced by courtesy of Dr Rena Yarom)

striations or a non-nucleated 'ghost' appearance of this muscle cell. (4) In a few cases large necrotic foci may be found in the myocardium and these are associated with marked cellular infiltration which consists of lymphocytes and monocytes. (5) Lipid stains show a fine fatty droplet deposition within muscle fibres (*Figure 17.8*). The deposition occurs in single fibres or in a group of fibres and is specially marked in the conduction fibres, and here may possibly involve the conduction system. There are also many fine droplets of lipid in the interstitial tissue. Sometimes these small lipid droplets have coalesced to form much larger lipid deposits, which are most commonly seen in the endocardium (*Figure 17.9*).

The intramyocardial blood vessels are generally unchanged, but occasionally arteries with an eccentric intimal thickening can be seen, especially when stained with Weigert's stain.

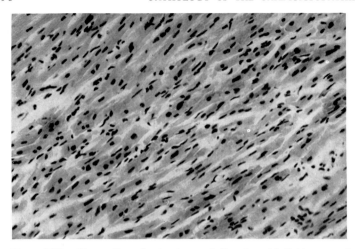

Figure 17.8. Myocardium showing intense infiltration with lipid, many of the myocardial cells being completely filled with lipid, while elsewhere lipid is present diffusely in the form of small droplets (haematoxylin and oil red 0 × 50, reduced to 6/10). (Reproduced by courtesy of Dr Rena Yarom)

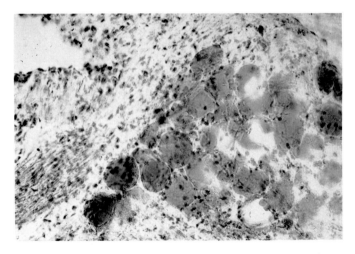

Figure 17.9. Scorpion sting cardiomyopathy showing numerous large globules of lipid in the slightly thickened endocardium at the base of an atrioventricular valve. There is also diffuse infiltration of that area with both acute and chronic inflammatory cells (haematoxylin and oil red 0 × 200, reduced to 6/10). (Reproduced by courtesy of Dr Rena Yarom)

The lungs of all patients show varying degrees of pulmonary oedema, accompanied by diffuse areas of alveolar haemorrhages. Pathological evidence of pancreatitis is only very rarely seen. Clinical evidence of acute pancreatitis, following a scorpion sting, has been found in some cases. Poon-King (1963) found that 29 of the patients whom he described as having evidence of myocarditis following a scorpion sting also had evidence of acute pancreatitis; 6 had hypoglycaemia and glycosuria and 16 had renal glycosuria.

DISCUSSION

The clinical picture as seen in these cases of scorpion bite of hypertension, anxiety, profuse perspiration and pulmonary oedema bears a marked resemblance to the effects of a sudden massive outpouring of pressor amines, as seen in phaeochromocytoma (Barsoum, Nabavy and Salama, 1954; Mohamed and Elkaremi, 1953; Rohayem, 1953). Indeed, the clinical picture and cardiac pathology are exactly similar to the catechol cardiomyopathy which has been described often as due to the accidental infusion of an overdosage of pressor amines (Szakacs and Mehlman, 1960, Ferrans et al., 1964).

Indeed, possibly the best study to show that these cardiac lesions are similar to those produced by catecholamines was that of Yarom and Braun (1969), who found exactly similar cardiac lesions in dogs injected with scorpion venom or isoproterenol.

The sympathomimetic origin of these cardiac lesions is further supported by the effect of pretreatment of some of these animals with adrenergic blocking agents prior to experimental venom injection, producing a remarkable reduction in the severity of the cardiac lesions.

References

Barsoum, G. S., Nabavy, M. and Salama, S. (1954). 'Scorpion poisoning, its signs, symptoms and treatment.' *J. Egypt. med. Ass.* **37**, 387

Ferrans, V. J., Hibbs, R. C., Black, W. C. and Weilbacker, D. G. (1964). 'Isoproterenol-induced myocardial necrosis. A histochemical and electron microscopic study.' *Am. Heart J.* **68**, 71

Gueron, M. and Yarom, Rena (1970). 'Cardiovascular manifestations of severe scorpion sting.' *Chest* **57**, 156

— Stern, J. and Cohen, W. (1967). 'Severe myocardial damage and heart failure in scorpion sting.' *Am. J. Cardiol.* **19**, 719

Mohamed, A. H. and Elkaremi, M. (1953). 'An antidote to scorpion toxin.' *J. trop. Med.* **56**, 58

Paterson, R. A. (1960). 'Physiologic actions of scorpion venom.' *Am. J. trop. Med.* **9**, 410

Poon-King, T. (1963). 'Myocarditis from scorpion stings.' *Br. med. J.* **1**, 373

Rohayem, H. (1953). 'Scorpion toxin and autonomic drugs.' *J. trop. Med.* **56**, 150

Stahnke, A. L. (1950). 'The Arizona scorpion problem.' *Arizona Med.* **7**, 23

Szakacs, J. E. and Mehlman, B. (1960). 'Pathological changes induced by l-norepinephrine: quantitative aspects.' *Am. J. Cardiol.* **5**, 619

Yarom, Rena and Braun, K. (1969). 'Cardiovascular effects of scorpion venom. Morphological changes in the myocardium.' *Toxicology* **8**, 41

— Gueron, M. and Braun, K. (1970). 'Scorpion venous cardiomyopathy.' *Pathologica Microbiol.* **35**, 114

SNAKE BITE

A valuable review of the whole subject of snake bite has been written by Reid (1968). The bite of *Viperis beris* is not uncommon in England. Walker (1945) reviewed 50 case reports from doctors in England and Wales; 7 deaths occurred from 'circulatory collapse'. Askanas (1959) reported a patient of 50 who developed posterior cardiac infarction, possibly from coronary thrombosis from hypotension. Brown and Dewar (1965), from Newcastle, reported the case of a patient bitten on the finger by a viper. Within fifteen minutes he was unsteady, in thirty he had abdominal colic, diarrhoea and vomiting, and within one hour he became hypotensive and unconscious. He was given saline infusion, hydrocortisone, noradrenaline, antivenom serum and tetracycline. His condition improved but at thirty hours he relapsed with hypotension, tachycardia, pulmonary oedema and syncope. Treatment was continued and recovery started but the electrocardiogram revealed T wave inversion and ST elevation and the SGOT rose to 106 units by the third day.

During convalescence he developed angina pectoris and although he had evidence of ischaemic heart damage $4\frac{1}{2}$ months later, eventually recovered fully so that he could undertake heavy manual work. Brown and Dewar suggested that the heart damage was due to dehydration, shock and hypotension from the action of the venom; they thought that the myocardial damage was probably due to infarction.

Cobra and Malayan viper venoms can damage the myocardium directly but viper venom does this by causing local coagulation and systemic anti-coagulation or, sometimes, thrombosis.

A boy of 14, described by Chadha, Ashby and Brown (1968) was bitten on the thumb, but despite being given antivenom and penicillin, developed enlarged axillary and cervical lymph glands, which subsided within four days. The electrocardiogram showed T wave inversion, probably due to toxic action on the myocardium and these changes persisted for more than two weeks.

SEA SNAKE (ENHYDRINA SCHISTOSA) POISONING

Sea snake venom is myotoxic, producing pain in the muscles and myoglobinuria, trismus and paresis; it may cause death from hyperkalaemia, acute renal failure or respiratory failure, and recovery is slow.

Reid (1961) described 4 cases and Marsden and Reid (1961) found that skeletal muscle necrosis and, as would be expected, renal damage were the chief lesions; plain muscle and myocardium seemed to be unaffected.

References

Askanas, X. (1959). 'Myocardial infarct in shock produced by snake bite.' (In Polish) *Polski Tygod. lek*. **14**, 1528

Brown, R. and Dewar, M. A. (1965). 'Heart damage following adder bite in England.' *Br. Heart J*. **27**, 144

Chadha, J. S., Ashby, D. W. and Brown, J. O. (1968). 'Abnormal electro-cardiogram after adder bite.' *Br. Heart J*. **30**, 138

Marsden, A. T. H. and Reid, H. A. (1961). 'Pathology of sea snake poisoning.' *Br. med. J*. **1**, 1290

Reid, H. A. (1961). 'Myoglobinuria and sea-snake bite poisoning.' *Br. med. J*. **1**, 1284

— (1968). 'Snakebite in the tropics.' *Br. med. J*. **3**, 359

Walker, C. W. (1945). 'Notes on adder bite (England and Wales).' *Br. med. J*. **2**, 13

ARGEMONE MEXICANA POISONING (EPIDEMIC DROPSY)

The syndrome of epidemic dropsy is characterized by oedema, its other chief manifestations being diarrhoea, pyrexia, anaemia, dyspnoea, tachycardia and elevated erythrocyte sedimentation rate. This disease is caused by Argemone poisoning.

It has been reported mostly from India and Burma, where mustard seeds or oils, which are often contaminated by this plant, are commonly eaten. The pathological changes in this disease are characterized by dilatation of capillaries.

CARDIAC CHANGES

These consist of increased vascularity of the myocardial capillaries, and oedema which separates the myocardial fibres, which are otherwise normal (Acton and Chopra, 1927).

Shanks and De (1931) confirmed these changes and noted that both ventricles are equally involved.

In the series of cases reported by Sanghvi, Misra and Bose (1960), however, cardiac enlargement was minimal and was mostly right ventricular in type, in contrast to other reports, where left ventricular enlargement has been described as common (Chopra and Basu, 1930).

Chopra and Bose (1933) noted that while cardiac involvement was the rule in epidemic dropsy, its severity was not uniform. They described three types of cardiovascular manifestations of the disease: (1) the acute fulminating and fatal type, resembling acute left ventricular failure; (2) the subacute or chronic type, and (3) formes frustes, with slight or no cardiac involvement. Congestive cardiac failure has been described by several writers and acute cardiac failure and acute dilatation of the heart has been reported to be the cause of deaths in this disease (Ghose, 1928).

References

Acton, H. W. and Chopra, R. N. (1927). 'Further investigations into the etiology of epidemic dropsy.' *Indian M. Gaz.* **62**, 359

Chopra, R. N. and Basu, V. P. (1930). 'Cardiovascular manifestations of epidemic dropsy and their treatment.' *Indian med. Gaz.* **65**, 546

— and Bose, S. C. (1933). 'Cardiovascular and other manifestations of epidemic dropsy.' *Indian med. Gaz.* **68**, 605

Ghose, G. (1928). 'An outbreak of epidemic dropsy in Allahabad in 1927.' *Indian med. Gaz.* **63**, 562

Sanghvi, L. M., Misra, S. N. and Bose, T. K. (1960). 'Cardiovascular manifestations in Argemone Mexicana poisoning (epidemic dropsy).' *Circulation* **21**, 1096

Shanks, G. and De, M. N. (1931). 'Pathology of epidemic dropsy.' *Indian J. med. Res.* **19**, 469

COBALT CARDIOMYOPATHY

In 1965 and 1966 cases of a fulminating cardiomyopathy producing severe heart failure occurred among heavy beer drinkers in Quebec (Bonenfant *et al.*, 1969; Morin and Daniel, 1967; Rona, 1968). Omaha (Sullivan, Parker and Carson, 1968; Rona, 1968), and Louvain (Kesteloot *et al.*, 1968). A further 28 patients with cobalt-beer cardiomyopathy admitted to the V.A. Hospital in Minneapolis from 1964 to 1967 were reported by Alexander in 1972. Detailed chemical and biological analyses of the beer consumed in Canada failed to reveal any known toxicants. Animals tolerated large quantities of beer without apparent adverse effects (Wiberg *et al.*,

1969). At autopsy the cardiac changes were considered to be those of a non-specific diffuse myocardiopathy or myocarditis.

CLINICAL PRESENTATION

This syndrome was characterized by acute dyspnoea and weakness followed by predominantly right-sided congestive heart failure.

Other findings were tachycardia, hypotension, electrocardiogram abnormalities, marked cardiomegaly and pericardial effusion. Laboratory findings in some patients indicated thiamine deficiency and lactic acid acidosis.

Pericardial effusion and polycythaemia were present in the majority of cases reported by Alexander (1972) and thereby suggested cobalt intoxication.

The ages of the patients varied between 20 and 70 years with a mean age of about 45 years, all being Caucasian, except for one American Indian. Those patients who died did so within 2–3 days of admission.

In Alexander's (1972) review from Minneapolis, death in the acute illness occurred in 18 per cent of cases but late deaths accounted for a total mortality of 48 per cent.

Some survivors continue to have abnormal disability and demonstrate abnormal electrocardiogram.

MORPHOLOGICAL OBSERVATIONS

Pericardium

In about 30 per cent of cases the pericardium was normal, but in another 40 per cent was distended by a large amount, 500–1,000 cc, of clear, yellow fluid. Histological examination of the pericardium in those cases which contained a pericardial effusion showed some slight degree of serosal cell swelling, but definite serosal cell proliferation was only seen where pericardiocentesis had been attempted and when pericarditis was present. This accumulation of pericardial fluid seemed to parallel the incidence of pleural and abdominal effusions. Peripheral oedema was not a noticeable finding.

HEART

Gross Examination

There was cardiac enlargement due to a combination of dilatation and hypertrophy.

Autopsy Findings

The heart was generally enlarged. The heart weight in Quebec ranged from 350 to 690 g and in the Omaha series from 425 to 600 g.

The average weight was 500 and 538 g respectively, with a combined average of 512 g. The cardiac enlargement was generally a function of a combination of cardiac hypertrophy and chamber dilatation but no single pattern was noted. It appeared, however, that the heavier the heart was the greater the degree of dilatation. This also correlated roughly with age, since the heart weight generally increased in proportion to the increasing age of the patient. The myocardium has a characteristic appearance. Loss of tone resulted in flabbiness to a degree that the heart generally resembled the form of the cupped hand. Flattening was instantaneous when the heart was placed on the examining table. The subepicardial venous vascular pattern was accentuated with exaggeration of the hair-like tributaries. In eight cases there was a moderate degree of atherosclerosis of the coronary arteries. In the smaller hearts the myocardium was pale brown but in the larger hearts it was pale grey-tan (grey-yellow). The myocardium also seemed to be soggy to the touch, as if waterlogged. Mural endocardial thrombi were present in six cases. In other cases the valvular and mural endocardium was delicate and translucent. Where cardiac dilatation was marked the trabeculae carneae were stretched and the intervening fenestrations were rendered quite prominent.

Thrombo-embolism was commonly seen, leading in six cases to haemorrhagic infarction of the lung.

Microscopic Study.—The general appearance of the myocardium showed some hypertrophy of myocardial cells and enlargement of intercellular spaces by oedema fluid (*Figure 17.10*). In the more mildly involved cases, the cytoplasm of muscle cells showed a pallor which had been imparted to it by delicate vacuolation due to hydropic degeneration (*Figure 17.11*) which might, on cursory examination, be presumed to be a post-mortem change. This vacuolation was present even when the interval between deaths and post-mortem fixation was short.

More distinctive, but not pathognomonic, degenerative changes involved myocardial cells in diffuse but focal patterns varying from case to case in the degree of involvement. The larger the heart the more striking the frequency, size and variety of cellular and interstitial changes. Examination of the myocardium revealed changes which could be classified under three headings.

(1) *Acute Myocardial Alteration.* Acute myocardial alteration, in the form of hyaline necrosis, has been seen in 14 cases. The lesions involved all the chambers equally; no specific subendocardial predilection, characteristic of anoxaemic myocardial necrosis, was noted. In three cases the necrosis was infarct-like and in eleven other cases was focal.

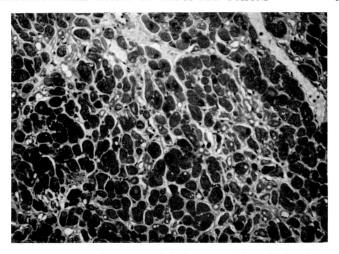

Figure 17.10. Diffuse myocardial changes and interstitial oedema (haematoxylin and eosin × 160) (Bonenfant et al., 1969)

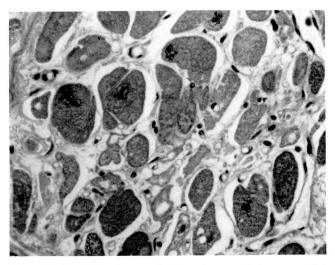

Figure 17.11. Hydropic vacuolization of some of the myocardial fibres (haematoxylin and eosin × 320) (Bonenfant et al., 1969)

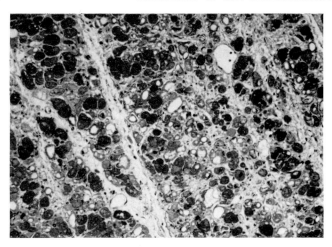

Figure 17.12.　Combination of acute and chronic myocardial changes with muscle fibres presenting dense basophilic cytoplasm and loss of cross striations (Phosphotungstic acid haematoxylin × 400). (Reproduced by courtesy of Dr G. Rona)

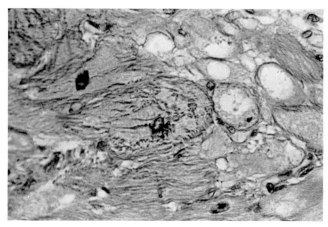

Figure 17.13.　Intracytoplasmic vacuoles situated along the longitudinal axis and leading to fusiform swelling of the muscle fibres (haematoxylin and eosin × 125). (Reproduced by courtesy of Dr G. Rona)

Although cellular reaction was insignificant, the site of the lesion was distinctly demarcated from the adjacent intact areas by cytoplasmic eosinophilia. In PAS stains there was disappearance of intracytoplasmic glycogen. PTAH stain revealed a loss of cross striations (*Figure 17.12*). The alteration of the contractile elements was more advanced than were the nuclear changes. The enlarged, irregular nuclei presented a condensation of chromatin; with

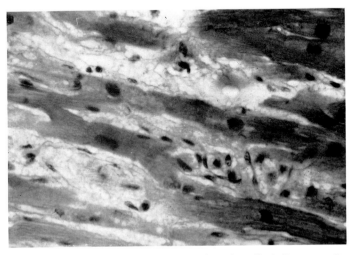

Figure 17.14. Myocardium diminution and loss of myofibrils (haematoxylin and eosin × 320) (Bonenfant et al., 1969)

progression of the necrobiotic process together with the contractile elements the nuclei also disappeared.

(2) *Vacuolar Degeneration.* This was the most conspicuous chronic myofibre change (*Figure 17.13*). The cytoplasmic vacuoles were generally multiple and particularly prominent on cross section, being less noticeable in longitudinal sections where there is no uniform pattern of localization, although the process may develop in the juxtanuclear zone.

The vacuoles were different in size and shape and produced a fusiform swelling of the muscle fibres. Often a vacuole (larger than the nucleus) was found on either side of a nucleus, compressing and disturbing it. A segment of certain muscle bundles, rather than certain specific layers of the myocardium, was effected.

(3) *Myofibre Degeneration.* Swelling, uneven staining of the cytoplasm and disorganization of the contractile elements could be

interpreted as evidence of myofibre dystrophy. This change involved the myocardial cell in a more uniform fashion than any of the changes listed above. Groups of enlarged fibres showed coarse irregular myofibrils. These fibrils presented a characteristic peripheral arrangement (*Figure 17.14*) leaving at the central portions of the distended muscle fibres a pale structureless basophilic area. Less frequently the contractile elements exhibited a dense basophilic cytoplasm. These myofibril changes were scattered throughout the cell in a diffuse fashion, the remaining sarcoplasm having a fine dust-like evenly dispersed granularity. There was an increase of lipochrome content of the fibres. The nuclei were irregular in shape and size and rich in chromatin. The nucleus might eventually appear to be centrally located in a relatively empty space at whose margins there was only a narrow zone of condensed cytoplasm.

Dystrophic and vacuolar fibres alternated. The fading fibres and empty sarcolemmal sheaths gave to the myocardium a moth-eaten appearance. In other foci, together with contractile elements and other cytoplasmic components, the sarcolemmal sheaths disappeared leading to myocytolysis (*Figure 17.15*).

It is common to find that the degenerative changes described above cause cellular drop-out involving only isolated cells or small clusters of cells producing a looseness and lack of cohesiveness in myocardial pattern. In some instances where large groups or even facicles of cells were involved, study of cross-cut sections revealed marked variation in myocardial cell bulk. Fat tissue replacement (lipomatosis) of the vanished myofibres completed the process. Frozen sections, stained for fat, all showed a fatty metamorphosis of varying intensity in the form of fine intracytoplasmic droplets (*Figure 17.16*). Lipochrome pigment could be seen freely dispersed among the stromal elements.

(4) *Lack of reactive changes in the myocardium.* This was remarkable. Associated with hyaline necrosis there were oedema and minimal cellular reaction, consisting mainly of mononuclear cells. Pronounced cellular reaction was recognized in one case only, which showed eosinophils, histiocytes and mast cells; this finding was regarded as exceptional. The apparent fibrosis in chronic cases resulted from myofibre collapse rather than from fibrous connective tissue proliferation. The scars contained enlarged capillaries.

A peculiar pathognomonic change was noted in the small myocardial arteries, arterioles and capillaries. The central portion was occupied by a watery substance which separated the intimal and adventitial layers apart and gave rise to the formation of a double contour image (*Figure 17.17*).

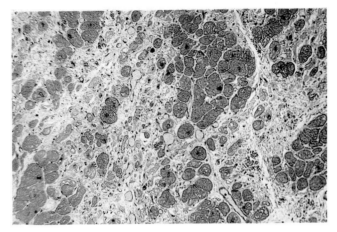

Figure 17.15.   Empty sarcolemmal sheaths and moth-eaten appearance of the myocardium. In some places the disappearance of myocardial fibres leads to collapse fibrosis (Phospho-tungstic acid haematoxylin × 125). (Reproduced by courtesy of Dr G. Rona)

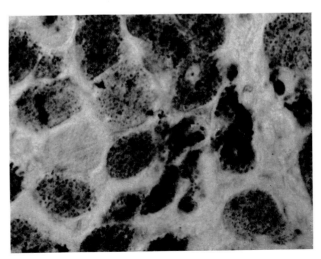

Figure 17.16.   Intracytoplasmic fat inclusions in myocardial cells. (Sudan V × 320) (Bonenfant et al., 1969)

The epicardium in most areas showed some degree of swelling of the serosal lining cells, and seemingly passive, isolated subepicardial aggregates of round cells suggested foci of ectopic erythropoiesis. When epicarditis occurred, as in those cases where a pericardiocentesis had been carried out, it was the typical fibrinous variety with a relatively mild inflammatory cell infiltrate.

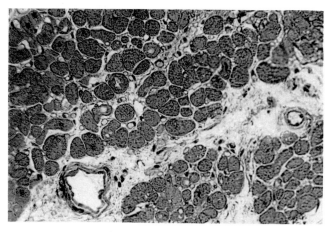

Figure 17.17. The characteristic double-contour image of a small artery formed by the compressed intimal and adventitial coats (phosphotungstic acid haematoxylin × 400). (Reproduced by courtesy of Dr G. Rona)

OTHER ASSOCIATED LESIONS

The most common organ to be infarcted was the lung. Infarction of the lung or other organs is due to mural thrombi—the emboli most commonly arising in the atrial appendages. The most frequent extracardiac lesion was widespread central or confluent hepatic necrosis associated with fatty metamorphosis and minimal cellular reaction.

AETIOLOGY

It was found that the onset of this disease and its subsequent disappearance coincided with the addition and later removal of cobalt sulphate, a foam stabilizer, from beer in the infected areas. Changes in the thyroid glands of fatal cases resembled those induced by cobalt hyperplasia (Morin and Daniel, 1967). Experimental studies were conducted therefore to determine the possible cardiotoxic effects of cobalt.

Rats given high levels of cobalt sulphate developed widespread degenerative and necrotic changes in myocardial cells with a reactive interstitial response (*Figure 17.18*) and occasional mural thrombi (Grice *et al.*, 1969). Administration of cobalt also markedly altered the electrocardiographic pattern especially in the older animals.

In experimental studies on rats (Rona, 1971) to investigate this cardiomyopathy the following features of the disease were elucidated.

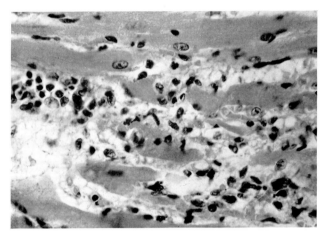

Figure 17.18. Section of heart from 7 month old rat killed 24 hours after receiving an intraperitoneal injection of 4 mg/kg cobalt. Necrosis of myofibres and infiltrations of inflammatory cells (haematoxylin, phloxin and saffron stains × 500). (Reproduced from Heggtoeit, Grice and Wiberg (1970) by courtesy of the authors and Editor of Pathologica et Microbiologia)

(1) All the chambers of the heart are affected with atrial predilection. The primary morphologic alteration is mitochondrial damage (*Figure 17.19*) that possibly reflects an enzymatic block of oxidative decarboxylation at pyruvate and ketogenic levels. Electron-dense intramitochondrial particles may be seen, representing cobalt protein complexes (*Figure 17.20*).

(2) In acute cobalt toxicity chelation of calcium may be a contributory factor, resulting in deficient utilization of high-energy phosphates.

Experimental cobalt cardiomyopathy requires preconditioning factors; protein deficiency appears to be one of them. Vegetative polypoid endocarditis (*Figure 17.21*) was an important accompaniment in these animals, suggesting that in rats (on a protein deficient

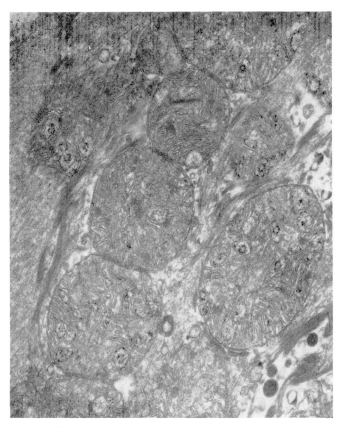

Figure 17.19.   Electromicroscopic presentation of swollen mitochondria, dilated sarcoplasmic reticulum and intrasarcoplasmic oedema (× 18,500)

diet) cobalt produced endothelial damage in addition to cardiocyte damage.

Cobalt ions were found to depress oxygen uptake in isolated rat heart mitochondria (Wiberg, 1968). It was therefore concluded that cobalt interfered with cardiac metabolism by complexing with the sulphydryl groups of alpha-lipoic acid and thereby prevented the oxidation of alpha-ketoglutarate and pyruvate. Since alpha-lipoic acid and thiamine act on co-factors (lipothiamide) in the tricarboxylic acid cycle and in association with pyruvate dehydrogenase the clinicopathological similarities between cobalt toxicity and acute cardiac beriberi are understandable (*Figure 17.22*).

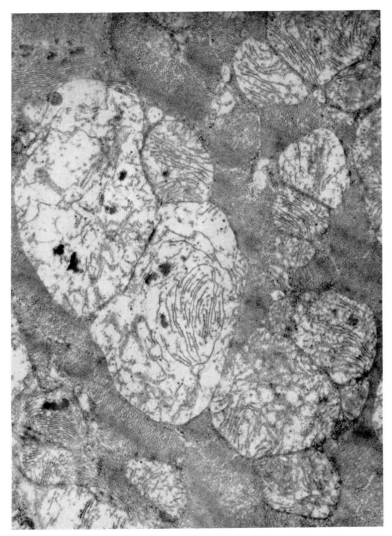

Figure 17.20. Myocardium electron-dense intramitochondrial particles which represent cobalt-protein complexes (× 16,300). (Reproduced from Rona (1971) by courtesy of the author and Editor of the British Heart Journal)

Cobalt ions, in effect, produce a biochemical block at precisely the same points in the myocardial metabolic pathways as thiamine deficiency would act. A number of factors, including the route of administration, affected the cardiotoxicity of cobalt. The incidence and severity of the lesions were greater in older rats, in rats with

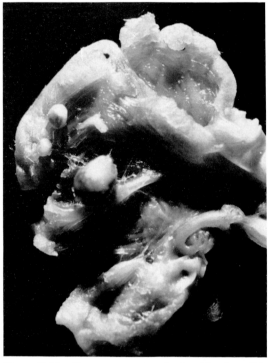

Figure 17.21.   Gross presentation of polypoid endocarditis in the mitral valve of a rat on protein-deficient diet treated with 12·5 mg/kg cobalt ion daily. (Reproduced from Rona (1971) by courtesy of the author and Editor of the British Heart Journal)

pre-existing heart damage and in animals having an unsatisfactory nutritional background.

Animals with a restricted thiamine intake or those maintained solely on beer were more sensitive to the cardiotoxic effects of cobalt (Grice *et al.*, 1969). The availability of a high quality protein diet afforded considerable protection against the acute and subacute toxicity of cobalt ions as they complex readily with both sulphydryl and amine groups. The protective effect of amino acids was probably related to the reduced absorption of cobalt from the gut (Wiberg *et al.*, 1969).

The so-called epidemics of cardiomyopathy in beer drinkers were probably multicausal in origin. A background of poor nutrition and chronic alcoholism (subclinical alcoholic or nutritional heart disease) apparently preconditioned these individuals to the metabolic consequences of cobalt ions which, perhaps along with some as yet unidentified factor, precipitated them into clinical heart failure.

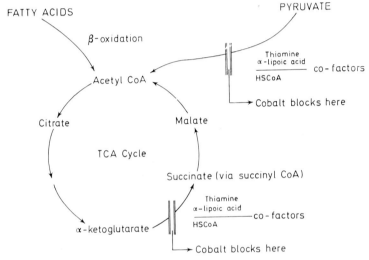

Figure 17.22. Effect of cobalt on cardiac energy metabolism. (Reproduced from Heggtoeit, Grice and Wiberg (1970) by courtesy of the authors and Editor of Pathologia et Microbiologia)

Barborik and Dusek (1972) have recently described the case of a metal worker, who had been exposed to cobalt for some time and had suddenly presented with congestive cardiac failure, dying suddenly two days after being admitted to hospital.

At necropsy the heart was found to weigh 490 g. Both the ventricles and atria were dilated and the myocardium of both ventricles was pale. A histological study of several areas from the ventricles showed that the myocardial fibres were mostly fragmented with focal vacuolar changes. The interstitial tissue, separating the muscle fibres, was diffusely increased and oedematous. The endocardium was also diffusely thickened with occasional small parietal thrombi. There was no inflammatory reaction in any of the areas studied. A sample of myocardium analysed for cobalt showed a high concentration of cobalt—140 μg/100 g of dry tissue (controls 10 μg/100 g of dry tissue). This case, therefore, seems to be the first report of cobalt cardiomyopathy from an industrial cause and not derived from drinking beer. This patient also had not had a high intake of alcohol or a poor nutritional history.

References

Alexander, C. S. (1972). 'Cobalt-beer cardiomyopathy.' *Am. J. Med.* **53**, 395

Barborik, M. and Dusek, J. (1972). 'Cardiomyopathy accompanying industrial cobalt exposure.' *Br. Heart J.* **34**, 113

Bonenfant, J. L., Auger, C., Miller, G., Chenard, J. and Roy, P. E. (1969). 'Quebec beer drinkers cardiomyopathy: Pathological studies.' *Ann. N.Y. Acad. Sci.* **156**, 577

Grice, H. C., Goodman, T., Munroe, I. E., Wiberg, G. S. and Morrison, A. B. (1969). 'Myocardial toxicity of cobalt in the rat.' *Ann. N.Y. med. Sci.* **156**, 189

Heggtoeit, H. A., Grice, H. C. and Wiberg, G. S. (1970). 'Cobalt cardiomyopathy.' *Pathologia Microbiol.* **35**, 110

Kesteloot, H., Roelandt, J., Willems, J., Class, J. H. and Joosens, J. V. (1968). 'An inquiry into the role of cobalt in the heart disease of chronic beer drinkers.' *Circulation* **37**, 834

Morin, Y. and Daniel, P. (1967). 'Quebec beer drinkers cardiomyopathy: Etiological considerations.' *Can. med. Ass. J.* **97**, 926

Rona, G. (1968). 'Endemic cardiomyopathy of beer consumers.' *Acta morph. hung.* **16**(i), 103

— (1971). 'Experimental aspects of cobalt cardiomyopathy.' *Br. Heart J.* **33**, Suppl. 171

Sullivan, J., Parker, M. and Carson, S. B. (1968). 'Tissue cobalt content in beer drinkers cardiomyopathy.' *J. Lab. clin. Med.* **71**, 893

Wiberg, G. S. (1968). 'The effect of cobalt ions on energy metabolism in the rat.' *Can. J. Biochem.* **46**, 549

Wiberg, G. S., Munro, L. C., Meranger, J. C., Morrison, A. B., Grice, H. C. and Heggtoeit, H. A. (1969). 'Factors affecting the cardiotoxic potential of cobalt clintoxical.' *Clin. Toxicol.* **2**, 257

PHYSICAL AGENTS

TEMPERATURE AND HUMIDITY

Hypothermia may occur in elderly people (living in ill-heated rooms), especially if they are debilitated, and the newborn baby is also very susceptible to exposure to cold. Kuhn (1956) demonstrated the occurrence of electrocardiogram alterations in healthy young men working in Arctic conditions.

Exposure to heat and high humidity can precipitate or aggravate congestive heart failure in patients with borderline function, but there is no evidence, at present, that such exposure will lead to heart disease in a normal person. Cellular injury or death occurs if tissue temperature is maintained at a level exceeding 5·5°C above or 15°C below that which is normal for blood. Circulatory failure occurs when the temperature of the circulating blood is reduced to approximately 20°C.

Systemic hypothermia produces no gross or histological changes that can be regarded as pathognomonic of death. The post-mortem findings usually consist only of dilatation of the right chambers of the heart and oedema of the lungs. Talbott, Consolazio and Peceria (1941) described a patient who died during therapeutic reduction of body temperature.

The pathological changes merely mentioned 'myocardial degeneration', but also stated that there was no marked coronary artery narrowing. Electrocardiogram evidence of widespread myocardial involvement was also observed.

Death during re-warming was thought not to be due to any organic damage to the myocardium but, by functional disturbances resulting from heat, induced vasodilatation and, aggravated by impaired gaseous exchange, sluggish circulation and acidosis. Duguid, Simpson and Stowers (1961) described 23 elderly cases with hypothermia.

Thirteen necropsies were performed: 3 of the patients had micro-infarcts in the myocardium of the ventricle and all had fatty changes in the myocardium. It was suggested that these lesions resulted from hypothermia, due to circulatory collapse, haemoconcentration, capillary sludging and depressed cell metabolism.

Read *et al.* (1961) reported two cases of hypothermia, one of whom died, and necropsy showed dilatation of the heart chambers, epicardial petechia and a subendocardial haemorrhage in the outflow tracts of the right ventricle. This outcome is heralded by generalized vasodilatation, rapid pulse, dilatation of the heart, impairment of cardiac frequency and respiratory irregularities.

EXPERIMENTAL STUDIES

Fisher, Febor and Fisher (1957) observed fatty degeneration in the hearts of dogs kept for several hours at about 23–24°C, but failed to detect any definite evidence of myocardial damage in sections taken from the left ventricle and including a portion of the conducting systems.

Short periods of hypothermia at about 30°C have been shown by Heinrich *et al.* (1960) not to result in producing any permanent myocardial damage.

In 1964 Sarajas carried out a detailed long-term study on the pathological changes found in the heart in dogs which had been cooled to $-27°C$ and kept hypothermic for a considerable time.

In the dogs cooled without subsequent rewarming, the changes consisted mainly of interstitial oedema, subendocardial haemorrhages, coagulation necrosis, and slight fatty necrosis of myocardial fibres.

References

Duguid, Helen, Simpson, R. G. and Stowers, R. G. (1961). 'Accidental hypothermia.' *Lancet* 2, 1213

Fisher, E. R., Febor, E. J. and Fisher, B. (1957). 'Pathological and histochemical observations in experimental hypothermia.' *Archs Surg.* 75, 817

Heinrich, G., Hove, G. E., Schavtz, R. and Helbid (1960). 'Der Einfluss des katrallierten Hypotherma auf das Herz und die parenchymatosie Organe.' *Archs clin. Chir.* 293, 513

Kuhn, L. A. (1956). 'The effects of arctic climate and different shelter temperatures on the electrocardiogram.' *Am. Heart J.* 51, 387

Read, A. E., Emslie-Smith, D., Gough, K. R. and Holmes, R. (1961). 'Pancreatitis and accidental hypothermia.' *Lancet* 2, 1219

Sarajas, H. S. (1964). 'Myocardial damage induced by immersion hypothermia.' *Am. J. Cardiol.* 13, 355

Talbott, J. H., Consolazio, W. V. and Peceria, L. J. (1941). 'Hypothermia. Report of a case in which the patient died during therapeutic reduction of body temperature, with metabolic and pathologic studies.' *Archs intern. Med.* 68, 1120

RADIANT ENERGY

Except for the effects of heat from the infrared end of the spectrum and the capillary damage caused by burns from the ultraviolet rays, radiant energy does not have any specific effect on the heart.

ELECTRIC CURRENT INJURY

In deaths from electric shock, the chief pathological lesion is blood stasis due to cessation of action of the heart.

Anatomical lesions of the heart are rare apart from rupture and fragmentation of myocardial fibres, which have been recorded. Disturbances of rhythm have been reported occasionally. Gossels (1949) found seven such cases in the literature and added another, that of a healthy man of 49 years who touched a high tension wire with an aluminium ladder. He was knocked unconscious; shortly afterwards the ventricular rate was 130 per minute, the pulse was weak and the blood pressure too weak to record; three hours later it rose to 80/60 mmHg, the pulse was 120 and the electrocardiogram showed atrial fibrillation and premature ventricular contractions.

He was treated with digitalis and by the third day the electro-cardiogram was normal and the blood pressure had returned to its normal level. Electric shocks are now used in defibrillating the heart, in pacemaking and in abolishing arrhythmias; if the apparatus is faultily designed, there is a danger of electrocution. Noordijk, Oey and Tebra (1961) described two such accidents in a boy of five years and a girl aged 15; the standard lead of the electrocardiogram, connected to the hand and foot, was earthed through the heart to the earth of a disconnected pacemaker apparatus. Both patients developed ventricular fibrillation as the electrocardiogram machine was connected; both patients recovered after cardiac massage.

Rivkin (1963) studied the cardiac burns produced by direct cardiac defibrillation shock in dogs; the degree was related to the energy of the defibrillating current and to the electrode contact; burns were less severe when good contact was made by saline moistened polythene pads on the electrodes. By contrast, external defibrillation through the chest wall did not produce lesions. Intraventricular and intramural temperatures were significantly raised by A.C. shocks of over 0·1 sec and by sparking from electrodes with D.C. shocks for 80 W-sec or more. Thirteen of the 33 dogs suffered deep myocardial burns after shocks of high thermogenic potential, 11 died in 24 hours with extreme myocardial necrosis.

References

Gossels, C. L. (1949). 'Auricular fibrillation caused by electric accident (effects of electric current on the human body).' *Expl Med. Surg.* **7**, 335

Noordijk, J. A., Oey, F. T. I. and Tebra, W. (1961). 'Myocardial electrodes and the danger of ventricular fibrillation.' *Lancet* **1**, 975

Rivkin, L. M. (1963). 'The defibrillator and cardiac burns.' *J. thorac. cardiovasc. Surg.* **46**, 755

IONIZING RADIATION

Schweizer (1924) reported that in humans irradiation of the chest in Hodgkin's disease produced atrophy of heart muscle and thickening of capillaries. Hartman *et al.* (1927), however, found no definite changes in the hearts of three patients receiving irradiation therapy, but no electrocardiograms were done on these patients.

Thibaudeau and Mattick (1929) examined the hearts from ten patients, who had received therapy for adjacent malignant disease, and found changes varying from slight interstitial fibrosis to hyaline and fatty degeneration of muscle fibres in sections of the lateral border of the ventricle between the apex and the mitral valve.

Ellinger (1957) regarded myocardial tissue to be amongst the most radioresistant tissues in the body. Leach (1943) has found that experimental animals must be exposed to at least 10,000 rads in a single dose in order to exhibit microscopic evidence of myocardial damage. The extent of the cardiac tolerance of human beings to irradiation is variously stated in the literature and Jones and Wedgewood (1960) have pointed out the paradoxic nature of the clinical reports alleging damage of the heart from doses which are relatively low in comparison with those required to produce lesions in experimental animals. Although electrocardiogram abnormalities were reported to have followed irradiation of the thorax, virtually all of them were of a transient nature and clinically insignificant. There are no records of electrocardiogram abnormalities indicative of a myocardial infarct that could be attributed to radiation. Warren (1942) who regarded the response of cardiac tissue to irradiation as non-specific stated, however, that the final effect is indistinguishable from that produced by conventional infarction. Damage from irradiation appears to be caused by its high absorption by the extra-cellular connective tissue, particularly collagen. Especially sensitive to such absorption are the walls of the blood vessels, wherein the changes are apparently secondary to the alteration and depletion of collagen. According to Rhoades (1948) the changes are most pronounced approximately two weeks after irradiation.

Liebow, Warren and Decoursey (1949) in a study of the victims of the atomic bomb explosions at Hiroshima and Nagasaki found haemorrhages, oedema, focal necrosis and infiltration with plasma cells and mononuclear cells in the hearts. Tullis (1949), however, found no significant changes in the hearts of the swine which had been exposed to the nuclear explosions at Bikini.

Windsor (1963) studied the heart of a man aged 62 who had received a total irradiation of 4,000 rads posteriorly and 5,250 rads anteriorly. At operation the right atrium tore through and this proved fatal. Histology showed patchy degeneration of muscle with swelling and eosinophils of the cytoplasm which appeared granular; there were a few areas of necrosis. Some vessels showed endothelial and fibroplastic proliferation and others fibrinoid necrosis. The pericardium showed thickening by hyaline collagen, with chronic inflammatory cell infiltrate.

Cohn (1967) of Stanford University School of Medicine reported on 25 patients who suffered heart disease following irradiation of the chest for various tumours. Total doses were 3,000 to 6,000 rads. Most common was acute pericarditis (in 15), often with effusion; chronic effusion (in 12) or constriction (in 10), sometimes with myocardial or endocardial fibrosis. The incidence was 3·4 per cent in patients with carcinoma of the breast and 5·8 per cent in those with malignant lymphoma. It was recognized that the disease itself might be associated with some of these complications.

Fajardo, Stewart and Cohn (1968) carried out a careful study on the myocardial changes found in 16 patients with radiation induced heart disease.

The myocardium was involved in the majority of these cases.

The most conspicuous change was the presence of diffuse interstitial fibrosis, frequently severe, which separated the myocardial fibres individually and rarely formed large areas of dense collagen.

Within the stroma occupied by collagen, capillaries were not easily seen and in large areas the myocardial fibres appear to be 'choked' by this endomyocardial fibrosis. Its extent and location varied widely.

Sometimes the myocardial fibres were small but, at other times, larger than normal and contained bizarre-shaped nuclei. Rarely vacuolation of some myocardial fibres was seen.

The endocardium is normally only slightly affected. It may show small patches of fibrosis but this endocardial thickening rarely contains elastic tissue fibres.

The small intramyocardial blood vessels were not usually found to show any consistent change but in about half the cases studied showed some endothelial proliferation.

EXPERIMENTAL CHANGES

Hartman *et al.* (1927) gave massive irradiation to the thorax of dogs and sheep. In the animals dying within 30 days there was pericardial effusion and swelling, indistinct striations or irregular staining of muscle fibres with engorgement of capillaries; the bundle of His appeared to be more resistant. In dogs surviving 3–5 months there was haemorrhagic infiltration of the right atrium, thickening of vessels and atrophy of ventricular muscle with vacuolization; the atrial muscle was largely replaced by areas of pink, homogeneous degenerative tissue; one animal died suddenly. Electrocardiograms revealed myocardial damage and also showed paroxysmal tachycardia, atrial flutter or fibrillation. Similar histological findings to these were found in the hearts of mice and rabbits by Warthin and Pohle (1929).

Animals exposed to high acute dosages develop lesions. Thus Phillips, Reid and Rugh (1964) after exposure of the canine heart to acute, high dosage of pre-cordial x-irradiation, observed microscopic changes varying from extravasation of red blood cells and hyaline alterations of connective tissue and muscle to marked destruction and fibrosis of muscle. Although the localized changes are not unlike those of acute myocardial infarct, the distribution of spared and damaged areas and the severity of reaction are inconstant and the overall picture unrelated to vascular distribution. Emphasizing the importance of dose-time relationships, Senderoff *et al.* (1959) reported that prior irradiation of the heart enhanced the ability of dogs to survive induced myocardial infarcts, owing to the expanded collateral circulation resulting from the dilatation of small coronary vessels. Careful examinations, as late as six months after the experiments, failed to show any harmful effects of irradiation on the heart.

Jones and Wedgewood (1960) have given a comprehensive review of the histological evidence of irradiation of the heart in animals.

ASSOCIATED MYOCARDIAL INFARCTION

It is thought probable that irradiation of the heart may cause coronary thrombosis. Pearson (1958) reported that two patients receiving deep x-ray therapy for mammary carcinoma developed extensive cardiac infarction six months later; they recovered and Dollinger, Lavine and Foye (1965) reported myocardial infarction following two months after irradiation of the lower mediastinum and oesophagus for Hodgkin's disease in a man of 31 years. Subsequently he suffered angina pectoris for 16 years and died of congestive failure. Necropsy showed virtual occlusion of the right ventricle and posterior septum. The occlusion was due to fibromuscular proliferation of the intima. The serum cholesterol was normal and there was no atheroma elsewhere.

Thomas and Forbus (1959) reported a man of 59 years who had received irradiation (180 rads) to the mediastinum for suspected lymphoma $2\frac{1}{2}$ years previously, followed by two further doses, one year and three months before death. At necropsy the aorta showed sharply defined thickening with wrinkled intima bearing thrombi, extending for about 10 cm distal to the origin of the left subclavian artery. Emboli were present in the kidneys and spleen although none were found in any coronary vessel. This case demonstrates that blood vessels may be so damaged that thrombosis is likely to arise in them, although it did not cause a myocardial infarction here.

Rarely, radiation seems to stimulate the production of atherosclerosis in the coronary arteries, as in the 15 year old boy reported by

Fajardo, Stewart and Cohn (1968), who died from a myocardial infarction shortly after being given a course of radiotherapy. At autopsy the coronary arteries, especially the left descending, were grossly atherosclerotic. In this case there was no family history of atherosclerosis or hyperlipidaemia (Fajardo, Stewart and Cohn, 1968).

References

Cohn, K. (1967). 'Heart damage tied to radiotherapy.' *Wld. Med.* June 6th 49

Dollinger, M. R., Lavine, D. M. and Foye, L. V., Jnr (1965). 'Myocardial infarction following radiation.' *Lancet* **2**, 246

Ellinger, F. P. (1957). *Medical Radiation Biology*, p. 945. Springfield Ill: Thomas

Fajardo, L. F., Stewart, R. J. and Cohn, K. E. (1968). 'Morphology of radiation induced heart disease.' *Archs. Path.* **86**, 512

Hartman, F. W., Bolliger, A., Doub, H. P. and Smith, F. J. (1927). 'Heart lesions produced by the deep x-ray: an experimental and clinical study.' *Bull. Johns Hopkins Hosp.* **41**, 36

Jones, A. and Wedgewood, J. (1960). 'Effects of radiation on the heart.' *Br. J. Radiol.* **33**, 138

Leach, J. E. (1943). 'Some effects of roentgen irradiation of the cardiovascular system.' *Am. J. Roentg.* **50**, 616

Liebow, A. A., Warren, S., and Decoursey, E. (1949). 'Pathology of atomic bomb casualties.' *Am. J. Path.* **25**, 853

Pearson, H. E. S. (1958). 'Incidental damages of x-ray therapy.' *Lancet* **1**, 222

Phillips, S. J., Reid, J. A. and Rugh, R. (1964). 'Electrocardiographic and pathologic changes after cardiac irradiation in dogs.' *Am. Heart J.* **68**, 524

Rhoades, R. D. (1948). 'The vascular system.' In *Histopathology of Irradiation from External and Internal Sources.* Ed. by W. Broom, p. 808. New York: McGraw-Hill

Schweizer, E. (1924). 'Über spezifische Roentgenschädigungen des Herzmuskel.' *Strahlentherapie* **18**, 812

Senderoff, E., Kanee, D. J., Johnson, R. J. R. and Baronowsky, I. (1959). 'Survival following acute coronary artery ligation subsequent to irradiation of the canine heart.' *Proc. Soc. exp. Biol. Med.* **100**, 1

Thibaudeau, A. A. and Mattick, W. L. (1929). 'Histological findings in hearts which have been exposed to radiation in the course of treatment of adjacent organs.' *J. Cancer Res.* **13**, 251

Thomas, Elizabeth, and Forbus, W. D. (1959). 'Irradiation injury to the aorta and lung.' *Archs Path.* **67**, 256

Tullis, J. L. (1949). 'The response of tissue to total body irradiation.' *Am. J. Path.* **25**, 829

Warren, S. (1942). 'Effects of radiation on normal tissues. VI. Effects of radiation on the cardiovascular system.' *Archs Path.* **34**, 1070

Warthin, A. S. and Pohle, E. A. (1939). 'The effect of roentgen rays on the heart. II. The microscopic changes in the heart muscle of rats and of rabbits following a series of exposures.' *Archs intern. Med.* **43**, 15

Windsor, R. (1963). 'Cardiac damage after radiotherapy.' *Br. med. J.* **1**, 382

Eighteen

Cardiomyopathies found in animals

While it is quite likely that cardiomyopathies are as common in animals as in man, few such cases have been reported. This is probably because of the infrequency with which veterinary neonatal deaths are investigated by necropsy or, if necropsies are carried out in older animals, then a detailed examination of the heart may be omitted once a cause of death has been found.

FIBRO-ELASTOSIS

Fibro-elastosis is possibly the most common type of cardiomyopathy to be found in animals, having been described in cattle by Smith and Jones (1967). This disease has also been reported in two puppies and a kitten (Eliot *et al.*, 1958; Krahwinkel and Coogan, 1971) in calves and in pigs (Nieberle and Cohrs, 1967; Hamlin, 1968). The apparent low incidence of this disease in animals is probably caused by the infrequency with which neonatal deaths in animals are investigated by necropsy.

Fibro-elastosis may sometimes be associated with congenital abnormalities, as in the puppy with congenital aortic stenosis, left ventricular hypertrophy and generalized cardiac enlargement (Eliot *et al.*, 1958).

Death usually occurs in the neonatal period in all species but some have survived to early adulthood (Smith and Jones, 1967). At necropsy the heart is usually found to be enlarged to two or three times its normal size. The right atrium and ventricle are dilated and the myocardium of these cavities is slightly hypertrophied.

When the heart is opened the endocardium is seen to be thickened and appears more grey and opaque than normal (*Figure 18.1*).

In one case (Krahwinkel and Coogan, 1971) the collagenous endocardial tissue in these areas was forming cartilage. There is no evidence of infiltration of the myocardium with lymphocytes or other

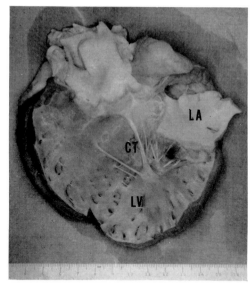

Figure 18.1. The left ventricle (LV) is dilated and its endocardium moderately opacified throughout, especially over the apex and inferior interventricular septum. The endocardium of the left atrium (LA) is also opacified. The mitral valve and chordae tendineae (CT) are thickened and fused. (Reproduced by courtesy of Dr D. F. Kelly)

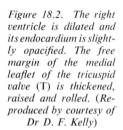

Figure 18.2. The right ventricle is dilated and its endocardium is slightly opacified. The free margin of the medial leaflet of the tricuspid valve (T) is thickened, raised and rolled. (Reproduced by courtesy of Dr D. F. Kelly)

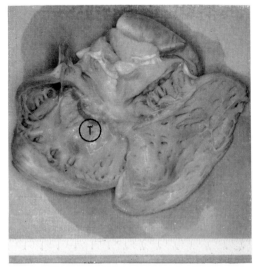

chronic inflammatory cells. In no cases have mural thrombi been found on the endocardial surface nor has evidence of a thrombo-embolic episode, the embolus originating from the heart, been noted.

The atrioventricular valves are usually dilated and the valves are often fused (*Figure 18.2*) and valve leaflets are thickened, especially along their free edges. These valvular thickenings consist of nodular masses of myxomatous tissue. These nodules are often confluent, producing a blunt rolled edge. The chordae tendineae may be thickened, fused and shortened as may the valvular annuli.

MYOCARDIUM

The left ventricle is, usually, more dilated than the right but is only slightly hypertrophied; the endocardium is usually thickened in all parts of the atria and ventricles, giving it a 'sugar icing' appearance. This thickening is most marked in the left side of the heart in the inferior portion of the interventricular septum.

MICROSCOPIC FINDINGS

The endocardium is seen to be thickened by a layer of cellular myxomatous fibrous tissue which is sometimes well marked, particularly in the region of the ventricular apices.

This endocardial layer is usually clearly demarcated from the myocardium. Strands of fibrous tissue may pass down into the underlying muscle and, in doing this, separate small fragments of muscle from the main mass of myocardial tissue.

The changes are best seen when a trichrome stain is examined and, in these sections, small deposits of fibrin are often found on the endocardial surface or in its more superficial layers (*Figure 18.3*).

When stained for elastic tissue the thickened endocardium is seen to contain a large number of thin, wavy, well-ordered elastic fibres within firm collagenous tissue. Often the most superficial part of the endocardium contains no elastic tissue (*Figure 18.4*).

References

Bajusz, E. (1969). 'Hereditary cardiomyopathy: A new disease model.' *Am. Heart J.* **77**, 686

Eliot, T. R. Jnr, Eliot, F. P., Lushbaugh, C. C. and Slager, V. T. (1958). 'First report of the occurrence of neonatal endocardial fibro-elastosis in cats and dogs.' *J. Am. vet. med. Ass.* **133**, 271

Hamlin, R. L. (1968). 'Prognostic value of changes in the cardiac silhouette in dogs with mitral insufficiency.' *J. Am. vet. med. Ass.* **153**, 1436

Krahwinkel, D. J. Jnr, and Coogan, P. S. (1971). 'Endocardial fibro-elastosis in a great dane pup.' *J. Am. vet. med. Ass.* **159**, 327

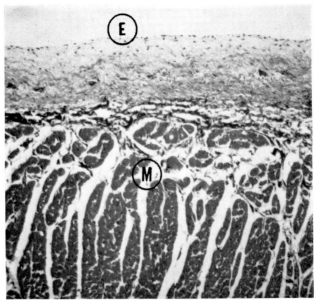

Figure 18.3. Section of apical endocardium and myocardium. Notice marked endocardial thickening (E) consisting of cellular myxomatous fibrous tissue. The elastic fibres are inconspicuous with this stain. The underlying myocardium is normal (M) (Masson's trichrome stain × 100)

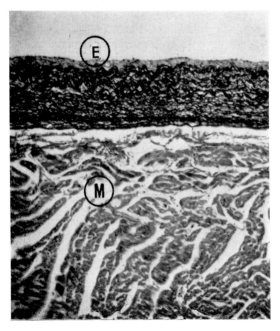

Figure 18.4. A section of apical endocardium (E). stained for elastic fibres. Notice abundant well-ordered elastic lamellae closely resembling elastic lamellae of the aorta. The underlying myocardium is normal (M)(Verhoeff's elastica stain × 100). (Reproduced from Krohwinkel and Coogan (1971) by courtesy of the authors and Editor of the Journal of the American Veterinary Medical Association)

Nieberle, K. and Cohrs, P. (1967). *Special Pathological Anatomy of Domestic Animals*. 1st English Edition, pp. 3–4. London: Pergamon

Smith, H. H. and Jones, T. C. (1967). 'Endocardial fibro-elastosis in cattle —first report of the condition.' In *Veterinary Pathology*, 3rd Edition, p. 791. Philadelphia: Lea and Febiger

CARDIOMYOPATHY IN SYRIAN HAMSTERS

A cardiomyopathy was first described by Homburger *et al.* (1962). It occurs in a strain of Syrian Hamster (Bio 14.6) and was developed

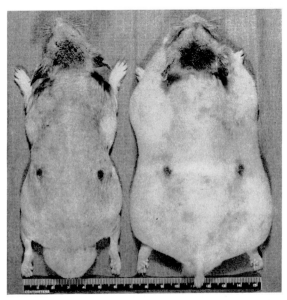

Figure 18.5. Cardiomyopathic hamsters show a normal physical appearance before generalized oedema becomes apparent. Comparison of two 138 day old female hamsters, one without appreciable oedema (left) the other highly oedematous (right), also indicates the variability that occurs in the progression of the spontaneous cardiac condition. Fluid accumulation gave rise to a difference in body weights amounting to 73 g (Bajusz, 1969)

by brother—sister matings. Some of these animals already had cardiomegaly. The spontaneous disease is characterized by the occurrence of focal myocardial degeneration resulting in congestive heart failure.

Myocardial degeneration occurs in all animals of both sexes within this inbred line. With the exception of a few cases (in which the

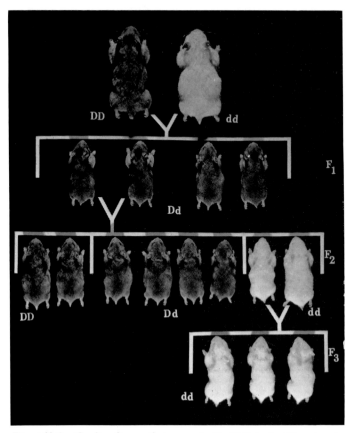

Figure 18.6.   Cardiac disease that occurs in Bio 14·6 strain of hamsters is transmitted by an autosomal recessive gene and, hence, new cardiomyopathic sublines may be developed by crossbreeding between healthy (DD) *and diseased* (dd) *strains. The carriers* (Dd) *in the* F_1 *and* F_2 *generations do not show any of the disease manifestations. In the* F_3 *generation, a* 100 *per cent incidence of cardiomyopathy is reached. There is no link between the inheritance of the disease and the colour of the coat: only white cardiomyopathic hamsters were selected for the purpose of the present photograph* (Bajusz, 1969)

disease runs a fulminating course leading to early death) the physical appearance and behaviour of the cardiomyopathic hamsters remain normal for a considerable time, despite the presence of heart muscle degeneration. Only when generalized subcutaneous oedema is obvious does the disease become apparent (*Figure 18.5*). In the terminal stages, the animals exhibit dyspnoea and cyanosis. Death usually occurs a few weeks after these signs are noted (Bajusz, 1969).

Progressive, chronic, congestive cardiac failure appears to be the ultimate cause of death in more than 90 per cent of the cardiomyopathic hamsters (Bajusz *et al.*, 1965).

This disease is transmitted by an autosomal recessive gene, and hence new cardiomyopathic sublines may be developed by cross breeding between healthy and diseased animals of the strain (*Figure 18.6*).

The condition shows a sex-dependent variative in the age of onset and severity of the cardiac lesions which subsequently develop, the females being affected much earlier and more severely (*Figure 18.7*).

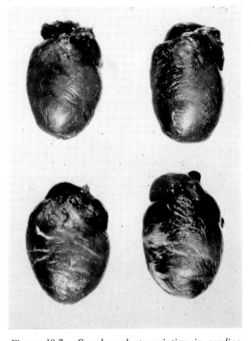

Figure 18.7. Sex-dependent variation in cardiac pathology of 60 day old Bio 14·6 myopathic hamsters. (Top) The hearts of males show no macroscopically visible cardiac damage. (Bottom) The hearts of females are already somewhat enlarged, revealing easily visible necrotic and calcified muscle fibres. The hearts with calcified fibres are obviously in an advanced stage of myocardial involvement. (Reproduced from Bajusz et al. (1965) by courtesy of the authors and Editor of the Annals of the New York Academy of Sciences)

GROSS PATHOLOGY

The autopsy findings depend largely, if not exclusively, on the duration and severity of the congestive cardiac failure. Significant pathological changes are usually not grossly detectable during the early stages of the disease, since the myocardial lesions are rarely visible by inspection of fresh specimens. Only when calcification of foci of degenerating muscle develop in the heart can lesions be clearly seen with the naked eye. When signs of generalized venous congestion become apparent, there is an appreciation in volume and weight of the heart, both the ventricles and auricles being affected by varying degrees of dilatation and hypertrophy (*Figure 18.8*(a)). During this phase of the disease, there is an increase in total ventricular mass ranging between 30 and 80 per cent (*Figure 18.8*(b)). Analysis of the ratio of the weights of left to right ventricles indicates that bilateral hypertrophy is present in the majority of animals: predominantly left- or right-sided hypertrophy is rarely seen. In a few cases the upper third of the free wall of both ventricles and the interventricular septum may be markedly hypertrophied, resembling the lesions of human subaortic muscular stenosis (Bajusz, 1967). During the terminal stages of the disease, when hypertrophy is no longer evident, auricular and ventricular mural thrombi are often found in the now greatly dilated and flabby hearts (*Figure 18.8*(c)). The hamsters with advanced degrees of cardiac enlargement exhibit variable amounts of subcutaneous oedema, ascites, hydrothorax and often hydropericardium. Pulmonary oedema of the acute or subacute type can be seen in the animals which die before reaching day 100 of life, i.e., in animals showing a rapidly fulminating course for the cardiac disease. Ventricular aneurysms and cardiac rupture in these hamsters are noted only during the advanced stages of the more common, slowly progressive variety of this cardiac condition.

HISTOLOGY

The first histologically detectable abnormality in the heart appears around day 30 of age in the female and about 10 days later in the male. By day 70–80 of age, the structurally damaged areas show a widespread distribution throughout the heart; by this time, the severity of the myocardial disease is comparatively uniform in all animals of both sexes. The myocardial lesions consist of focal myolysis by primary dissolution of myofibres in the absence of any significant cellular infiltration, resulting in the disappearance of sarcoplasm (*Figure 18.9*). The formation of small vacuoles, often observed in the initial muscle fibres, resembles hydropic vascular

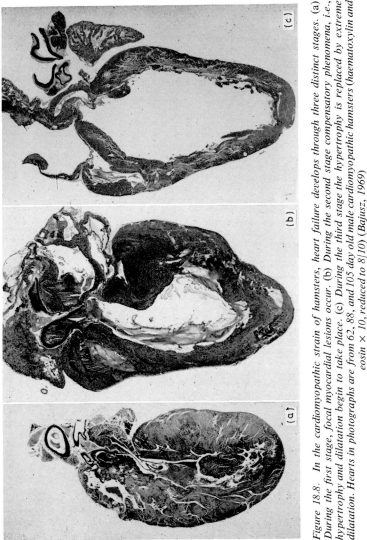

Figure 18.8. In the cardiomyopathic strain of hamsters, heart failure develops through three distinct stages. (a) During the first stage, focal myocardial lesions occur. (b) During the second stage compensatory phenomena, i.e., hypertrophy and dilatation begin to take place. (c) During the third stage the hypertrophy is replaced by extreme dilatation. Hearts in photographs are from 62, 88, and 105 day old male cardiomyopathic hamsters (haematoxylin and eosin × 10, reduced to 8/10) (Bajusz, 1969)

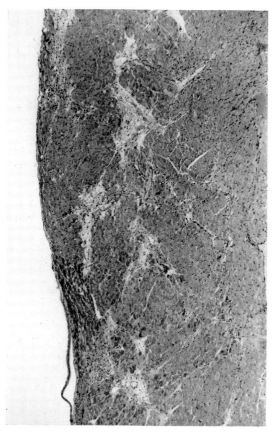

*Figure 18.9.   Focal lesions without secondary calcification
in the subepicardial and middle two thirds of the free wall
of left ventricle in a 76 day old male cardiomyopathic
hamster (von Kossa and haematoxylin and eosin × 40)*
(Bajusz, 1969)

degeneration. The myofibrils usually disappear and the sarcolemmal
remnants are indistinguishable from the endomysial connective tissue.
The myolytic foci are randomly distributed throughout the walls of
both ventricles and auricles, the intraventricular septum being the
least affected.

As the disease progresses, the number of myolitic foci increase and
the foci, in various stages of myolysis, are intermixed with necrotic
muscle cells.

Although a cellular infiltration is absent (*Figure 18.10*) in the

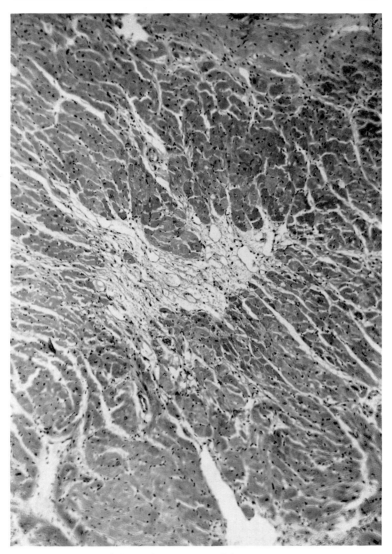

Figure 18.10. Morphologic characteristics of focal myolysis in the heart of a 50 day old male, Bio 14·6 hamster. Myocardial degeneration proceeds in the absence of cellular invasion; sarcolemmal remnants and free muscle nuclei are left behind by the disappearing muscle fibres (haematoxylin and eosin × 450, reduced to 9/10) (Bajusz, 1969)

areas affected by myolysis, some foci show increased vascularity, histiocytic proliferation and fibroplasia; while others exhibit calcification and fibrosis. The majority of the cells are of muscle cell origin but occasionally histiocytes, fibroblasts and round cells may also be seen. Newly-formed and healing lesions are often seen in the same heart. The disintegrated muscle fibres within the smaller foci are replaced by connective tissue. Mineral deposits of calcium phosphate are not seen in lesions in advanced stages of healing. The final result is the formation of a collagenous fibrous scar. Valvular and endocardial changes are rare, and although atrial mural thrombi do occur during the late stages of the disease, there is no correlation between the presence or absence of atrial mural thrombi and the severity of congestive heart failure.

References

Bajusz, E. (1967). 'Cardiomyopathies.' *Science, N.Y.* **156**, 16
— (1969). 'Hereditary cardiomyopathy: A new disease model.' *Am. Heart J.* **77**, 686
— *et al.* (1965). 'The heart muscle in muscular dystrophy with special reference to involvement of the cardiovascular system in the hereditary myopathy of the hamster.' *Ann. N.Y. Acad. Sci.* **138**, 213
Homburger, F., Baker, J. R., Mixon, C. W. and Whitmey, R. (1962). 'Primary generalised polymyopathy and cardiac necrosis in an inbred line of Syrian hamsters.' *Med. Exp.* **6**, 339

'WHITE MUSCLE' DISEASE

Systemic waxy muscular degeneration of muscles in animals is a disease which has been known for many years. Stoll (1886) first described it in Austria in young calves, and later Hobmaier (1925) reported on a field outbreak of a similar disease in rabbits and in lambs (Hobmaier, 1926).

It has also been found to occur in ewes, goats, pigeons, and a wide variety of other domestic and wild animals and birds.

At first assumed to be a single entity, 'white muscle disease' must now be considered to be the response of voluntary or cardiac muscle to a variety of injurious stimuli.

CLINICAL PRESENTATION

The animals may be found dead, sudden cardiac arrest having occurred. Alternately, animals when first affected may be in considerable pain and have difficulty in moving the limbs, the term 'stiff-limb' disease being used in describing lambs so affected.

The lesions consist of areas of skeletal muscle, which are white, or practically white, in colour.

The affected areas in the heart muscle are less regularly and less sharply outlined than in voluntary skeletal muscle, because of the anatomical arrangement of the fibres.

Affected hearts show fairly distinct pale or white areas in the ventricular walls or septum, or in the papillary muscles.

These areas are located throughout the musculature and vary greatly in size, sometimes a few are hardly visible while white streaks appear under the epicardium, at other times almost the entire musculature is affected (a waxy, greyish-yellow with a border merging diffusely into the surrounding normal myocardium). There seems to be no predictable site for the lesions, except for a region near either the epicardium or endocardium.

The musculature of the atria is, however, only affected in about five per cent of cases.

MICROSCOPIC CHANGES

The severity of the muscle changes varies greatly; in some sections a few fibres with pathological changes can be seen, while in others almost every fibre is severely affected. Often an affected fibre is surrounded by completely normal fibres, the change within the affected portion of the muscle fibre being sharply demarcated from the remaining portion.

The affected fibres become swollen, form thick whorls, and lose their cross striations in areas where degeneration occurs, but other parts may be intact. The sarcoplasm of the muscle cells contains clumps of cloudy and homogeneous or floccular and granular masses. Sometimes the contents of a cell have been completely lost, leaving only the cell wall.

This process is accompanied by the presence of numerous macrophages and lymphocytes. There are also attempts at regeneration by the muscle fibres, although these seldom succeed in more than the production of highly-bizarre, syncytial nuclei.

Persistent endomyosial connective tissue may be augmented by mild fibrous tissue proliferation in those areas where whole muscle fibres have disappeared. Early foci of calcification may be seen in some of the affected muscle fibres.

AETIOLOGY

The first type of 'white muscle' disease to be carefully studied was that which occurs with some frequency in calves (Anderson, 1960), lambs and chickens, and which appears to be caused by a deficiency of α-tocopherol.

Goettsch and Pappenhemier (1931) while studying the requirements of vitamin E for reproduction in guinea-pigs and rabbits, observed extreme degeneration of voluntary muscle.

Azzone and Aloisi (1958) have produced this condition by withholding vitamin E and curing it by supplying this vitamin.

Telford, Wiswell and Smith (1954) and Day, Young and Dennings (1957) have reported vitamin E deficiency in monkeys, and cattle, sheep and goats are all known to be susceptible. Turkeys, chickens, and other birds have been shown to develop manifestations of vitamin E deficiency.

What is apparently an entirely different 'white muscle disease' is common in lambs and calves in Oregon and other parts of the western USA, where it has been extensively investigated by Muth *et al.* (1959). The mothers of the affected animals have been fed, during pregnancy, on alfalfa or clover hay which has been grown in certain areas known to produce 'white muscle disease' year after year.

In these animals α-tocopherol has no protective action but when selenium, 0·1 parts per million of the total feed, is given in the form of sodium selenite, it is found to be an almost perfect preventative.

It has been shown that at least two types of plants produce poisons characterized by whiteness of muscle, together with some areas of necrosis. Microscopically the affected muscle fibres may show hyalinization and/or fragmentation. There was also an increase in glutamic oxalo-acetic transaminase due to the associated muscle cell necrosis. The plants responsible are *Karwinsha humboltiane* and coffee senna (*Cassia occadentialis*), both natives of the south western parts of the United States of America.

Dotta, Balbe and Guarda (1968) have also reported another detailed study on calves with 'white muscle disease', the histological and enzyme findings being identical with those previously reported and which responded to vitamin E and selenium.

Some of their other cases, however, also died suddenly, without showing prodromal symptoms. Usually these animals presented with severe clinical symptoms such as pulmonary oedema, intense dyspnoea and weak, frequent and irregular pulses.

The SGOT and SGPT levels were lower than in the other group of animals described.

At necropsy the hearts were small, and the ventricular wall was thinned.

Histologically the myocardium showed dystrophic and necrotic changes in some muscle fibres, small foci of inflammatory cells and some areas where the myocardial fibres had been replaced by fibrous tissue. Similar changes were also seen in the conducting system.

Treatment of these animals with selenium and vitamin E was without effect.

It is not known if these latter cases represent another type of 'white muscle disease' but this seems probable.

References

Anderson, P. (1960). 'Nutritional muscular dystrophy in cattle.' *Acta Path. microbiol. scand.* Suppl. 134, **48**, 39

Azzone, G. F. and Aloisi, M. (1958). 'Changes produced by antaminosis E with protein of rabbit muscle extract.' *Biochem. J.* **69**, 161

Day, P. L., Young, D. E. and Dennings, J. S. (1957). *Fedn. Proc.* **16**, 383

Dotta, V., Balbe, T. and Guarda, F. (1968). 'The cardiac types of muscular dystrophy in calves.' *La Nouva Vet.* **199**, 255

Goettsch, M. and Pappenheimer, A. M. (1931). *J. exp. Med.* **54**, 145

Hobmaier, M. (1925). *Arch. wiss. prakt. Tierheilk.* **52**, 38

— (1926). *Arch. wiss. prakt. Tierheilk.* **54**, 213

Muth, O. H., Oldfield, J. E., Schubert, J. R. and Remmert, L. F. (1959). 'White muscle disease in lambs and calves. Effect of selenium and vitamin E in lambs.' *Am. J. vet. Res.* **20**, 231

Stoll, A. (1886). *Österr. Wschr. Tierheilk.* **11**, 25

Telford, I. R., Wiswell, D. B. and Smith, E. L. (1954). *Proc. Soc. exp. Biol. Med.* **87**, 162

GOUSIEKTE

Gousiekte is a toxic congestive cardiomyopathy in ruminants characterized by a latent period of about 2–6 weeks followed by sudden death. (The word gousiekte, when translated from the Afrikaans means 'sudden death'.)

AETIOLOGY

The disease is caused by ingestion of five different plants of the family Rubiaceae, namely: *Pachystigma pygmaeum* (Schltr.) Robyns (*Figure 18.11*); *Pachystigma thamnus* Robyns, *Pavetta harborii* S. Moore (*Figure 18.12*); *Pavetta schumaniana* F. Hofm (*Figure 18.13*); and *Fadogia monticola* Robyns (*Figure 18.14*). The distribution of the five plants causing gousiekte in Southern Africa is shown in *Figure 18.15*.

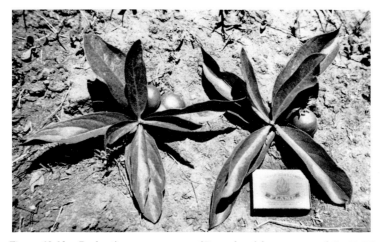

Figure 18.11. Pachystigma pygmaeum. (*Reproduced by courtesy of Dr T. W. Naude*)

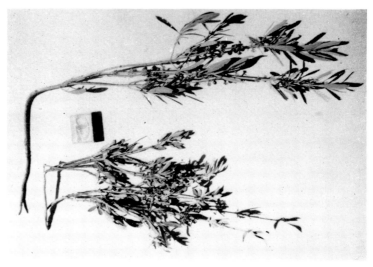

Figure 18.12. Pavetta harborii. (*Reproduced by courtesy of Dr T. W. Naude*)

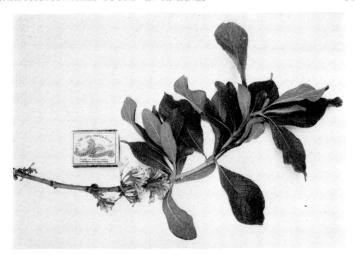

Figure 18.13. Pavetta schumaniana. (*Reproduced by courtesy of Dr T. W. Naude*)

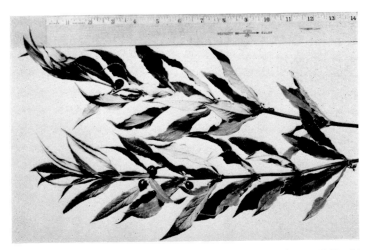

Figure 18.14. Fadogiam onticola. (*Reproduced by courtesy of Dr T. W. Naude*)

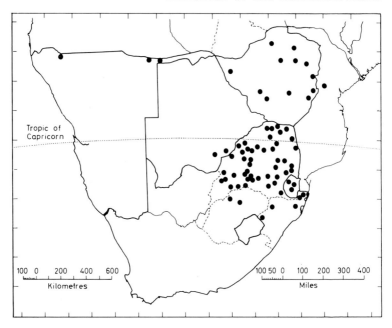

*Figure 18.15. The distribution of the five plants of the family Rubiaceae known
to cause gousiekte. (Map supplied by courtesy of Dr de Winter)*

If the affected animals are examined *clinically* they are often found
to show a conspicuous increase in sinus arrhythmia and the occurrence of ectopic heart beats is frequent during the latent period of the
disease. Gallop rhythm and bundle branch block may also be present.

PATHOLOGY

Post-mortem examination shows that there are severe congestion
and oedema of lungs, so that very often (*Figure 18.16*) the trachea is
filled, and often obstructed by an accumulation with frothy mucinous
fluid.

There may be an associated hydrothorax, due to a traumatic rupture of the visceral pleura of a lung and to strenuous attempts at
respiration—usually in the terminal stages of this disease (*Figure
18.17*).

At autopsy the hearts are found to be dilated, floppy and larger
than normal (*Figure 18.18*). When the heart is opened the myocardial
walls are seen to be greatly thinned. The cardiac cavities may contain
ante-mortem thrombi, some of which may be found to be adhering

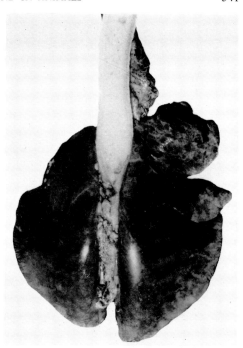

Figure 18.16. Severe congestion and oedema of the lungs with foam accumulation in the trachea in a sheep that had died from eating Fadogia monticola. *(Reproduced by courtesy of Dr T. W. Naude)*

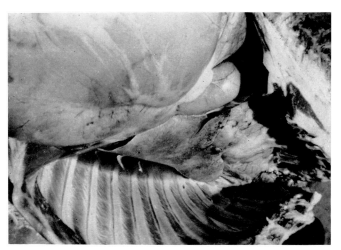

Figure 18.17. Hydrothorax in a sheep that died from Fadogia monticola *poisoning. (Reproduced by courtesy of Dr T. W. Naude)*

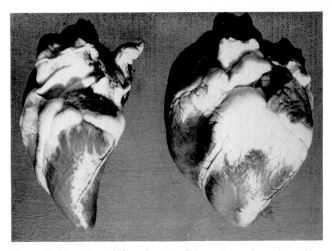

Figure 18.18. *Normal sheep heart on left and heart from sheep that died of* Pavetta schumaniana *poisoning on right. Note dilatation and failure to go into rigor mortis.* (*Reproduced by courtesy of Dr T. W. Naude*)

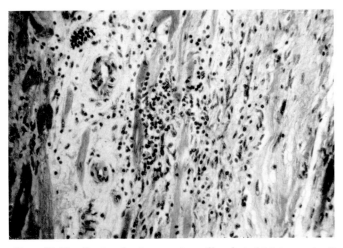

Figure 18.19. *Section showing prominent fibroplasia* (*right*), *round-cell reaction* (*centre*) *with accompanying hyaline necrosis* (*left*) (*haematoxylin and eosin* × *150, reduced to 6/10*). (*Reproduced by courtesy of Dr T. W. Naude*)

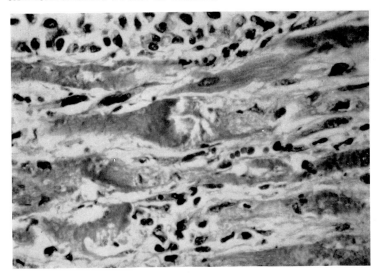

Figure 18.20. Acute stage of myocardial lesion showing hyaline necrosis of muscle fibres. Lymphocytic and mononuclear reaction at top. Early fibroplasia in interstitium (haematoxylin and eosin × 150, reduced to 6/10). (Reproduced by courtesy of Dr T. W. Naude)

to the underlying endocardium. The endocardium itself will be seen to be greyish in colour and slightly thickened. A pathognomonic chronic focal myocarditis is seen histologically (*Figure 18.19*).

Hyaline necrosis of fibres, mononuclear reaction, round-cell infiltration and interstitial fibrosis (*Figure 18.20*) are also seen.

The myocardium is found at post-mortem to be extremely flabby. At autopsy, the heart is found not to be in rigor mortis. This is due to the muscle fibres being so involved by the toxic process that they are unable to respond to any stimuli, even that of death.

HISTOLOGICAL FINDINGS

In the acute stage of these myocardial lesions, many of the muscle fibres show hyaline necrosis with loss of the normally occurring muscle striations (*Figure 18.19*). In many places the myocardium is diffusely infiltrated with mononuclear cells and small lymphocytes (*Figure 18.20*). Fibrous tissue hyperplasia in the interstitium between the muscle fibres begins to take place at the same time.

As this disease progresses the amount of fibrous tissue present becomes much more marked (*Figure 18.21*) and the accompanying round cells may have aggregated themselves with small, but definite

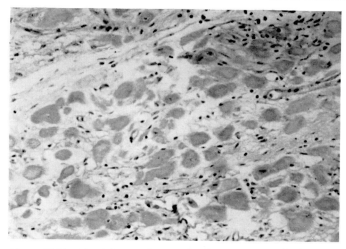

Figure 18.21. Gousiekte cardiomyopathy showing an acute hyaline myocarditis with destruction of many of the myocardial cells and loss of nuclei and increase of interstitial tissue oedema and infiltration with polymorphs and lymphocytes (haematoxylin and eosin × 50, reduced to 6/10). (Reproduced by courtesy of Professor Jacobson)

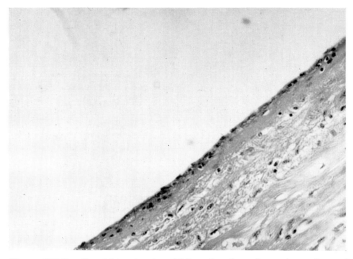

Figure 18.22. Gousiekte showing thickened endocardium, the surface of which is covered by a layer of fibrin that appears to be undergoing organization. The endocardium and myocardium are diffusely infiltrated with lymphocytes and polymorphs (Martius' Scarlet Blue × 50, reduced to 6/10)

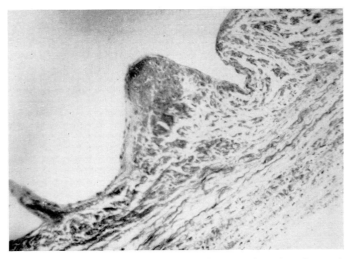

Figure 18.23.   Gousiekte showing deposit of fibrin in the endocardium and subendocardial connective tissue. (Martius' Scarlet Blue × 50). (Reproduced by courtesy of Dr Johannesson)

foci, while the accompanying hyaline necrosis is more marked. If this disease process is not immediately followed by sudden death, marked fibrous thickening of the endocardium follows (*Figure 18.22*). This thickening of the endocardium is produced by (1) organization of fibrin thrombi (*Figure 18.23*), which are commonly present on the endocardial surface and (2) the associated hyperplasia of fibrous tissue in the endocardium and superficial myocardium.

Electronmicroscopy has shown some evidence of myofilament dissolution, but nothing else of note.

The cause of death in these animals is, therefore, seen to be acute heart failure, the peripheral organs in all the affected animals showing the changes of acute or chronic congestive failure.

Walker (1908–9) reported outbreaks of this disease in the Transvaal, South Africa, where cattle died suddenly and at post-mortem were found to have died with congestive heart failure.

This disease has a high incidence among sheep on the high veldt during very dry seasons (Watt and Breyer-Brandwijk, 1962).

References

Walker, J. (1908–9). 'Gauwziekte—A disease of sheep.' In *Report of Government Veterinary Bacteriologist* Transactions of the Department of Agriculture, South Africa

Watt, J. M. and Breyer-Brandwijk, M. G. (1962). In *The Medical and Poisonous Plants of Southern and Eastern Africa*. 2nd Edition, pp. 901–903. London and Edinburgh: Livingstone

IDIOPATHIC CARDIOMYOPATHY (PRIMARY MYOCARDIAL DISEASE)

The large breeds of dogs, such as boxers, bulldogs or great danes may develop an idiopathic cardiomyopathy which is characterized by biventricular cardiac dilatation, with distention of the atrioventricular valve rings leading to valvular incompetence and thereby producing marked atrial dilatation. Atrial fibrillation is often present when this condition is first recognized.

PATHOLOGY

Extensive pathological descriptions of this condition have not been reported—the best, at present, being that of Ettinger and Suter (1970).

Grossly, the heart is generally enlarged, and there is dilatation of all chambers. In addition, the atrioventricular valve rings are both dilated, producing valvular incompetence.

Left atrial thrombi are sometimes found late in the disease and may be responsible for thrombo-embolic episodes, resulting in systemic, usually peripheral, infarctions.

Microscopic examination of the ventricular myocardium does not demonstrate lesions which can be considered pathognomonic for this cardiomyopathy.

Sections of the right and left ventricular myocardium may, however, reveal small focal areas of fibrosis. These are neither extensive nor consistent, and they do not help in differentiating animals with this disease from normal animals.

Reference

Ettinger, S. J. and Suter, P. F. (1970). 'Idiopathic cardiomyopathy.' In *Canine Cardiology* pp. 392–400. London: Saunders

ISCHAEMIC CARDIOMYOPATHY

The occurrence of small, ventricular myocardial infarctions has been reviewed by Detwéiler *et al.* (1968). These small focal areas of myocardial necrosis and fibrosis are a relatively common finding in dogs with acquired disability (Luginbühl and Detwéiler, 1968). These lesions vary in size from those which can be seen only microscopically to others which may be a few millimetres in diameter.

Macroscopically, visible foci are reddish brown or grey in colour and opaque; they vary in consistency from soft and friable to being firm and fibrotic.

Microscopically, various stages of myocardial degeneration and necrosis, resorption and reparative fibrosis can be found. In some cases dystrophic fibrosis may occur in the areas of myocardial necrosis.

Many of these sequelae to focal myocardial damage are seen in the vicinity of those smaller intramyocardial arteries which show hyaline arteriolosclerosis or intimal fibro-elastic proliferation, which greatly narrow or almost completely occlude the lumen. Presumably, the resultant reduction of the blood supply is sufficient to account for the ischaemic necrosis of the myocardium.

The lack of severe arteriosclerotic changes in the intramural coronary vessels in a given area, with these myocardial changes, may be explained on the grounds that the scarred or necrotic areas in the myocardium may represent the terminal fields of blood supply of an artery, the diseased segment of which is situated proximally.

The lesions occur almost exclusively in the left ventricular wall, especially in older dogs with chronic mitral valvular fibrosis or in younger dogs with congenital subaortic stenosis (Flickinger and Patterson, 1967).

Intramural arteriolosclerosis and subsequent left ventricular fibrosis may contribute to the frequency of heart failure in older dogs. Hamlin (1968) has used the term 'microscopic intramural myocardial infarction' to describe this condition and has stressed its importance in valvular heart disease in the dog.

References

Detwéiler, D. K., Luginbühl, H., Buchanan, J. W. and Patterson, D. F. (1968). 'The natural history of acquired cardiac disability of the dog.' *Ann. N.Y. Acad. Sci.* **147**, 318

Flickinger, G. L. and Patterson, D. F. (1967). 'Coronary lesions associated with sub-aortic stenosis in the dog.' *J. path. Bact.* **93**, 133

Hamlin, R. L. (1968). 'Prognostic value of changes in the cardiac silhouette in dogs with mitral insufficiency.' *J. Am. vet. med. Ass.* **153**, 1436

Luginbühl, H. and Detwéiler, D. K. (1968). 'Cardiovascular lesions in dogs.' *Ann. N.Y. Acad. Sci.* **147**, 517

INTRACARDIAC THROMBOSIS

Meier and Hoag (1961) have reported the occurrence of spontaneous thrombosis in the left auricle of some mice. Consistently the left auricle is greatly enlarged, haemorrhagic and filled with either one large thrombus or many small thrombi.

Prothrombin levels in these animals were found to be 20–25 per cent above those in normal animals. It is said to be caused by a post partum 'prothrombin rebound'—a phenomenon which is commonly found to occur after pregnancy.

The animals present clinically with dyspnoea caused by severe pulmonary congestion and, in most instances, sub-cutaneous oedema.

Microscopically, focal areas of necrosis present in the myocardium and progressively increase in size. The sites of attachment of the thrombi to underlying muscle fibres are lost and replaced by fibrous tissue. Dystrophic calcification of the myocardium may occur. Much more rarely cartilagenous metaplasia may be seen at the site of attachment of the thrombus, but not elsewhere in the myocardium.

At necropsy, the left auricle is usually grossly dilated (3–5 times its normal size) and contains one or two large thrombi. In younger mice, small thrombi are often found loosely attached to the endocardium, but, usually, in these cases no symptoms are observed.

AETIOLOGY

From the evidence described above, it would seem that the thrombus is primary, as it is formed quickly. Endothelial change is believed to be secondary since even in those mice with small thrombi no endothelial abnormality can be observed or demonstrated.

Meier and Hoag believe that the thrombus is due to post partum hyperprothrombinaemia, as all these animals were found to have been pregnant on numerous occasions. No males or virgin females were affected and they were found to have a plasma prothrombin level of 20–25 per cent above that of the other unaffected mice.

It is believed that the post partum hyperprothrombinaemia might be explained as a 'rebound phenomenon' following parturition recovery; prothrombin rebound has been observed in mice and experimentally in animals in response to dicoumarol therapy (Miller and Bayer, 1961).

The identical condition of unknown aetiology was previously reported (Fry, Hamilton and Lisco, 1960).

SUMMARY

Left auricular thrombosis occurs with a high incidence—about 66 per cent—among older breeding females and current breeders of the BALB/C strain of mice. Deficiencies in certain coagulant clotting factors appear in the last days of pregnancy and are followed by a 'prothrombin rebound', consquent to recovery after parturition. Hormonal imbalance and strain predisposition (auricular blood flow and stagnation) may be accessory factors.

References

Fry, R. J. M., Hamilton, K. and Lisco, H. (1960). 'An unusual spontaneous cardiac lesion of unknown etiology in mice.' *Fedn Proc.* **19**, 109

Meier, M. and Hoag, W. C. (1961). 'Studies of left auricular thrombosis in mice.' *Exp. med. Surg.* **19**, 317

Miller, K. B. and Bayer, W. C. (1961). *Fedn Proc.* **20**, 135

PARASITIC INFECTIONS

CHAGAS' (*T. cruzi*) MYOCARDITIS

Infection with *Trypanosoma cruzi* is common in certain animals residing in the southern parts of the USA and in certain parts of Central and South America.

The disease has been reported in the armadillo, racoon, opossum, wood rat, mouse, dog, cat, domestic pig, house rat, skunk and red uakari (Kolfoid and Donat, 1933; Hunter, Mackie and Worth, 1954; Woody and Woody, 1955; Woody and Woody, 1961; Lasry and Sheridan, 1965).

Diagnosis of trypanosomiasis usually has to be made initially from an examination of a blood film but post-mortem examination is necessary to show that the degree of infestation is compatible with the chronic phase of Chagas' disease.

Clinical Presentation

Evidence of cardiac damage may be present and various forms of arrhythmia which may be fatal before other signs of the disease present themselves, may be seen. In other cases marked disturbances in rhythm and conduction and all degrees of congestive heart failure may be present. Myocardial damage and resultant heart failure usually herald the terminal illness.

In animals the heart is usually seen to be grossly dilated and flabby (*Figure 18.24*).

Microscopically, the myocardial fibres are usually well preserved but the nuclei are enlarged and irregular, while the cytoplasm may contain small vacuoles. The arteries of the heart are often surrounded by small areas of perivascular fibrosis; areas of replacement of the muscle with fibrous tissue represent areas of chronic inflammation which have healed following muscle destruction. Some parasites, which can be identified as *T. cruzi*, are present in the myocardium.

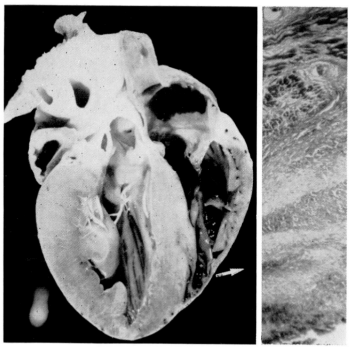

Figure 18.24.   Dog heart (LXI, P8) as seen from its posterior aspect. Duration of T. cruzi *infection, 2½ months. Marked dilatation of the RV chamber, and, in lesser degree, of the RA are seen. Thinning of the wall at the inferior aspect of the anteriolateral surface of the RV. Intramural thrombus adhered to the endocardium. Extensive fibrosis consisting of collagenous connective tissue and muscular islets. Fibrotic plaques became confluent near the subepicardium (Gomori trichrome × 125, reduced to 9/10) (Reproduced from Anselmi* et al. *(1965) by courtesy of the author and Editor of the* American Heart Journal)

Anselmi *et al.* (1965) while studying experimentally infected dogs with *T. cruzi* found two spontaneous cases of the disease in mongrel (semi-wild) dogs. Their findings are described below.

In the first animal the heart was enlarged and globular. Bright whitish plaques of different sizes appeared all over the endothelial surfaces of both ventricles. The right ventricular wall was very thin and speckled greyish yellow in appearance, because of small zones of fibrosis and there was a small organised thrombus at the tip of the right ventricle. Microscopically a severe inflammatory cell infiltrate, together with areas of severe fibroplastic proliferation was seen in many parts of the myocardium, together with some foci of muscle fibre degeneration.

In the second case, which these workers described, there was dilatation of all the cardiac cavities, but mainly of the right ventricle.

Microscopically sections of myocardium from all the cardiac chambers showed a diffuse infiltrate with inflammatory cells, mainly lymphocytes and monocytes, but also certainly some polymorphs, together, in some areas, with a diffuse proliferation of fibrous tissue. There were also many damaged or necrotic myocardial fibres.

Bullock, Wolf and Clarkson (1967) reported the presence of myocarditis associated with *T. cruzi* infection in a Cebus monkey which had been taken to Florida for experimental purposes. The only sign it presented with was a right-sided bundle branch block, but it was then killed. Significant lesions at autopsy were found only in the heart, but there was no evidence of cardiac hypertrophy and the heart was of normal size—7 per cent of body weight. The pericardium was slightly thickened and opaque. In the myocardium many randomly isolated foci of myocarditis were seen. The inflammatory cells were typically mononuclear. Nests of the leishmania form of *T. cruzi* were found in the muscle fibres of the right ventricle and in the intraventricular septum.

In another animal, which had been experimentally infected with *T. cruzi* five years previously, the heart was found to be enlarged— 280 g. When placed on the autopsy table, before fixation in formalin, it collapsed and folded like a piece of cloth.

Small foci of fibrosis were seen, both on the epicardial surfaces of the ventricles and over the endocardium lining the ventricles, particularly in the region of the trabeculae carneae.

Incidence

Two studies have been done on the frequency of finding *T. cruzi* in primates found in South America. In the first study (Dunn, Lambrecht and Du Plesis, 1963) *T. cruzi* (or *T. cruzi*-like) trypanosomes were found in the blood of 8 of 23 non-human primates from South America while Marinkelle (1966) investigating 85 primates from Columbia found 7 infected with *T. cruzi* and a further 12 with *T. cruzi*-like organisms.

References

Anselmi, A., Pifano, F., Svare, A., Dominguez, A., Diaz, Vazqvez, A. and Anselmi, G. (1965). 'Experimental *T. Cruzi* myocarditis.' *Am. Heart J.* **20**, 638

Bullock, B. C., Wolf, R. H. and Clarkson, T. B. (1967). 'Myocarditis associated with trypanosomiasis in a cebus monkey (*Cebus albifrons*).' *J. Am. Vet. Med.* **151**, 920

Dunn, F. L., Lambrecht, P. J. and Du Plesis, R. (1963). 'Trypanosomes of South American monkeys and marmosets.' *Am. J. trop. Med. Hyg.* **12**, 524

Hunter, G. W., Mackie, T. T. and Worth, C. B. (1954). *Manual of Tropical Medicine*, 2nd. Edition. Philadelphia: Saunders

Kolfoid, C. A. and Donat, F. (1933). 'South American trypanosomiasis of the human type, occurrence in mammals of the United States.' *Calif. West Med.* **38**, 245

Lasry, J. E. and Sheridan, B. W. (1965). 'Chagas' myocarditis and heart failure in the red nakari—*Cacajoo rubicandus.*' *Int. Zoo. Yb.* **5**, 182

Marinkelle, C. J. (1966). 'Observations on human, monkey and bat trypanosomes and their vectors in Columbia.' *Trans. R. Soc. trop. Med. Hyg.* **60**, 109

Woody, N. C. and Woody, H. B. (1955). 'American trypanosomiasis (Chagas' disease). First indigenous case in the United States.' *J. Am. med. Ass.* **159**, 676

—— (1961). 'American trypanosomiasis (I)—clinical and epidemiological background of Chagas' disease in the United States.' *J. Pediat.* **58**, 568

SCHISTOSOMIASIS

In those parts of the world where this disease affects humans, it is also commonly found to infect the indigenous animals of the region, particularly primates and the various forms of deer and larger herbivores. I have seen intramyocardial schistosomal ova in both hippopotamus and a Thompson's Gazelle in Uganda.

Perhaps the damage observed in the so called bilharzial myocarditis found in some of these animals may result from toxins produced by schistosomal ova actually present in the cardiac muscle, although later destroyed by phagocytes. This is the explanation given for the fact that many of the affected hearts contain, at autopsy, no schistosomal ova to account for the diffuse myocarditis often seen (Bruce, Warren and Sadun, 1963). Sometimes a few ova may be found in the myocardium in the same way, as has been described in Chapter 11 for the ova in man.

Reference

Bruce, J. I., Warren, K. S. and Sadun, E. H. (1963). 'Observations on the pathophysiology of *Schistosomiasis mansoni* in monkeys.' *Exp. Parasital.* **13**, 194

DIROFILARIA IMMITIS

The canine heart worm also affects many other types of animal—it has been described in ten different species by Levine (1968). The adult worm normally affects the right ventricle and pulmonary arteries, but is sometimes found in the right atrium (Henninger and Ferguson, 1957).

In a few cases emboli from dead parasites may produce thrombosis and infarction of small branches of the coronary arteries. The ensuing tissue reaction may result in the formation of circumscribed nodules and granulomas (Luginbühl and Detwéiler, 1968).

References

Henninger, G. R. and Ferguson, R. W. (1957). 'Pulmonary vascular sclerosis as a result of dirofilaria immitis infection in dogs.' *J. Am. Vet. Med. Ass.* **131**, 336

Levine, N. D. (1968). *Nematone Parasites of Domestic Animals and Man.* Minneapolis: Burgess

Luginbühl, H. and Detwéiler, D. K. (1968). 'Cardiovascular lesion in dogs.' *Ann. N.Y. Acad. Sci.* **147**, 517

SARCOSPORIDIOSIS

Sarcosporidiosis is a common parasitic infection of skeletal and cardiac muscle in many species of birds, reptiles and mammals. It is found most commonly in cattle (*Sarcocystis blanchardia*), sheep (*S. tenella*), horses (*S. bartrani*) and swine (*S. miescheriana*), but may be found in many other animals, for example in camels (El-Etreby, 1970).

Sarcocysts are found in the cardiac muscle in nearly 100 per cent of cattle, in about 90 per cent of horses and swine, and in 70 per cent of sheep (Ratz, 1910; Bergman, 1913; Stroh, 1921).

Clinically, this disease has been found to produce symptoms of myositis, heart block and congestive cardiac failure.

No lesions are seen, macroscopically, in the hearts which may be supposed to be caused by the parasite, except in a few cases where small foci of thrombosis are seen within the myocardium.

Microscopically, these sarcocysts are found, almost invariably, in the papillary muscles of the left ventricular wall, but also in the wall of the right ventricle in about 40 per cent of cases and, rarely, in Purkinje fibres.

The cysts are usually tubular, vary greatly in size and are filled with basophilic crescentric bodies about 4×8 μm in size. The cyst wall is distinctly hyaline and bears, on its inner surface, many fine strands which divide the cyst into numerous compartments wherein the spores lie. Smaller cysts are in muscle fibres wherein they displace the sarcoplasm but the larger cysts are in the interstitial connective tissue. It appears that as the cysts enlarge the muscle fibres eventually rupture and set the cyst free.

Most affected hearts are free from any degenerative or inflammatory changes but in a few cases sarcocysts are found in foci of myocardial necrosis and themselves appear degenerated.

The fibrous connective tissue around some of these foci is infiltrated with fibroblasts, lymphocytes, plasma cells, macrophages and eosinophils.

In some areas of the myocardium there are no inflammatory cells but an increase in the interstitial connective tissue spreads the myocardial fibres apart. Foci of proliferation of sarcolemmo nuclei occur in this connective tissue.

What effect, if any, cysts in Purkinje fibres have on the conduction of cardiac impulses, even when the infection is heavy, is unknown (Jones, 1961), but Agnese (1950) believed that a disturbance of conduction did occur in a calf and a goat as a result of myocardial sarcosporidiosis. Jones (1961) reported a granulomatous reaction to degeneration sarcocysts in bovine hearts.

References

Agnese, M. O. (1950). 'Sarcosporidiose cardisea como une das possiveis causas da doenca de Adams-Stokes,' p. 363. Proceedings of the fourth Congress bras. vel. Sao Paulo, 1950

Bergman, A. M. (1913). 'Beitrag zur Kenutivis des Vorkommens der Sarkosporidien bei den Haustieren.' 2 *Fleisch-Milelbyg* **23**, 169

El-Etreby, H. F. (1970). 'Myocardial sarcosporidiosis in the camel.' *Path. Vet.* **7**, 7

Jones, T. C. (1961). In *Veterinary Pathology*. Ed. by Smith, H. A. and Jones, T. C. 2nd Edition. Philadelphia: Lea and Febiger

Ratz, V. I. (1910). 'Über die Struktur der Sarkosporidien—Schläuche.' *Arch. wiss. prakt. Tierheilk.* **36**, 573–589

Stroh, G. (1921). 'Sarkosporidicubefunde in gesunden und Klauenseache degenerierten Rinderherzen sowie in weiteren Maskelpartien des Rindes.' *Münch. tier. Wschr.* **72**, 725

TOXOPLASMOSIS

The toxoplasma parasite is commonly found to infect domestic animals, particularly dogs (Luginbühl and Detwéiler, 1968), and may cause a chronic myocarditis. Diffuse areas of infiltration with lymphocytes are usually seen in the myocardium, together with scattered areas of fibrosis. Some focal areas of inflammation may, however, be present.

There are few reports on the disease in wild animals but where it has been studied the disease appears to be fairly common (Alcaino, 1964)—the cardiac lesions being similar to those found in domestic animals.

References

Alcaino, H. (1964). 'Toxoplasmosis en animales domesticos.' (In Portuguese) *Boln chil. Parasit.* **19**, 21

Luginbühl, H. and Detwéiler, D. K. (1968). 'Cardiovascular lesion in dogs.' *Ann. N.Y. Acad. Sci.* **147**, 517

MYOCARDITIS

Inflammatory changes in the myocardium may accompany acute bacterial or virus diseases and are sometimes observed in mild form following relatively minor surgical procedures in domestic animals. Myocarditis may also be associated with a relatively local infection, such as an abscess, and in animals dying from various other causes such as uraemia, nephritis or poisoning with heavy metals.

When an exhaustive study is made to confirm the clinical diagnosis of myocarditis lesions are often found. Therefore, histological evidence of myocarditis may very frequently be missed and great care should, therefore, be taken in examining histological material.

CLINICAL PRESENTATION

Sudden death, particularly in young animals, is often found to be due to myocarditis, which is often unsuspected until discovered at necropsy. These animals may, however, present with an arrhythmia or congestive heart failure. On the other hand, extensive myocarditis may give rise to no clinical signs but may be discovered fortuitously on histological examination of cardiac material.

The most detailed study of myocarditis in monkeys is that of Soto *et al.* (1964) who found evidence of myocarditis, at post-mortem, in 18 of 20 apparently healthy rhesus monkeys. The animals had recently been imported from India.

These workers, however, found no bacteria in heart extracts and no viruses could be isolated from mice injected with heart extracts.

It seems that, in dogs, evidence of myocarditis is found, at post-mortem, in about 10 per cent of all hearts studied. Luginbühl and Detwéiler (1968) diagnosed acute or subacute myocarditis in 30 of 314 dogs which they examined for cardiac disease. In only two of these animals, however, was myocarditis thought to be the primary cause of death.

AETIOLOGY

Agents known to cause myocarditis in animals are few and are generally restricted to viruses and parasites. The viruses known to cause myocarditis in monkeys often belong to the encephalomyocarditis (EMC) family (Warren, Smadel and Russ, 1949).

Coxsackie viruses have been used in the experimental production of myocarditis in monkeys (Hamilton and Syverton, 1951; Leu, Wenner and Kamitsuka, 1960), but have rarely been isolated from the tissues of normal or sick monkeys. In cynomolgus monkeys, however, they apparently cause no noticeable infection (Plager, 1962). Coxsackie viruses frequently produce severe myocarditis in birds, the myocardium being usually diffusely infiltrated with lymphocytes while many of the myocardial cells are necrotic and are being replaced with fibrous tissue.

Bacteria have been used to produce myocarditis (Hamilton and Syverton, 1950) and the results indicate that killed streptococci can produce an inflammatory picture similar to that seen in viral infections. Grossly the heart usually appears normal.

Various specific granulomatous diseases may cause myocardial lesions in animals including tuberculosis, actinomycosis, nocardiosis, blastomycosis and coccidiomycosis.

PATHOLOGY

Macroscopic evidence of myocarditis is found only in very severe cases. Changes are normally only found microscopically and are usually focal rather than diffuse in distribution. The accompanying cellular infiltrate consists predominantly of lymphocytes, large mononuclear cells and an occasional eosinophil or plasma cell. Necrosis is not a constant feature but, when present, is minimal and seen only where the myocarditis is marked. When the cellular accumulates are moderate or interstitial they are accompanied by oedema. Enlargement of many of the nuclei of myocardial fibres may be seen in areas adjacent to the most severe areas of myocarditis. Foci of inflammation are sometimes seen in the septum and both ventricles but mainly in the left ventricle. In addition, no bacteria, viral occlusion bodies, or parasites can be seen. These findings are similar to those previously reported by Vanace (1960) in 18 of 36 asymptomatic monkeys. The monkey has been studied most in recent years although there are numerous references to myocarditis in dogs, cats and birds.

In an earlier study Lapin and Yakovleva (1963) found that, in the hearts of 90 monkeys, aged between $2\frac{1}{2}$ years and 'senility' (? age) studied over a 10 year period, 9 showed myocardial scars which were thought to represent old myocarditis.

Neither viral inclusion bodies nor parasites were found in the cardiac muscle. No bacteria grew from culture of the cardiac muscle, nor could any antibodies to bacteria be detected in it. It was, therefore, concluded that the aetiological agent was unknown.

In a third report on chronic myocarditis in monkeys, the following results were found. Two hundred and eighty free-range Howler monkeys were studied by Maruffo and Malinow (1967), the animals being killed in the wild state in the northern part of Argentina. All the hearts were normal in size and weight. Myocarditis was observed in 19 (8·4 per cent) but, in all of these animals, except two, the changes were minimal; and none were seen in any of these hearts macroscopically. In only one animal was the myocarditis marked and in this case there was well-marked necrosis of muscle cells. The lesions were extensive and numerous. Enlargement and margination of many of the myocardial cell nuclei were observed in adjacent areas. There were also some areas of fibrosis in the myocardium and lipofuchsine was seen in many myocardial cells, as also in many of the less severe cases of myocarditis.

References

Hamilton, T. R. and Syverton, J. T. (1950). 'Experimental studies in cardiovascular disease, rheumatic type.' *Bull. Univ. Minn. Hosp. Med. Found.* **21**, 173

—— (1951). 'Carditis and pulmonary arteritis in monkeys.' *Fedn. Proc.* **10**, 357

Lapin, B. A. and Yakovleva, L. A. (1963). 'Diseases of the cardiovascular system.' In *Comparative Pathology in Monkeys*, pp. 152–174. Springfield, Ill: Thomas

Leu, T. Y., Wenner, H. A. and Kamitsuka, P. C. (1960). 'Experimental infections with Coxsackie viruses II, myocarditis in cynomolgus monkeys infected with B4 virus.' *Arch. Virusforsch.* **10**, 451

Luginbühl, H. and Detwéiler, D. K. (1968). 'Cardiovascular lesions in dogs.' *Ann. N.Y. Acad. Sci.* **147**, 517

Maruffo, C. A. and Malinow, M. R. (1967). 'Pathologic changes in the heart in free ranging Howler monkeys (*Alucutta carsysi*. Haubolt, 1912).' *Am. J. Vet. Res.* **28**, 237

Plager, H. (1962). 'Coxsackie viruses.' *Ann. N.Y. Acad. Sci.* **101**, 390

Soto, P. J., Beall, F. A., Nakamura, R. M. and Kuffenberg, L. L. (1964). 'Myocarditis in rhesus monkeys.' *Archs Path.* **78**, 681

Vanace, P. W. (1960). 'Experimental streptococcal infection in Rhesus monkeys.' *Ann. N.Y. Acad. Sci.* **85**, 910

Warren, J., Smadel, J. E. and Russ, S. B. (1949). 'Family of encephalomyocarditis, columbia SK, MM and mengo encephalomyocarditis viruses.' *J. Immun.* **62**, 387

CARDIAC TUMOURS

There are only a very few reports of cardiac tumours in animals. Smith and Jones (1961), for example, list only one primary tumour of the heart in a dog, a rhabdomyosarcoma, in 5,854 canine neoplasms which they listed. Later studies have shown, however, that both primary and metastatic cardiac tumours, although very uncommon, are not so rare as this in dogs (Detwéiler, 1962).

Luginbühl and Detwéiler (1968) reviewed the cardiac tumours previously reported in their laboratory as well as those reported elsewhere. They listed the following primary tumours: haemangioendothelioma, mixed-cell sarcoma, spindle-cell sarcoma, round-cell sarcoma, lymphangioendothelioma, haemangioma, fibroma, rhabdomyoma, chondroma, fibromyxoma, myxoma and teratoma.

Tumours occupying space within the cardiac cavities are usually haemangioendotheliomas, these tumours having a predilection for the right atrium (Stünzi and Mann, 1970).

From what little can be gained from a survey of the veterinary literature, cardiac tumours seem to be of similar types to those occurring in man.

Myxoma of the heart has been described in a dog by Roberts (1959). At necropsy the tumour was found to be lying freely in the right atrial cavity, but attached to the base of the interatrial septum by a pedicle. The neoplasm was soft and friable, presenting a pale pink semi-translucent surface when cut.

A microscopic examination showed that the tumour consisted of mesenchymal tissue in which the component cells were separated by loose, faintly-staining myxomatous material. In most areas the cells were spindle shaped and often showed centrally placed, hyperchromatic nuclei, while the cytoplasm sometimes contained clear vacuoles. Many of the larger vessels of the lungs were filled with neoplastic tissue. There was some extension of the tumour into the adjacent pulmonary tissue.

This tumour is identical histologically with similar tumours seen in man, but unusual in that it metastasized into the lung.

Contrasting with the apparent infrequency of primary haemangiosarcoma of the heart in man, only about 20 cases having been reported to date, this tumour was found to be the only primary cardiac tumour affecting dogs necropsied at the Angel Memorial Hospital in Boston (Kleine, Zook and Munson, 1970). Sixty-one dogs with haemangiosarcomas were necropsied in this hospital between 1954 and 1967; 31 of these tumours were considered to have originated in the heart. In half these dogs the haemangiosarcoma was located in the auricle just above the atrioventricular junction. The tumours ranged in size from 0·5 to 13 cm in greatest diameter, but most were between 2 and 4 cm. Histologically these tumours do not differ from those seen elsewhere in man or animals, being very cellular and composed of spindle-shaped cells with large elongated nuclei in a vascular, sparsely-collagenous stroma.

Cardiac haemangiomas in dogs have also been reported by Geib (1966) in two dogs. In both cases these neoplasms were histologically found to contain channels lined by endothelial cells. Many of these cells were round and lay free in the lumen, others were attached to the basement membrane by a thin pedicle of cytoplasm.

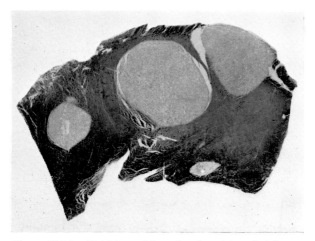

Figure 18.25. Multiple nodules of pale-staining rhabdomyo-matous tissue in wall of left ventricle (haematoxylin and eosin × 3). (Reproduced from Omar (1969) by courtesy of the author and Editor of Pathologia Veterinaria)

There is also one report of a reticulum cell sarcoma originating in an animal (dog) (Colby and Collins, 1965). It involved the heart but also spread extensively into the area surrounding the media-stinum and into both lungs. It is not, therefore, possible to say with certainty that this was a primary tumour.

RHABDOMYOMA

Since the publication by Von Recklinghausen in 1962 there have been few reports of so called Rhabdomyomatosis of the heart. This lesion, in which the large vacuolated cells contain glycogen, is also called 'nodular glycogenic infiltration' or 'congenital glycogenic tumour' (*Figure 18.25*).

Vink (1969) described the finding of 22 cases of rhabdomyomatosis in a study of 1,400 guinea-pigs. Subsequently, 5 other cases were found when another 200 normal guinea-pigs were killed.

In only a very few of Vink's cases (three) could these glycogenic tumours be seen with the naked eye. The lesions were found exclusively in the wall of the left ventricle and were located subendocardially, subepicardially or intramurally.

Macroscopically, these altered areas vary in appearance and are very rarely sharply circumscribed; the adjacent muscle does not show pressure atrophy. The lesions consist of a spongy network of enlarged cardiac myocytes, each of which contains a centrally located, somewhat poorly-defined nucleus, surrounded by a narrow rim of cytoplasm in which, sometimes, some cross striations are observed (*Figure 18.26*). Round, oval or tube like structures are sometimes seen in the meshes of the network formed by the cell walls.

In some cases there is a rounded mass of cytoplasm in these cellular 'cavities', which sometimes contain a nucleus.

The typical 'spider cells' found in human cases, vacuolated cells with a centrally located nucleus which is connected with the cell wall by slender cytoplasmic threads, are not found in these animal 'tumours'.

In only a few of these 'tumours' is it possible to demonstrate the presence of glycogen in these vacuoles, even if this material has been initially fixed in absolute alcohol.

In the border region between normal and altered muscle tissue transitional changes are observed in some cases. Only very rarely are fine droplets of fat seen in the cytoplasm of the affected cells. These tumours are rarely found in animals, other than guinea-pigs. According to Rooney (1961), who encountered 24 cases out of 193 guinea-pigs in a closed colony, the condition is rather common in this species. From brief mentions in reviews by Cotchin (1956), Hadlow (1962) and Moulton (1961) it appears that this condition has been described 20 times in other animals.

Eleven of these cases were in domestic swine, all of the reports being in the non-English literature. Other reports of this disease in swine have been those of Kast and Hanichen (1968) and Omar (1969).

In the pig, grossly, the walls of the ventricles contain multiple, discrete, yellowish-grey nodules which vary in size from 1 mm to 1 cm.

Microscopically, the nodules in the ventricular wall consist of large myoblastic cells with varying degrees of cytoplasmic vacuolation; for the most part they were well demarcated, though not encapsulated, from the surrounding normal myocardium.

A few small nodules contained largely non-vacuolated cells which resembled the Purkinje fibres of the heart. The cells are large and contain open nuclei with 1 or 2 prominent nuclei (*Figure 18.26*). The

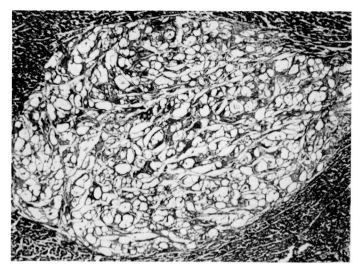

Figure 18.26. A rhabdomyomatous nodule of highly-vacuolated cells, well demarcated from the surrounding myocardium. There is no limiting capsule (Masson's trichrome stain) (Reproduced from Omar (1969) by courtesy of the author and Editor of Pathologia Veterinaria)

cytoplasm stains faintly and in some cases is granular. The vacuoles have hazy outlines; the degree of vacuolization being highly variable. In extremely vacuolated cells, only a peripheral margin of cytoplasm remains; in other cells the cytoplasmic margin is connected by slender cytoplasmic processes to a small quantity of perinuclear cytoplasm giving rise to 'spider cells'.

Sometimes cross striations may be seen in PTAH-stained cells.

The term 'glycogenic' is inappropriate in discussing these tumours as they do not actually produce glycogen.

Furthermore, it confuses the condition with the cardiac form of glycogen storage disease, which is a separate and hereditary entity which is transmitted as a recessive character (Di Sant'Agnese, 1959). This disease is dealt with in the following section on glycogen storage disease.

References
Colby, E. D. and Collins, W. G. (1965). 'Reticulum-cell sarcoma with cardiac involvement.' *Vet. Med.* **60**, 1021

Cotchin, E. (1956). 'Neoplasms of the domesticated mammals.' *Commonwealth Bureau of Animal Health*, Review Series. No. 4, p. 20

Detwéiler, D. K. (1962). 'Wesen und Häufigkeit von Herzkrankheiten bei Hunden.' *Zeitbl. Vet. Med.* **9**, 317

Di Sant'Agnese, P. A. (1959). 'Diseases of glycogen storage with special reference to the cardiac type of generalised glycogenosis.' *Ann. N.Y. Acad. Sci.* **72**, 439

Geib, L. W. (1967). 'Primary angiomatous tumors of the heart and great vessels: A report of two cases in the dog.' *Cornell Vet.* **57**, 292

Hadlow, W. J. (1962). 'Diseases of skeletal muscle.' In *Comparative Neuropathology*, p. 274. Ed. by J. R. M. Innes, and L. L. Saunders. New York: Academic Press

Kast, A. and Hanichen, T. (1968). 'Rhabdomyoma in Schweineherzen.' *Vet. Med.* **15**, 140

Kleine, L. J., Zook, B. C. and Munson, T. O. (1970). 'Primary cardiac haemangiosarcoma in dogs.' *J. Am. Vet. Med. Ass.* **157**, 326

Moulton, J. E. (1961). *Tumours in Domestic Animals*, p. 65. Berkely: University of California Press

Omar, A. R. (1969). 'Congenital rhabdomyoma in a pig.' *Pathol. Vet.* **6**, 469

Roberts, S. R. (1959). 'Myxoma of the heart in a dog.' *J. Am. Vet. Med. Ass.* **134**, 185

Rooney, J. R. (1961). 'Rhabdomyomatosis in the heart of a guinea pig.' *Cornell Vet.* **51**, 388

Smith, H. A. and Jones, T. C. (1961). *Veterinary Pathology*. 2nd Edition, pp. 176 and 1250. Philadelphia: Lea and Febiger

Stünzi, H. and Mann, M. (1970). 'Pathologisch-anatomische Befunde beim Hämoperikard des Hundes.' *Schweiz. Archs Tierheilk.* **112**, 233

Vink, H. M. (1969). 'Rhabdomyomatosis (nodular glycogenic infiltration) of the heart in guinea-pigs.' *J. Path.* **97**, 331

Von Recklinghausen, F. D. (1862). *Mschr. Geburtsk. Frauenkrankh.* **20**, 1

GLYCOGEN STORAGE DISEASE

Glycogen storage disease rarely seems to involve animals. There are only three papers written on this subject in the veterinary literature (Bardens, Bardens and Bardens, 1961; Bardens, 1966; Mostafa, 1970), and in only one, that of Mostafa, is there a report of this disease affecting the heart.

The case was that of a male Lap dog, aged 1½ years, in whom a diagnosis of cardiac dilatation, due to myocarditis, had been made and who, subsequently, died suddenly. At autopsy, the heart was found to be markedly enlarged to about three times its normal weight. The cardiac hypertrophy was symmetrical and the myocardium appeared fibrous.

The microscopic picture was as follows. In sections stained with haematoxylin and eosin, enormous vacuolization was observed. The cell boundaries were mostly marked by delicately striated or vacuolated rims. Higher magnification revealed an incomplete cytoplasmic meshwork in some of the cells, while others were dilated and contained two or three large vacuoles which were separated by thin cytoplasmic walls; some others, although greatly hypertrophied, presented an intact cytoplasm with insignificant vacuolization or striations.

The nuclei were comparatively large, rounded or elliptical in shape and mostly situated in the centre of the vacuoles. Delicate cytoplasmic strands connected them with the rest of the cytoplasm.

A representative amount of glycogen was stainable—by the PAS method—and was seen to be diffusely distributed in the different vacuoles. The vacuoles were not completely filled with glycogen but this may have been due to the heart having been originally fixed in formolsaline, glycogen storage disease not being suspected.

References

Bardens, J. W. (1966). 'Glycogen storage disease in puppies.' *Vet. Med.* **61**, 1174

— Bardens, G. W. and Bardens B. (1961). 'Clinical observations on a Von Gierke-like syndrome in puppies.' *Allied Vet.* **4**, 7

Mostafa, T. E. (1970). 'A case of glycogenic cardiomegaly in a dog.' *Acta vet. scand.* **11**, 197

DYSTROPHIC CALCIFICATIONS OF THE MYOCARDIUM

Hummel (1961) has reported examples of dystrophic calcification of the myocardium and testicular blood vessels appearing in an inbred strain of mice (3 HeBFe). Lesions were seen in 100 per cent of breeding females and, when severe, the whole striated muscle was also involved. Only a few males and virgin females were involved, and, in these, the lesions were less severe. Two other strains of mice (DDA/1 and DBA/2) were similarly affected and this disease was thought to be hereditary. Calcific cardiomyopathy in which myocardial degeneration and necrosis are associated with extensive fine dystrophic calcification of cardiac muscle cells has also been reported in a wide range of other animals, the aetiology being nutritional in origin.

These cardiac lesions have been well documented in several species of domestic mammals and found to be due to vitamin E deficiency. These lesions have also been produced experimentally by vitamin E deficiency in several laboratory animals (Mason, 1941; Blaxter and Brown, 1952; MacKenzie, 1953).

The occurrence of similar lesions in non-domesticated animals, and, in particular, in Camelidae, is less well documented, although there are a few relevant papers (Heck, 1941; Kraft, 1961; Finlayson, Keymer and Manton, 1971). At necropsy the myocardium may be partly discoloured, usually being yellowish and sometimes hyperaemic. Part, or all, of the affected muscle initially may show extensive hyaline degeneration and necrosis of cardiac muscle fibres.

Histologically, the muscle cell in some parts of the myocardium may show a loss of cross striations with varying degrees of nuclear pyknosis and karyolysis. The cell borders are preserved but many of the affected muscle cells show intense haematoxyphilic streaking and spotting of the cytoplasm. These basophilic structures are coloured brown or black by von Kossa's stain and the histological appearances are those of discrete, multiple small foci of intracellular calcifications.

References

Blaxter, K. L. and Brown, F. (1952). 'Vitamin E in the nutrition of farm animals.' *Nutr. Abstr. Rev.* **22**, 1

Finlayson, R., Keymer, I. F. and Manton, V. J. A. (1971). 'Calcific cardiomyopathy in young camels (Camelus Spp.).' *J. comp. Path.* **81**, 71

Heck, H. (1941). 'Das Tier und Wir, 3.' Cited by Stünzi, H. (1947). *Schweiz. S. Path. Bakt.* **10**, 219

Hummel, K. P. (1961). Personal communication to Dr. D. K. Detwéiler (1964) Cited in *Circulation* **30**, 114

Kraft, H. (1961). *Kleintier-Prax* **6**, 64

MacKenzie, G. G. (1953). 'The physiological role of certain vitamins and trace elements.' In *Symposium on Nutrition.* ed. by R. M. Herridt. Baltimore: Johns Hopkins Press

Mason, K. E. (1941). 'Das Tier und Wir, 3.' Cited by Stünzi, H. (1947) *Schweiz. S. Path. Bakt.* **10**, 219

SPONTANEOUS MYOCARDIAL NECROSIS

Prichard and Bullock (1965) reported the finding of spontaneous myocardial necrosis in a young male squirrel monkey (*Sakmiri sciurus*).

The animal had normal physical findings and base-line laboratory tests (except for an increased number of platelets found on examination of the blood film). Seven days later he was found moribund in his cage and died the next day. Autopsy showed a 20 per cent loss of body weight and extensive myocardial necrosis, mostly left ventricular, together with extensive fatty metamorphosis of muscle fibres and coagulation necrosis of some of these affected fibres, together with a neutrophilic exudate in most areas. All the coronary arteries were normal. A small collection of coccoid bodies were found in a right ventricular muscle fibre.

It is worth remembering that local and diffuse necrosis of myocardial muscle, as a result of extreme thiamine deficiency has been described by Ashburn and Lowry (1944) and may, therefore, be a possible explanation for the development of necrosis in this animal.

References

Ashburn, L. L. and Lowry, B. C. (1965). 'Development of cardiac lesions in thiamine deficient rats.' *Archs Path.* **37**, 22

Prichard, R. W. and Bullock, B. C. (1965). 'Spontaneous myocardial necrosis in a squirrel monkey.' *Fedn Proc.* **24**, 310

INTRA-ATRIAL THROMBOSIS

Meier and Hoag (1961) have reported the occurrence of left atrial thrombosis in an inbred strain of mice (BALB/C). This disease process was restricted to breeding females and was attributed to post partum hyperprothrombinaemia.

A similar report of this condition in mice had previously been made by Rye, Hamilton and Lisco (1960). It is not understood why the left atrium should be particularly implicated in this disease.

References

Meier, H. and Hoag, W. G. (1961). 'Studies of left auricular thrombosis in mice.' *J. exp. Med. Surg.* **19**, 371

Rye, R. J. M., Hamilton, K. and Lisco, H. C. (1960). 'Intra-auricular cardiac thrombosis of unknown etiology.' *Fedn Proc.* **19**, 109

FOOT AND MOUTH DISEASE

Foot and mouth disease is highly contagious to cloven-hoofed animals, especially cattle, sheep, goats and pigs. It is occasionally transmitted to man, causing a self-limiting febrile illness, but without any known cardiac involvement or sequelae.

Myocardial changes are reported as having been produced in guinea-pigs and suckling mice, both of which are particularly susceptible. In the heart, Holz (1943) found areas of myocardial necrosis, together with infiltrates of inflammatory cells, lymphocytes and neutrophils and deposits of calcium in the myocardium. In an electron microscopic study Lubke (1960) noted multiplication of the virus in infected mice during the first day of infection; on the second day severe fatty change and marked intracellular oedema with liquefactive dissolution of mitochondria were seen in some myocardial fibres. This worker believed that the intracellular oedema was the primary change in this virus infection.

References

Holz, K. (1943). 'Über Myokardschaden bei der Maul- und Klauen-seuche des Rindes.' *Virchows Arch. path. Anat. Physiol.* **310**, 257

Lubke, A. (1960). 'Electron microscopy of myocarditis caused by foot and mouth disease.' *Virchows Arch. path. Anat. Physiol.* **333**, 487

MULBERRY HEART DISEASE

Mulberry heart disease designates a poorly understood syndrome which causes the death of young healthy pigs in a matter of hours. The whole heart at death is in a state of firm contraction and is spotted with haemorrhages, this suggesting the appearance of a mulberry. Oedema is the most impressive lesion, however, with hydropericardium, limited hydroperitoneum and marked pulmonary oedema. The cause is not known although it is thought to be due to an unknown toxic substance in the food, although research has, so far, failed to reveal it.

Macroscopically, the whole heart at death is found to be in a state of firm contraction. The pericardial surface is spotted with small haemorrhages, these haemorrhages suggesting the appearance of a mulberry. Oedema is found to be the most impressive lesion. However, there is often an associated hydropericardium, a limited hydroperitoneum and marked pulmonary oedema. The oedema fluid may clot, owing to its high protein content.

Microscopically, the myocardium is found to be markedly oedematous. Many of the myocardial fibres are widely separated by the increased amount of oedema fluid which is present in the interstitial tissue of the myocardium. A diffuse infiltration of the myocardium with lymphocytes is also seen. Throughout the myocardium the intracardiac myocardial blood vessels are all intensely congested and dilated. In a few areas below the endocardium some of these blood vessels have ruptured, the liberated erythrocytes lying in the interstitial tissue or sometimes immediately below the pericardium.

AETIOLOGY

The cause is not known but may be due to an unknown toxic substance in the food, although a limited amount of experimental work has failed to reveal it.

A relationship to enterotoxaemia, with or without hypersensitivity, has also been suggested.

ROUND HEART DISEASE

Round heart disease has been used in the United States to describe a syndrome in pigs and poultry in which the heart is in severe contraction at death, there having previously been considerable dilatation of the ventricles to produce the rounded shape.

Little is known of its cause or pathogenesis. Smith and Jones (1957) state that this is a disease which commonly occurs in swine, goats and sheep. At death the heart is found to be severely contracted. Before death there has been severe ventricular dilatation and, consequently, a round cardiac shape is produced.

Blackland and Markson (1947) had previously described 'round heart disease' of poultry. The affected birds died suddenly, having previously appeared normal, although they had not at that time been laying well. These birds often died suddenly, often while running for their food, although, previously, they had been off their food.

At autopsy the hearts were enlarged in all cases, both in size and weight. On section the myocardium often appeared to be fatty and necrotic.

MICROSCOPY

Many of the myocardial cells showed clearly swelling of the cytoplasm and fragmentation of some muscle fibres. Some of the muscle fibres also showed loss of striations in their cytoplasm, together with the presence of a few small intracytoplasmic vacuoles.

There was a little cellular infiltrate of the myocardium with lymphocytes, but little fibrosis was seen. No other changes were found in these animals at autopsy. Bacteriological examination of cardiac material has shown nothing. No nutritional cause for this disease has been found.

A study of 216 outbreaks of 'round heart' disease showed that 184 (80 per cent) occurred in chickens kept in built-up litters which suggested that this disease may have an infectious cause. In a study carried out, 2 out of 4 piglets died 24 and 45 days after they had been placed with fowls in a deep litter in which the disease was occuring. Experimental attempts to isolate the causative organism were, however, unrewarding and no organism could be found.

References

Blackland, J. D. and Markson, L. M. (1947). 'Toxic heart degeneration or "round heart disease" of poultry.' *Vet. J.* **103**, 401

Smith, H. A. and Jones, T. C. (Eds) (1957). *Veterinary Pathology.* 2nd Edition. Philadelphia: Lea and Febiger

MYOCARDIAL LESIONS DUE TO MINERAL DEFICIENCIES

A variety of metallic element deficiencies may produce cardiac lesions. Some are briefly listed below.

In 1937 Neal and Amman described small degenerative lesions in the hearts of calves who had suffered from 'cobalt' deficiency. This condition they termed 'enzootic marasmus'.

Thomas, Mylon and Winternitz (1940) in studies on many animals subsisting on a potassium deficient diet showed that this often had a marked cardiotoxic effect.

Bennets, Beck and Harley (1948) later described 'falling disease' in cattle and showed that, in these animals, 'copper' deficiency caused atrophy and fibrosis of cardiac muscle.

Most recently Blaxter, Rook and MacDonald (1954) have shown, experimentally, that 'magnesium' deficiency will cause small foci of necrosis in the myocardium in calves.

References

Bennets, H. W., Beck, A. B. and Harley, R. (1948). 'On the pathogenesis of "falling disease".' *Aust. Vet. J.* **24**, 237

Blaxter, K. L., Rook, L. A. F. and MacDonald, A. H. (1954). 'Experimental magnesium deficiency in calves.' *J. comp. Path.* **64**, 157

Neal, W. M. and Amman, C. F. (1937). 'The essentiality of cobalt in bovine nutrition.' *J. Dairy Sci.* **20**, 741

Thomas, R. M., Mylon, E. and Winternitz, I. M. (1940). 'Myocardial lesions produced by dietary deficiency of potassium.' *Yale J. biol. Med.* **12**, 345

CARDIAC LESIONS BELIEVED TO HAVE TOXIC AETIOLOGY

Henson *et al.* (1965) have shown that at least two types of plants produce poisons which affect cardiac and skeletal muscle. The plants responsible for this disease are coyotillo (*Karwinsha humboltiane*)

and coffee senna (*Cassia occadentialis*), both native to the south-western parts of the USA. Animals (goats) which have eaten the coyotillo plant have a marked increase in SGOT and a slight increase in SGPT.

Macroscopically, the affected cardiac muscle appears white. Microscopically, there is found to be widespread cardiac muscle degeneration with hyaline change in many of the myocardial fibres, loss of striations, and myocardial fragmentation of other cardiac muscle fibres. Similar changes are also present in many of the skeletal muscles.

There is also a marked increase (up to 18-fold) of SGOT due to myocardial cell necrosis.

In *Karwinsha humboltiane* poisoning there is widespread hyaline and granular degeneration of cardiac muscle fibres. There is disruption of the sarcoplasm in some muscle fibres into fragments.

Dolta, Balbe and Guarda (1968) further reported a detailed clinical, as well as pathological, study of the hearts of 22 calves which presented with the cardiac type of muscular dystrophy.

These cases could, however, be divided into two groups. The first type was characterized by presenting as severe myocarditis while the second type presented as congestive heart failure.

Treatment of the animals in the first group with vitamin E and selenium produced a complete cure, but was not completely effective in the second group.

This latter group of animals also showed, at necropsy, a small heart, and that there was marked thinning of the ventricular wall.

Microscopically, the myocardial cells showed small foci of necrosis which were surrounded by small foci of lymphocytes.

Many of the myocardial cells also showed dystrophic changes, being smaller than normal with loss of striations and often with pyknotic nuclei. In some places there were areas of fibrosis which had replaced myocardial cells. Similar changes were also seen in the conduction system.

It is not known, although it is suggested, that these cases represent other examples of the diseases originally described by Henson et al. (1965).

References

Dolta, V., Balbe, T. and Guarda, F. (1968). 'The cardiac types of muscular dystrophy in calves.' *La Nouva Vet.* **199**, 255

Henson, J. E., Dollahitt, J. W., Bridges, C. W. and Rao, R. R. (1965). 'Myodegeneration in cattle grazing Cassia species.' *J. Am. Vet. Ass.* **147**, 142

COYOTILLO

The fruit of the coyotillo plant (*Karwinsha humboltiane*) has been shown to cause, in sheep and goats, a disease called 'limberleg' which is manifest by progressive weakness of the legs, muscular incoordination and death (Marsh, Clawson and Roe, 1928). The lesions found in cardiac and skeletal muscle are as follows.

In the myocardium disseminated focal lesions of coagulation necrosis involve a few muscle fibres in each location. A few fibres lose their sarcoplasm.

In skeletal muscle, any or all muscles may be involved and the microscopic lesions are typical Zenker's necrosis. The isolated muscle fibres are swollen, eosinophilic, often fragmented and occasionally associated with infiltration of lymphocytes, macrophages and proliferation of sarcolemmal cells.

Associated with these lesions are marked increases in the serum concentrations of glutamic oxaloacetic transaminase and a moderate increase in glutamic pyruvate transaminase.

References

Dewan, M. L. (1965). 'Toxic myodegeneration in goats produced by feeding mature fruits from coyotillo plant (*Karwinsha humboltiane*).' *Am. J. Path.* **46**, 215

Marsh, C. D., Clawson, A. B. and Roe, G. C. (1928). 'Coyotillo (*Karwinsha humboltiane*). Poisoned Plants.' *U.S.D.A. Tech. Bull.* 29

ENCEPHALOMYOCARDITIS

The virus of encephalomyocarditis (EMC), which produces disease in man, was isolated by Helwig and Schmidt (1945) and Schmidt (1948) from anthropoid apes and chimpanzees dying of interstitial myocarditis. Intracerebral inoculation of the various strains of the virus group into mice produces encephalitis and myocarditis. Warren, Smadel and Russ (1949) observed it to be extremely neurotropic in mice, but by reducing the infective dose in the inoculum administered to these animals delayed their death and induced myocarditis. From a group of patients with similar encephalitic symptoms Koch (1950) isolated the virus from the blood, the cerebrospinal fluid and from the faeces from one patient. Of the group the one who died also had interstitial myocarditis. In instances wherein Saphir (1952) noted evidence of both encephalitis and myocarditis at autopsy, although viral studies proved negative, the myocarditis was similar to that observed with another neurotropic virus, poliomyelitis (Jungeblut and Edwards, 1951). These findings thus suggested that both the encephalitis and myocarditis were produced by the same virus. One of the four cases cited by Fiedler as isolated myocarditis may have been caused by the EMC virus (Schmidt, 1948; Saphir, 1952). Neutralizing antibodies have been demonstrated in the serum of many patients suggesting that human infection does occur (Jonkers, 1961).

It has been shown by Gajdusek (1955) that encephalomyocarditis virus infection in childhood is found in different parts of the world. He carried out a series of observations on the sera of adolescents of an Indian tribe in Mexico and found that 4 out of 56 children examined had neutralizing antibodies of the EMC virus.

Craighead (1966) studied the sequential pathological alterations in the hearts of 12–14 week old mice which were sacrificed at various intervals during a period of 45 days after intraperitoneal inoculations of two variants of the virus, one myocardiotropic (M) and the other encephalotropic (E). The earliest changes in the myocardium were recognized four days after inoculation of the M strain and consisted of focal myocytolysis localized almost exclusively to the subendocardial myocardium and the atria. By the tenth day the myocardial necrosis was extensive, and variable numbers of histiocytes, lymphocytes and unidentified histiocytes had appeared. Late in the course of the experiments focal areas were noted in which only the myocardial stroma persisted, associated with scattered histiocytes and a few lymphocytes. Fibroblasts and sprouting blood vessels were abundant but healing fibrosis was not prominent. All parts of the myocardium were affected, most frequently that of the left ventricle. Later mononuclear cells and fibroblasts appeared and after 12–14 days numerous Anitschkow cells.

It is interesting to note that no case of myocarditis being caused by the EMC virus has ever been proved in human subjects, merely suspected as in the case reported by Saphir (1952). It seems possible, therefore, that although the EMC virus may cause myocarditis in mice, this may be a species specificity.

References

Craighead, J. E. (1966). 'Pathogenicity of the M and E variants of the encephalo-myocarditis (EMC) virus. I. Myocardiotropic and neurotropic properties.' *Am. J. Path.* **48**, 333

Gajdusek, D. C. (1955). 'Encephalomyocarditis virus infections in childhood.' *Pediat.* **16**, 902

Helwig, F. and Schmidt, E. C. H. (1945). 'A filter-passing agent producing interstitial myocarditis in anthropoid apes and small animals.' *Science, N.Y.* **102**, 31

Jonkers, A. H. (1961). 'Serosurvey of encephalomyocarditis virus neutralizing antibodies in Southern Louisiana and Peruvian Indian populations.' *Am. J. trop. Med.* **10**, 593

Jungeblut, C. W. and Edwards, J. E. (1951). 'Isolation of poliomyelitis virus from the heart in fatal cases.' *Am. J. clin. Path.* **21**, 601

Koch, F. (1950). 'Die Encephalomyocarditis (EMC) und ihre Abgrenzung von der Poliomyelitis.' *Z. Kinderheilk.* **68**, 328

Saphir, O. (1952). 'Encephalomyocarditis.' *Circulation* **6**, 843

Schmidt, E. C. H. (1948). 'Virus myocarditis: pathologic and experimental studies.' *Am. J. Path.* **24**, 97

Warren, J., Smadel, J. E. and Russ, S. B. (1949). 'The family relationship of encephalomyocarditis. Columbia SK, M.M. and Mengoencephalomyelitis viruses.' *J. Immun.* **62**, 387

Author Index

In this Index to authors the number shown in italic type denotes the page on which full details of the reference are given.

Subject Index